The Child in His Family

CHILDREN IN TURMOIL:
TOMORROW'S PARENTS

VOLUME 7

*YEARBOOK OF THE INTERNATIONAL
ASSOCIATION FOR CHILD ADOLESCENT
PSYCHIATRY AND ALLIED PROFESSIONS*

EDITOR-IN-CHIEF—E. JAMES ANTHONY, M.D. (U.S.A.)
CO-EDITORS—CYRILLE KOUPERNIK, M.D. (FRANCE)
COLETTE CHILAND, M.D., Ph.D. (FRANCE)

Volume 1   The Child in His Family

E. James Anthony and Cyrille Koupernik, Editors

**Volume 2   The Child in His Family:
The Impact of Disease and Death**

E. James Anthony and Cyrille Koupernik, Editors

**Volume 3   The Child in His Family:
Children at Psychiatric Risk**

E. James Anthony and Cyrille Koupernik, Editors

**Volume 4   The Child in His Family:
Vulnerable Children**

E. James Anthony, Cyrille Koupernik, and Colette Chiland, Editors

**Volume 5   The Child in His Family:
Children and Their Parents in a Changing World**

E. James Anthony and Colette Chiland, Editors

**Volume 6   The Child in His Family:
Preventive Child Psychiatry in an Age of Transitions**

E. James Anthony and Colette Chiland, Editors

**Volume 7   The Child in His Family:
Children in Turmoil: Tomorrow's Parents**

E. James Anthony and Colette Chiland, Editors

The Child in His Family

CHILDREN IN TURMOIL:
TOMORROW'S PARENTS

VOLUME 7

Edited by
E. JAMES ANTHONY, M.D.
St. Louis, Missouri, U.S.A.

and

COLETTE CHILAND, M.D., Ph.D.
Paris, France

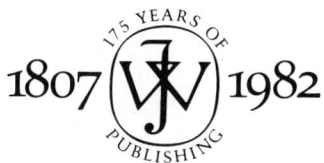

A WILEY-INTERSCIENCE PUBLICATION

JOHN WILEY & SONS
New York • Chichester • Brisbane • Toronto • Singapore

Copyright © 1982 by John Wiley & Sons, Inc.

All rights reserved. Published simultaneously in Canada.

Reproduction or translation of any part of this work beyond that permitted by Section 107 or 108 of the 1976 United States Copyright Act without the permission of the copyright owner is unlawful. Requests for permission or further information should be addressed to the Permissions Department, John Wiley & Sons, Inc.

Library of Congress Cataloging in Publication Data:

Main entry under title:

Children in turmoil.

(The Child in his family; v. 7) (Yearbook of the International Association for Child and Adolescent Psychiatry and Allied Professions, ISSN 0277-6790; v. 7)
  "A Wiley-Interscience publication."
  Includes index.
  1. Child psychopathology.   2. Mental illness.
3. Parent and child.   4. Psychiatry, Transcultural.
I. Anthony, E. James (Elwyn James), 1916–
II. Chiland, Colette.   III. Series.   IV. Series: Yearbook of the International Association for Child and Adolescent Psychiatry and Allied Professions; v. 7)

RJ499.A1C42 vol. 7 [RJ499]   618.92′89s   82-8421
ISBN 0-471-86873-6   [618.92′89]   AACR2

Printed in the United States of America

10 9 8 7 6 5 4 3 2

To *Doris Diephouse,* who has been my right arm for twenty-five years and made my administrative role a sinecure

Contributors

E. James Anthony (M.D.), Blanche F. Ittleson Professor of Child Psychiatry, Director, Edison Child Development Research Center, Washington University School of Medicine, St. Louis, Missouri, U.S.A.

Ayo Binitie (M.D.), Professor of Mental Health and Head, Department of Mental Health, University of Benin, Benin City, Nigeria

Michael Bohman (M.D.), Professor, Department of Child and Youth Psychiatry, University of Umeå, Umeå, Sweden

Katherine Canavan (M.D.), World Health Organization, Geneva, Switzerland

Gerald Caplan (M.D.), Professor, Department of Child Psychiatry, Hadassah–Hebrew University Hospital, Jerusalem, Israel

Marianne Cederblad (M.D.), Head, Child and Adolescent Psychiatric Clinic at Regionjukhuset, Linköping, Sweden

Peter de Chateau (M.D.), Department of Child and Youth Psychiatry, University of Umeå, Umeå, Sweden and the Department of Pediatrics, Karolinska Institute, Stockholm, Sweden

Colette Chiland (M.D., Ph.D.), Professor of Psychology, Clinique à L'Université Rene Descarte de Paris (Sorbonne), Paris, France

John A. Connolly (M.D.), Consultant Psychiatrist, Health Care and Psychosomatic Unit, Irish Foundation for Human Development, Dublin, Ireland

John Cullen (M.D.), Consultant Psychiatrist and Director of Research, Health Care and Psychosomatic Unit, Irish Foundation for Human Development, Dublin, Ireland

Phillip Graham (M.D.), Professor of Psychological Medicine, Hospital for Sick Children, Great Ormond Street, London, United Kingdom

Christopher M. Green (M.B.), Clinical Director and Staff Psychiatrist, Regional Psychiatric Center, Saskatoon, Saskatchawan, Canada

Lionel Hersov (M.D.), Consultant Psychiatrist, The Maudsley Hospital, London, United Kingdom

Borje Höök, Child and Adolescent Psychiatry Clinic at Regionjukhuset, Linköping, Sweden

R. Olukayode Jegede (M.D.), Senior Lecturer and Consultant Psychiatrist, Department of Psychiatry, University College Hospital, Ibadan, Nigeria

Reimer Jensen (Ph.D.), Professor, Dansk Selskab for Bornepsykiatri og Klinisk Bornepsykologi Med Tilknyttede Faggrupper, Copenhagen, Denmark

Ragnar Jonsell (M.D.), Overlakare Med. Dr., Barnkliniken, Vanersborg, Sweden

Richard Lansdown (Ph.D.), Principal Psychologist, Department of Psychological Medicine, The Hospital for Sick Children, London, United Kingdom

Serge Lebbvici (M.D.), Professeur Associe de Psychiatrie de l'Engant a l'Université de Paris (Sorbonne), and Directeur, Centre Alfred Benet, Paris, France

Norman V. Lourie (M.A., Ph.D.), Treasurer, Department of Public Welfare, International Association for Child and Adolescent Psychiatry and Allied Professions, Harrisburg, Pennsylvania, U.S.A.

Karen Madsen (MSW), Child Guidance Clinic, Birkerod, Denmark

Liz McWhirter (Ph.D.), Department of Psychology, Queen's University of Belfast, Belfast, Northern Ireland

Klaus K. Minde (M.D.), Director of Psychiatric Research, Hospital for Sick Children, Toronto, Ontario, Canada

Regina Minde (Ph.D.), Educational Consultant in the Toronto, Ontario area, Toronto, Ontario, Canada

Seggane Musisi (M.D.), Resident in Psychiatry, University of Toronto, Toronto, Ontario, Canada

Peter B. Neubauer (M.D.), Director of Child Development Center, New York, New York, U.S.A.

Ulf Otto (M.D.), Assistant Professor and Director, Department of Child Psychiatry, Kristiansstad, Sweden

Per-Anders Rydelius (M.D.), Department of Child and Youth Psychiatry at Karolinska Institute, St. Gorans Hospital, Stockholm, Sweden

A. O. Sanda (Ph.D.), Head, Social Development Division, Nigerian Institute of Social and Economic Research, University of Ibadan, Ibadan, Nigeria

Soren Sigvardsson (Ph.D.), Department of Child and Youth Psychiatry, University of Umeå, Umeå, Sweden

Albert J. Solnit (M.D.), Professor, Departments of Pediatrics and Psychiatry, and Director, Child Study Center, Yale University School of Medicine, New Haven, Connecticut, U.S.A.

Karen Trew, Queen's University of Belfast, Belfast, Northern Ireland

Britt Wiberg, Psychologist, Department of Child and Youth Psychiatry, University of Umeå, Umeå, Sweden and the Department of Pediatrics, Karolinska Institute, Stockholm, Sweden

Preface

In this seventh volume of the series *The Child in His Family*, which began a dozen years ago in Jerusalem, the International Association and its scientific arm—the International Study Group—have turned their attention to still another significant clinical area, the transformation of the child of today into the parent of tomorrow. To have done this adequately from a rigorous research point of view, we would have needed to carry out a variety of "follow along" studies requiring a minimum of two decades, and the ISG had only four years at its disposal. We therefore did what we were best equipped to do, which was to blaze still another crosscultural trail for other investigators to follow. Our task, as we defined it, was first of all to illuminate different aspects of the total problem and present them to those attending the Congress as well as to the many thousands of our colleagues who were unable to participate in Dublin. We saw three parts to the overall question implied in the transformational process. If the child is father or mother to the parent, and if there is a solid clinical connection involved, our inquiries could take the following forms:

1. What kind of parents do disturbed children make?
2. What kinds of children do disturbed parents make?
3. What kinds of disturbed parents and children do different cultures make?

Readers will perceive from the text that we are by no means married to an exclusively genetic or environmental causal hypothesis, but we subscribe to a more generalizable Waddington–Piaget–Erikson epigenesis. In the general section we look at some prospective and retrospective investigations. In Sweden, the prototype of the developed country, we examined a society that seemed almost utopian in structure and therefore least likely, it would seem, to generate disturbed children, but readers will discover for themselves that this is far from being the case. When we turned for contrast to a developing country like Nigeria, we went there with some innocent Rousseau-like assumptions that a peaceful, more-or-less conflict-free development would be characteristic of Nigerian children. Once again, the findings of our colleagues confuted our expectations. Unlike Dr. Pangloss in *Candide,* clinicians the world over were not looking for the best of all possible worlds to prevent psychiatric disorder in children, but the least detrimental (to quote Solnit, Freud, and Goldstein out of context): neither the welfare state nor the extended family could guarantee prevention. We have also proven to ourselves that single country studies, like single case studies, can be equally misleading for international child psychiatry and that alleged universal mechanisms and manifestations frequently fail to cross borders. The one message that we hope will come through from our series of seven volumes is that child psychiatry is an international field, and that to solve its problems, we must continue to foster international exchange.

Our first lot of thanks are due to the Grant Foundation and the Commonwealth Fund, which have supported the work of the ISG. Our second vote of thanks goes to all the countries that have accepted us as visiting colleagues who wish to cooperate with them in solving some of the general problems that beset children all over the world. In the past four years, Sweden and Nigeria have been the host countries and have carried out their functions with exemplary zeal and scientific honesty. Our last, but by no means least vote of thanks goes to Mrs. Crisanne Roberts, who, working in her ivory tower in St. Louis, Missouri, helped to put Volume VII together and prepare it for publication.

E. JAMES ANTHONY, M.D.

St. Louis, Missouri

COLETTE CHILAND, M.D., Ph.D.

Paris, France
June 1982

Contents

Introduction

In Search of the Little People: The Elaboration of an Irish Fantasy of the Past, Present, and Future of Our Child Patients   3
E. James Anthony (U.S.A.)

Making Connections

The Formation of Maternal Filicidal Impetus from Childhood Incestuous Experiences   27
Christopher M. Green (Canada)

Yesterday's Children in Turmoil—Today's Parents   35
Per-Anders Rydelius (Sweden)

Infants Under Stress: Tomorrow's Adults   43
John Cullen and John A. Connolly (Ireland)

Children in Northern Ireland: A Lost Generation?   69
Liz McWhirter and Karen Trew (Northern Ireland)

The Gällöfsta Conference

Introductory Remarks   85
Albert J. Solnit (U.S.A.)

Sweden—A Society in Turmoil?   93
Marianne Cederblad (Sweden)

Long-Term Effects on Mother−Infant Behavior of Extra Contact During the First Hour Postpartum IV. Study Design and Methods 105
Britt Wiberg and Peter de Château (Sweden)

Daycare for Three-Year-Olds—An Interdisciplinary Experimental Study 129
Marianne Cederblad and Börje Höök (Sweden)

Psychosocial Risk Factors in Children 145
Ragnar Jonsell (Sweden)

Drug Abuse and Alcoholism Among Children and Youth in Sweden 153
Per-Anders Rydelius (Sweden)

Suicidal Behavior in Childhood and Adolescence 163
Ulf Otto (Sweden)

Adoption and Fostering as Preventive Measures 171
Michael Bohman and Sören Sigvardsson (Sweden)

A Site Visit to the Family Village at Skå-Edeby in Stockholm 181
Karen Madsen (Denmark)

Discussion of Papers Presented at Gällöfsta 185
Chairman: Lionel Hersov (U.K.)

The Ibadan Conference

The Mental Health of Children in Developing Countries 197
Phillip Graham and Katherine Canavan (U.K.)

Some Aspects of Disruption of the Attachment
 System in Young Children: A Transcultural
 Perspective ... 215

 *Klaus K. Minde (Canada), Regina Minde (Canada)
 and Seggane Musisi (Nigeria)*

The Nigerian Family in Transition ... 235

 A. O. Sanda (Nigeria)

Effects of Rapid Socioeconomic Change on the
 Nigerian Family ... 251

 R. Olukayode Jegede (Nigeria)

Clinical Aspects of Adolescent Problems in Nigeria ... 261

 Ayo Binitie (Nigeria)

Discussion of Dr. Graham's Presentation ... 277

 Chairman: Norman V. Lourie (U.S.A.)

Discussion of Dr. Minde's Presentation ... 281

 Chairman: Peter B. Neubauer (U.S.A.)

Discussion of Dr. Sanda's Presentation ... 285

 Chairman: Colette Chiland (France)

Discussion of Dr. Binitie's Presentation ... 287

 Chairman: Lionel Hersov (U.K.)

General Comments ... 291

 Colette Chiland and Serge Lebovici (France)

Site Visits

Aro: Village of the Past, Present, or Future? ... 299

 Reimer Jensen (Denmark)

A Home for Motherless Babies at Ibadan: A Site Visit
by an International Study Group 305
Colette Chiland (France)

Epilogue

The Essential Human Child and His Cultural
Counterparts: An Epilogue for an International
Congress 309
E. James Anthony (U.S.A.)

The Child in His Family

CHILDREN IN TURMOIL:
TOMORROW'S PARENTS

VOLUME 7

INTRODUCTION

In Search of the Little People

THE ELABORATION OF AN IRISH FANTASY
OF THE PAST, PRESENT, AND FUTURE
OF OUR CHILD PATIENTS
(THE EMERGENCE OF THE CHILD AS A PSYCHIATRIC AND
PSYCHOTHERAPEUTIC PATIENT AND OF THE CHILD PSYCHIATRIST
AS A SPECIALIZED PHYSICIAN)

E. James Anthony, M.D. (U.S.A.)

The title of this presentation refers to an unusual and intriguing project carried out by the poet W.B. Yeats toward the end of the last century [8]. He traveled around Ireland "in search of the little people" (the leprechauns) and questioned a variety of informants in faraway villages about their knowledge, or the knowledge of their fathers and grandfathers, especially when this involved alleged encounters. Who had seen them? Who had spoken with them? What were they like? How accessible were they? Were they easy to deal with? And on and on. The answers he obtained were very mixed. There were many different kinds of little people, and none of them were alike. They differed in mood, in size, in shape, in sociability, and, most important, in the degree to which they allowed people from outside their small world to know and understand them. Some seemed isolated, some fearful, some mischievous, and some compulsively industrious (the little shoemakers). Some wanted to be helped (offering good luck in exchange); others insisted on being left alone and threatened violence if their privacy was violated.

These leprechauns of Ireland are a good example of the absorbing interest that "big people," like us, have maintained for centuries (and possibly since the species first evolved) in the fantasied intermediate construct of the childlike adult or the adultlike child. The composite creations reflect the admired, envied, and sometimes feared qualities of child and adult: the inhabitants of Middle Earth or Lilliput are imagined to be able to think like men, feel like women, and act like children—a truly powerful combination. Hobbits, for instance, have many different facets: they are good natured, amiable, and disinclined to wear shoes; they can move rapidly, hide easily, and recover marvelously from bumps and bruises; and they also have sharp eyes and ears that take in a good deal more than seems possible, and a fund of wisdom that "big people," like us, forgot long ago. This saves them from becoming pompous or taking themselves too seriously—a common failing, unfortunately, of the "big people."

"Big people" tend either to idealize them, derogate them, or mix the two defenses in a mainly unconscious ambivalence. On a more rational plane, we need to remember their limitations: they are inclined to be self-absorbed, self-centered, greedy, envious, and certain that the sky arches over them and that the sun and moon follow them slavishly around. As Gandalf says to a remarkable Hobbit, Bilbo Baggins: "You are a fine person, Mr. Baggins, and I am very fond of you; but you are only quite a little fellow in a wide world after all!" This is the perspective that we need to keep on the "little people"; fine persons, but only little after all!

I might add parenthetically that we treated primitive people with the same admixture of condescension and reverence until the anthropologist Levi-Strauss taught us otherwise, insisting that the primitive world was populated by people very much like ourselves, in some ways better, in some ways worse, and that a genuine encounter could enhance the depth and complexity of both the civilized and the uncivilized. For one to dub the other special is essentially alienating. Rather, they need to work together and conceive a cooperative vision of human coexistence.

I have been talking analogically, but, like Yeats, I too have tried over the past 25 years as a professional child psychiatrist to get in touch and keep in touch with the thousands of "little people" who visit our clinics every year. I wanted to find out what they were really like before the adult reconstructed and mythologized them: how closely could one get to know them; what sort of patients they made; and whether the private psychological inquiry was the best entrance into their minds and lives. Like Levi-Strauss, I felt that a genuine encounter between adult and child could contribute to the depth, complexity, and creativity of the human world as a whole. We could learn from each other by discovering each other.

At the start of my investigation I had two aims: to capture the perceptions of the child who sees everything in its newness before convention dictates what is to be seen; and second, to turn this pre-Adamite eye, still relatively uncontaminated by the thick gloom of common existence, on to the therapeutic meeting between the child and adult. In a sense, I wanted to rediscover childhood at first hand (before I read about it), convinced that this was where one had to begin to break new ground in an established field. I am reminded here of Picasso, who lived an almost ageless life, remarking in his latter years that the secret of genius lay in the constant rediscovery of the past, and that as he grew older, he continually grew younger until he eventually recaptured the visual perspectives of childhood before it succumbed, alas permanently, to the tyranny of representation.

The First Child Psychiatric Patient

In my reading of history, I find that the first child psychiatric patient, in the fullest and most modern sense, was Victor, the wild boy who was found in the forests of Aveyron 170 years ago. When he first presented himself to Itard [5], he looked like an abused child, covered with scars. He was as challenging a patient as any adventurous clinician might wish to treat, and Itard was not only adventurous and courageous but able to approach a novel clinical situation in a creative and innovative manner. He was motivated by almost a Frankenstein fantasy: he wanted to make a new child out of an animal; to humanize him and domesticate him; to teach him to become aware of the world around him, to think, to feel, and to talk. He achieved all this except the last; nevertheless, Victor was finally able to communicate his needs in an appropriate manner, respond to demands, and exchange thoughts. In every way, it was a miraculous transformation of wolf into boy, and it brought about a renaissance in the treatment and care of the retarded. By the end of his short life, Victor was experiencing gratitude for kindness shown him and remorse for bad behavior on his part. He was forming affectionate relationships, the most important of which was the strong therapeutic alliance that was built up between him and his doctor, which weathered many tempestuous setbacks.

I believe (with the understandable bias of a therapist) that the most crucial insights obtained from the management of this early psychiatric patient are first, the connection that Itard observed between affect and intelligence, namely that whenever the patient's feelings were involved either in the psychiatrist or in the task, his intellectual development sped along in leaps and bounds; and second, the realization that the psychiatrist's counteraffects could be remarkably informative on what was occurring in the patient. This knowledge led Itard at times to manipulate Victor's emotional state. For example, he would reproach the boy for wasting his time and would tell him that he could go to a mental institution for all he cared. Although he had never responded to language, Victor would sadden and tears would roll down his cheeks. As his emotional life broadened and deepened, his problem solving improved. On another occasion, he had been working industriously and accurately on a number of tasks and expected his usual measure of praise and reward. Instead he was met by disapproval and punishment. At first he was bewildered, then resistive, and finally he bit his mentor hard and deservedly on the hand. Itard was delighted. "At that moment," he said, "I would have given anything to have been able to have made my patient understand my act and to have told him that the very pain of his bite filled me with satisfaction and more than rewarded me for my pains . . . the bite was a legitimate act of vengeance . . . and incontestable proof that the idea of justice and injustice . . . was no longer foreign to his mind . . . I had revived a savage boy to the full stature of a moral individual." You will hear this same cry of satisfaction echoed by Freud a hundred years later. I would add, having had my own hand bitten, that it is possible to react to a bite with pleasure only if the attack is part of a creative and understandable process of treatment. It seemed to me that the bite signified that Victor had become a real psychiatric patient, the first child in history to do so, in that he had developed a reciprocal relationship with his psychiatrist.

The First Psychotherapeutic Patient

All roads in child therapy lead back to little Hans [3]. He has become the best known child patient in the world, and it was a sheer act of genius that led Freud, with no therapeutic experience of children whatsoever, to undertake the first analysis of a little five-year-old boy. He also happened to be the first child patient to be treated completely by his father—in itself a daring innovation. It was something new in 1909 to designate a disturbance in a child as neurosis and not naughtiness; it was something new at the turn of the century to look at the symptoms, the dreams, and the play of a small child and try to understand them in symbolic terms; it was something new, prior to the advent of ego psychology and child observation, to examine the total ecological setting of the child; to look at infantile sexuality and the development of the Oedipus complex not retrospectively but prospectively as they unfolded in the child; it was something entirely new to conduct a follow-up on a case many years later and to establish the protocol for the reevaluation of the case; to demonstrate what an integral part the parents played in the development and resolution of the Oedipus complex in the child, their own reaction to the oedipal crisis, and the reactivation of oedipal conflicts in themselves; and it was something new to have therapeutic supervision for any kind of case, let alone a child case. The treatment of little Hans was therefore a therapeutic cornucopia from which endless good things poured and continued to pour in the decades that followed. Having said all this, I quote a contemporary review of the case (1908). It is entitled Psychiatry of the Young with Moral Degeneracy and Social Imbecility [7].

> Acquaintances of Freud working under his direction have studied a remarkable case of sexual precocity in a boy who, at the age of three, began to be interested, above all things, in his widdler (the child's name for his penis). He was avidly concerned as to whether animals, men and women, etc., possessed this part, and his incessant preoccupation and conversation on the topic could not be restrained. The child was plainly hereditarily tainted but was cured by hypnotic treatment modified in form to be applicable to children.

Let me describe how Freud himself saw this first child patient. As far as he was concerned, there was nothing degenerate or imbecilic about Hans, nor was he manifestly condemned by any heredity. On the contrary, he was a physically robust, cheerful, amiable, and mentally alert young fellow whom it was a pleasure to meet. There was no doubt that he was sexually precocious, conceded Freud, but he cited research that indicated that American boys (who else?) tended to show heterosexual interests at a similarly early age. He frankly admitted his partisan attitude toward infantile sexuality but surmised that sexual precocity might well be correlated with intellectual forwardness, and therefore was not to be thoughtlessly repudiated. It was a package deal.

What was surprising to the world of 1909 was not only the demonstrable fact that even very small children were fascinated by sex wherever and whenever they had access to it but that they were also so articulate and logical about it. Once again the interplay of logic and affect can be illustrated brilliantly from the text. One day Hans and his father went out together, although the little boy had resisted at first because of his phobia. It was Sunday and so there was not much (horse-drawn) traffic, and Hans remarked, "How sensible! God's done away with horses now," which was a fine counterphobic observation tinged with grandiosity. (Piaget would have chalked up this egocentric remark as appropriately preoperational.) While they walked, his father (who took every opportunity to rub things in) explained to him very earnestly that his little sister had not got a widdler like him. Hans immediately asked: "Have you got a widdler?" and the father, duly affronted by the sound of it, replied, "Of course. What else would you suppose?" After a thoughtful pause, Hans said, "But then how do little girls widdle if they have no widdlers?" The father answered, "They don't have widdlers like yours. Haven't you noticed this already when your sister was being given her bath?" He obviously had and put it out of mind, and the reminder depressed him. That same night he awoke with a nightmare that Freud correctly diagnosed as a masturbation fantasy. "I saw Mummy quite naked in her chemise, and she let me see her widdler." His father was quick to point out the logical contradiction: how could his mother be both naked and in her chemise at one and the same time? "She was in her chemise," said the little boy very simply, "but the chemise was so short that I saw her widdler." (At that time in Vienna "baby doll" nightwear would not have passed the censors, so a certain amount of wish fulfillment was involved in the syllogism.) The final logical encounter between father and son once again involved the problematical new sister whom Hans ardently wished would drop dead. Having elicited the death wish, the father goes on ponderously to remark, "A good boy doesn't wish that sort of thing, though," to which Hans replied with sublime directness, "But he may think it." "But that isn't good," says the father defensively. "If he thinks it," responds Hans, "it is good all the same, because you can write it to the professor." (And presumably get some needed supervision!) When Freud heard this, he was enchanted and exclaimed (in a footnote), "Well done, little Hans! I could wish for no better understanding of psychoanalysis from any grown-up." And no better example of early operational thinking, Piaget would have added. What was more was that the "widdler" was here to stay, with a permanent niche in the psychiatric literature.

Thus this first child patient in psychotherapy showed that five-year-olds can reason with a subtle logic of their own, transact with adults on an equal footing, and develop blazing insights. After Hans, children could never again be treated with high and mighty superiority. One could claim that following on the footsteps of little Hans, children came into their own as patients. As each decade passed, new psychopathological possibilities were found for them: they could now become recognizably autistic, psychotic, neurotic, psychosomatic, oppositional, developmentally deviant, anxious, and depressed. Their clinical functioning was determined by their age and stage of development, their intellectual and linguistic capacities, their genetic endowments, their cultural and social environments. Every 10 years, or even less, it seemed, a new diagnostic classification would be proposed, growing in length and complexity and culminating in the GAP classification of 1966 [4], which covered 75 pages of responses, disorders, reactions, and syndromes, matching the worst of the psychiatry of adults. The child was not only father to the man but progenitor to all his ills as well.

The Task of Becoming a Patient

Becoming a patient is not an easy task by any means, and child patients range widely in their competence to present their problems and obtain help. In addition to innate deficiencies and acquired inadequacies, resistances and defenses more than anything can impede this development. Unless children become patients, it is very hard to treat them except by manipulating their behavior or giving them medication. The trouble is that child patients in the making are as much affected in their roles as the child psychiatrist or therapist by the state of the art. This was demonstrably true of analytically oriented child psychotherapy. As emphasis was laid in turn on the pathogenetic influence of the primal scene, the withholding of sexual knowledge, the suppression of aggression, the constrictions brought about by anxiety, and the tensions induced by guilt, child patients in psychotherapy were shuffled out of parental bedrooms (which children have occupied carte blanche for centuries), offered advanced *ad hoc* courses in sexual education, allowed a free hand with their destructive urges, handled with extreme permissiveness, and subjected to no prohibitions whatsoever. All this resulted not in the production of free, blithe spirits but of tense, deeply troubled and conscience-stricken youngsters who almost demanded and certainly provoked the setting of limits and a more careful consideration of the strengths and weakness of their developing egos. There is no doubt that such historical shifts in emphasis leave both patients and their doctors equally confused and unsure of themselves. Anna Freud has spoken sympathetically of the therapists "faced by nothing but enigmas with no certainty about the therapeutic possibilities," and one could apply this equally to the child patient caught up in such fluctuations. However, children in general adapt to mystification and accept it as part of the inscrutable universe to which they have been accustomed since infancy.

The child patient, like his or her adult counterpart, is, therefore, affected by a host of presenting factors in the psychiatrist—appearance, personality, ethnic origins, age, sex, theoretical orientation, and, most significantly, comfortableness in the presence of children. I am sometimes struck by how many young child psychiatrists experience an awkwardness when so exposed, sometimes amounting to a kind of "cultural shock." I can only assume that they have been brought up under sociocultural conditions of two discontinuous societies: adults and children.

There are other subtle elements that might interfere with the orderly transition of child into patient, but we still know little of such metamorphoses. To mention just one, there has been some empirical work carried out in Britain suggesting that a mismatching of body build (and presumably temperament, if we are to accept Shelden's thesis) can bring about failures in treatment. In most clinics, the only variable manipulated is the sex of the therapist in relation to the sex of the child.

It often has been claimed, with some justification, that child patients (especially those who refuse to accept the patient role) can occasion more counteraffect than the average adult patient. Certainly it is harder to make sense of what goes on, since much of it takes place on a nonverbal, preoperational, and amorphous level. The child is overtly diabolical in the use of resistances and chooses the more unpleasant of these: mutism, boredom, hypermobility, physical aggressiveness, plain silliness, negativism, and even planned craziness to control and defeat the often hard-working, well-meaning, good-enough doctor. What children lack in sophistry, they make up for in truculence. (It is often a pleasurable relief to leave this arena and retreat behind the couch with a quietly resistant adult patient—and even conducive to a brief nap!)

An important question needs to be raised. Are we witnessing a significant change in the patient status of children today? I think we are. The impact of the media seems inordinate and yet so subtly effected. Children are constantly absorbing ideas about psychology, psychiatry, mental health, and the patient–doctor relationship that were unknown even to their parents a few years ago. Children in the middle phase are beginning to ask for treatment and even refer themselves. As a sign of the times, Robert Coles reported in 1961 on an eight-year-old girl who walked alone into the emergency ward of the Children's Hospital in Boston and asked to talk to a psychiatrist about her worries.

Society's attitudes to mental health and mental treatment are certainly shifting (again, with the help of the media), and children are beginning to experience less shame in being referred to the "shrink." For some children, as with some adults, it is even becoming something of a status symbol. Patients are also discovering that the secondary gains more than compensate for any embarrassments. Once they are officially defined as card-carrying attendants at a clinic, their failures are underplayed and their badness is exonerated. They cannot be faulted since they are patients. If they are giving their families hell, it is because of their problems, and what parents (under the monitoring eye of the clinic social workers) can dare to reproach them, let alone discipline them? The child patient consequently is afforded a diplomatic immunity unavailable to unlabeled siblings and can sit back and enjoy the spectacle (especially if he has been previously scapegoated) of rough and ready discipline being meted out to them.

Becoming a patient, therefore, can provide some ill-used and needy children with a tantalizingly attractive solution to their life problems and a means of escape from the exacting obligations that accrue to their lot with maturation. They are no longer compelled to be their ages. Whether the gains are appreciable enough to make them permanent patients only time can tell.

The home environment does play an important role in the making of a child patient. It can and often does provide a competent or incompetent model of patient behavior through parents and siblings. The smaller the home and the more nuclear the family is in its functioning, the more intense and focused the conflict becomes. "Only" children sometimes appear to carry the whole emotional load of the family on their shoulders. If large families are inclined to make neglected children, small families, in which there is little "shock absorption," are potent in producing conflicted children, as a loose general rule.

The patient's way of life is both spontaneously generated and, in its external form, learned, together with the language that goes with it, introspections that need to be developed, symbolisms that have to be translated, early memories that have to be reactivated, and dreams that have to be remembered and understood. For the ordinary child, who becomes the ordinary adult, such penumbral phenomena are hardly even considered and certainly not seriously. (It is, therefore, difficult to treat an ordinary child, and when I have tried to do so for research reasons, I have failed. Either the child drops out of treatment or I do.)

One can pick out potential child patients from a general population of children because of giveaway signs. They show up like "sore thumbs" against the general background of ordinary, good-enough children. They react too much or too little to the routine things of life. Here, for example, is a school girl writing an account of going to bed for her teacher [5a]. (Contrast what follows with the brief account of another child who wrote succinctly: "When I go to bed, I go to sleep.") Our potential patient writes:

> Before I go to bed, I look under the bed, and I look inside the closet because I think there might be a man, and then I look out the backyard and look at the trees and say to myself the way the days go by and I am wasting them, soon I'll die and my children will waste them too. I go to bed, then I start thinking about boys and about the future, and then I turn off the light, and I dream of all black. Once I had a dream, and I woke up crying. And the other day I was dreaming that I was with my father, and these two were looking for him to kill him, and then I got in the way, and they stabbed a knife at me. Then all of a sudden I wake up and call my brother and tell him it's time to go to school. And that is what I do before I go to bed.

That, I predict, is a future patient. (I should add that children of psychiatrists, psychoanalysts, and child psychiatrists often give "false" positives and are not to be taken seriously. They are probably just on the way to becoming psychiatrists, psychoanalysts, and child psychiatrists!)

Here is another response from a potential patient who was asked to write about anger by his teacher [5a]. As a contrast to what follows, an ordinary child wrote, "When I'm angry, I'm mad, and then I hit somebody whom I don't like, and then I'm better." Our potential patient writes:

> It feels like all the hatred in the world has gone into you, and you just have to blow up. So you just have to let it out, so you scream and kick to let it out. But always there will be a little left in you.

And another potential patient in the classroom has this to say about fear [5a]:

> I fear other people might kidnap me or something like that. Or that the wind will push me into the slush, or I'll slide right into a car. Sometimes I think that the bus driver is under a threat and that the bus will explode.

Another intriguing question relates to the amount of practice children obtain in the art of becoming patients. "Learning the ropes," as usual, begins in play that from time immemorial has attracted all children and fascinated a few that are potentially, depending on activity—passivity drives, therapists or patients. Doctor games, nurse games, dentist games are rich training grounds for future clients and practitioners, and it sometimes depends on the chance turn of the developmental wheel which role is to be undertaken, not excluding the possibility of both roles!

Here is an account by a child of the dentist game, giving some indication of how things might subsequently turn out [5a]:

> The night before I went to the dentist's my sister and I were playing at the dentist. She stamped on the floor that made the chair go up. She then switched on a light. She used a pair of pliers out of my tool set for the pinchers. She used my bubble hat for the gas mask. She used a pudding dish for the thing that you spit your blood into. She used a poker for the drill and a glass of water for the mouthwash. She tied me to the chair with some thick string and tied a hanky around my neck. She got a lolly stick and pressed my tongue back to see which tooth to pull out. She put a bit of rock in my mouth to keep it open and put my bubble hat on me. She took it off and got the pair of pliers and pretended to pull my tooth. She took a look at it and gave me the water, and I pretended to wash my mouth out. She untied the hanky, but she didn't untie me from the chair. She hit me about ten times and then ran off. I shouted to Mom to come and untie me. However, the next time we play, she's definitely going to be the patient. (an eight-year-old boy)

One wonders about the outcome. I have a feeling that the future dentist did the tying and running.

The Development of the Child as a Psychiatric Patient

It is always assumed, erroneously I think, that patients, like the goddess Athena, leap forward fully fashioned at whatever stage of development one first encounters them. From my experience as a therapist and child psychiatrist, I would say that being a patient is a complex matter involving the interplay of a large number of facilitating and resisting factors apart from endogenous predispositions that put the child immediately at risk. I believe that it takes almost the whole of childhood development to become a patient in the fullest sense of the term, and this includes the growth of understanding.

It has always been taken for granted that understanding is what the therapist gives to the individual when he or she becomes a patient. I want to consider very seriously what part understanding plays in the process of getting better. Does the patient get better through understanding better, or through being better understood, or because someone is trying to understand? "You don't understand me" is what one-half of the world always seems to be saying to the other half, and "I'm trying to understand you, but you don't make it easy" is what the other half of the world is saying in response.

Dr. Edward Glover once said, in considering the interpretations made to child patients two and three years of age by certain analysts, that he was sure that simply making nonsensical sounds would work wonders if the effects were right. There are several problems connected with being understood. It reminds me of the interchange between the Spanish ambassador and Queen Elizabeth I of England. Her Majesty had just made a statement about what her fleet would do to the Spaniards if they got any more bellicose. The Spanish ambassador said, "I quite understand you, Madame"; the queen, drawing herself up to her full stature, said, "We are not to be understood." I think what she meant was that it was presumptuous for a mere ambassador to attempt to decipher the mind of a queen of England. For many individuals, being understood contains a certain amount of threat. Being understood can mean being disarmed or vulnerable. On the other hand, not being understood can be aggravating, frustrating, and worrying. One can feel abandoned and alone.

What I think is consistently therapeutic is the process of the therapist trying to understand and the patient trying to feel understood. It is this experience that I think makes both the therapist and patient feel better, and this, in turn, makes the treatment better. The question to be considered is whether it is important for both therapist and patient to feel better for therapy to be successful.

This can be illustrated with a 16-year-old's account of the vicissitudes of the therapeutic situation over developmental time.

I first saw Debbie on her mother's lap at the age of 10 months. She was being demonstrated to a child development class. Compared to other babies that we were observing at the time, she was inactive, apathetic, uninterested in interesting sights, slow to respond, apparently bored by objects, and very quick to withdraw inside herself at the slightest hint of pressure. The mother's interest in her was fleeting and quickly turned to irritability so that the ambivalence was at times mutual. At the time, I labeled her a "difficult baby," predicting that she would have a difficult development and adjust only with difficulty to stressful events in her environment. Today, with more experience and understanding, I would have labeled her a vulnerable child at high risk for emotional disturbances during childhood and more serious disturbances at adolescence and adult life, and I would have suggested that she be convoyed through parts of her development.

The mother brought her to see me when she was a toddler, describing her as a "real headache." She often gave her mother a headache, and at times her mother confessed to hating her. "I think we are bad for each other. It's a love–hate business. I make her depressed, and she makes me depressed. I can't stand her demanding ways, and I suppose she can't stand my demands on her." I did my best to woo her. I broke my golden rule of therapy (which is never to leave the chair I sit in), and I sat with her on the carpet. At first she withdrew from me, and when I got closer, she hit me, and then failing to take the hint, I got still closer and she bit me. I withdrew to my chair and began interpreting to her at a safer distance. She paid no attention to me at all. I saw her about five or six times, on each occasion with her mother present. The mother, saying the child was much better, stopped coming. She was not in the least bit better in my room and continued to treat me with studied indifference. She never again bit me for the simple reason that I never again gave her a chance to do so. She returned for about three sessions at the age of five because she was having nightmares and phobias. One of her fears included men, but oddly enough, she showed no fear of me, and the mother remarked on this. She wondered whether it was due to the fact that she had known me since infancy. At this stage, she approached me very spontaneously, climbing on my lap several times. On one occasion when she was so located, she whispered to me that she saw bad people at night when she was sleeping and that this frightened her. I said that I was glad she had told me because I wanted to help her. She said she wanted to tell me something else but she first wanted her mother to leave. The mother looked a little hurt and then went out. Debbie said, "She is mean to me." I said, "Why couldn't you tell her that when she was here with us?" "Because she'd hit me," Debbie replied. Later I asked the mother whether she beat her child, and she said vehemently: "Never," adding, "it would make me feel too guilty. I sometimes want to very much, but I can't." I saw Debbie once again before she began grade school, and the phobias and nightmares had stopped. However, she remained somewhat quiet and apprehensive, and the kindergarten teacher said she really had no friends. She preferred to play by herself.

She was brought again during the second latency phase, aged nine. She was much less positive toward me and only just tolerated being in the room alone with me. She was sullen, uncooperative, uncommunicative, and showed some of her toddler negativism. The more I pressed her, the more she became silently defiant, and I detected underlying depression so I said to her in a friendly way, "I have known you since you were a baby," to which she replied uninterestedly, "I know." There was certainly no answering enthusiasm. I asked her if she would like to come and see me regularly, and she immediately said no. I asked her what objection she had to coming, and she was unequivocal about this: "I don't like you." I asked her if she was scared of coming, and she said, "I am scared of you." She would not enlarge on this, but in a later session she said, "Whenever I'm bad, Mom brings me to see you. If I do anything naughty, she tells me that she is going to tell you about it and that you would do something." I asked the mother afterward if she was using me as a disciplinary person, and she said, rather shamefacedly, that she was. "I'm afraid I've really made you into a big bad wolf." I told the mother that Debbie did not want to come to see me regularly, and the mother said that she agreed with this. "We get the best out of it coming to see you from time to time. I don't think she's ready to see you regularly." "How will you know when she is ready?" I asked. "I think she'll know," the mother answered.

At the age of 14 Debbie started to menstruate and was very upset. She said repeatedly that she did not want to grow up and that the blood made her feel sick. She hated everybody. "I feel like shit." "I never did anything bad. Why did God make this happen to me?" She was still very angry when she saw me, and she became angry with me. "You're supposed to be a doctor. Why can't you make me feel any better. I hate myself, and I hate everyone, and I hate you. I don't want to live, but I am afraid to die. I know there is something wrong with me or this wouldn't happen." She was referring to her menstruation, and I talked to her sensibly about this and said that it was a universal experience and part of growing up. She said savagely to me, "You don't bleed," and lapsed into a gloomy silence. I asked her again whether she would like to see me on a regular basis. She said that whenever she did come to see me she felt much worse. "You've always made me feel bad ever since I was a baby." I said that I knew she was unhappy and that she needed friends and that I would like to be her friend. She said, "I want a real friend, not a doctor friend. Doctors just pretend to be your friends because they are paid to be friendly." I said to her again, "I've known you since you were a baby," to which she responded with a toss of her head, "So what."

When she was 16½, she referred herself to me. She was having difficulties with friends, led a somewhat reclusive life, had many private hobbies, and was given to bursts of silent weeping for no apparent cause. As she entered my office she said, somewhat shyly,

"Well, here I am again," and I replied, "And here I am again." I asked her why she had come, and she said, "Because I have problems. I can't get on with anybody or anything, and I want you to help me." I said that I would do what I could, but then asked her why she had come to see me and not someone else. She answered: "Because I've known you since I was a baby. You're the only one who has always been there, and I wouldn't know who else to go and see." A little later she said, "I'm sorry that I used to give you such a hard time in the past. Didn't I bite you once? I really feel so bad and stupid the way I've treated you all these years. I wish I could make up for what I did." I said to her, smiling, that she was certainly trying to do just that, that she'd had a lot of feelings boiling in her in those days, and so I got some of it. Perhaps it had been useful to her to have somebody she could get angry with. I said to her, "Growing up can sometimes be a tough business," and she said quickly. "You can say that again. I've hated every minute of it. Thank goodness I'm almost finished with it." She reminisced a little about the past. "I'm not sure whether you couldn't help me or whether I just couldn't be helped. I know I was never a real patient. I never knew what you wanted me to do. I always felt trapped. Now I want to be a real patient." I asked her what a real patient was. "I don't know, but I feel more like a patient. I think a patient is someone who knows there is something the matter with him and wants to get over it and comes for help to get over it." I said that I thought that was a very good definition and welcomed her to treatment as a real patient.

I asked her why it had taken such a long time for her to become a real patient. She considered this seriously. "Perhaps it always takes that long. Perhaps little children can't be real patients. They try to be patients because their mothers want them to be, but they really don't know how, and they never learn. I have only just begun to understand about myself and about you and about what happens here, but when I was small, I just thought you were there to tell me that I must behave myself because that was what my mother wanted." I asked her what she had thought of me when she was a child. "I thought that you could do magic things—that you would just wave your pencil over my head to make things different and that you didn't like me and wouldn't. The funny thing was that even though I didn't like you at all, I used to feel quite different after seeing you. That's what made me come back now. I used to feel worse when I saw you but much better when I went away. I never connected this, but I think this is the reason I've come now. I also came because you're a kind of father because you've seen me since I was a baby and you know all about me. You've seen me when I've been very bad, and you've seen me when I've been good. I suppose that counts. In a way I feel like your child." A little later in the session, she asked whether I would have liked her to have been my child, so I asked her what she thought about this, and she said: "Who would want me? I don't think my parents ever really did, and now I'm certain they didn't. I have a feeling that my mother would have liked an abortion, but it was against her religion. Who would want me? I have such a dreadful personality [she paused a bit tearfully]; I suppose they had something to do about it. If I had been your child, I would have been wonderful and everyone would have liked me." I said lamely, "Parents often do the best they can. They're human. They make mistakes." She said hurriedly, "I'll tell you what's different. Ever since I've known you all this long time, you've been the same. I keep changing, but you stay the same and that makes me feel safe. My parents change even more than I do. They are never the same from one day to the next. I think that's the main reason why I came to see you."

She had taken 17 years to become what she called a "real patient"; she had been a patient in the making all these years. No one had told her how to become a patient, and she had gradually perceived the role for herself. I would add that she became a real patient in every sense of the word, and perhaps the most important sense: she made me feel at long last like a real therapist. Looking over the years, I could see that I was treating her in an *ad hoc* fashion, and it was only when she came to me herself that I knew what I had to do. It is my conviction that one needs to learn in every case how to treat each patient, no matter how many patients one has treated before.

Conclusion

When one goes searching for the "little people," one does not find them immediately under the first toadstool. It takes a lifetime of gradual, patient investigation, step by step, before one finds them—they must learn to trust you and you must learn to trust them.

The same developmental process of "gradualism" is at work when the "little people" become patients; they do not immediately become patients in the full grown-up sense with all its attendant array of signs and symptoms, diagnosis and prognosis, treatment planning, and methods of treatment. It takes time to become a "real" patient in this structured sense. As child psychiatrists and child therapists, we are often treating nonpatients and patients in the making, and we sometimes get impatient (especially if we recently have come from adult psychiatry) that our patients do not behave exactly like real patients (meaning adult patients). If we remember this, we will be less demanding of ourselves and less demanding of our cases. We must remember that they are, like Mr. Bilbo Baggins, fine people, but only little people in a wide world and that we should not expect too much or too little. In either case, we will be disappointed.

As big people, if we wish to be successful in our treatment, we must try to change the image that adult life forces on us, and that image is sometimes hard to change. As one of the little people once said to me (when I asked him about differences), "A little person is someone who starts something and a big person is someone who comes along and stops it." We must alter this image: a little person is someone who starts something, and a big person is someone who helps to make it go.

We have observed how the child psychiatrist of the past was gradually equipped to deal with children as psychiatric and psychotherapeutic patients; to understand them cognitively and emotionally, and to make use of their natural propensities for work and play in the service of treatment. When the problem of delinquency arose in the 1920s, it became clear that the model in use required expansion and elaboration. Some delinquents had brain dysfunctions; some had early privational experiences; some had neurotic problems, and some were well on the way to becoming people with character disorders. There was also a larger group that had been reared under such grossly disadvantageous circumstances that sociopathic strategies appeared to be the only logical ones for the purposes of survival.

The next generation of child psychiatrists began to become familiar with the social conditions, the cultural anomalies, and the devastating impact of poverty on the child's physical and psychological development. They began to appreciate how difficult it was to lead middle-class lives and cultivate middle-class virtues in ghetto surroundings. The environment clearly stamped the child as indelibly as the gene. The ecological approach added a new dimension to clinical practice, and the science of ekistics, which deals with the matching of the human habitat with human developmental needs, is fast becoming an area for the future child psychiatrist to explore.

The child psychiatrist of today is suffering from some degree of scientific backlash as a result of earlier experiences. Set as he is now within the schools of medicine, he is gaining increasing consciousness of himself as a physician, more widely trained than most. He is now mourning his lost stethoscope and his dormant medical skills and knowledge, and, following his prodigal use of multiple social and psychological talents, he is finding the way back to the laboratories, to the technologies of modern medicine, and to the new and so much more effective pharmacopoeia. The earlier enchantments with the mind and personality of the little people had led today's child psychiatrist increasingly away from the soma, but he is now realizing that his interdisciplinary training has advantages in bridging age-old mind–body gaps.

At national conferences, the child psychiatrist is still in a curious stage of transition. He can enter one auditorium and listen to the pathetic story of little Johnny, whose parents were divorced, who was reluctant to go to school, and who wanted nothing better than to get into bed with his mother of a morning and let the horrors of the classroom go by. He can enter another auditorium and listen to discussions on evoked potentials, the neurochemical correlates of depression, the perceptual anomalies associated with minimal brain dysfunction, and the reduced brain weights of African infants dying of malnutrition. At the end of such conferences, he may emerge in a state of semiconfusion with the feeling that his identity is a little muddled. He would be attempting to synthesize data from three different parts of a complex model—and not always successfully.

There is little doubt in my mind that if child psychiatry is to remain a thriving medical entity, it will need to adopt the biopsychosocial model described by Engel [2] and constantly reexamine the child patient in the light of recent knowledge deriving from neurobiology, social science, and systems theory. Whatever his biases (and the psychotherapeutic one is the most noticeable), the conditions of life today almost certainly impose a new look on his perspective. He needs to adapt to the changing system of health-care delivery, to the change in setting where care is being carried out, to the change in the heterogeneity of the population that requires care, to the change in social and cultural conditions that have important causal repercussions on the mental health of children and their families, and to the changes stemming from new work in the biological determinants of behavior. At this point, we cannot afford to be locked into a particular system until we have gained experience with these changes and until we have integrated them into our total approach.

Freud anticipated all this when he talked of the biochemist standing behind the analyst and gradually moving in on his preserves so that where psyche was, soma will be. Piaget had a more comprehensive viewpoint. In 1974 [6] he said that he was looking forward "with great expectation to the emergence of developmental psychopathology as a new discipline still struggling to organize its own relevant field of knowledge." He felt that "in spite of all the obstacles in the way and the huge amount of creative effort required for the purpose that this science will constitute itself of an interdisciplinary basis as wide as possible and on a common language that helps to unify what is precise and generalizable."

As if to supplement these powerful ideas, the National Institute of Mental Health of the United States has set up the Center for the Study of Child and Adolescent Psychopathology with two primary tasks: the grooming of future child psychiatric investigators and the exploration of psychopathological phenomena by current child psychiatric researchers in conjunction with other behavioral and biomedical scientists.

Let me, however, address a cautionary word to future child psychiatrists, still unborn, still untutored, and still wide open to all available influences. I would ask them not to forget their past or whence they came, and I would urge them to keep the understanding of the individual child in the forefront of their professional interest. I would ask them to bear in mind the remarks made by one of the leading clinicians and researchers of our time, Professor Manfred Bleuler [1], who, in conjunction with his father, has followed the families of schizophrenics from generation to generation so that his spectrum of clinical knowledge covers grandparents, parents, children, and grandchildren. Bleuler pointed out that if he had taken a purely scientific look at the schizophrenic disorder of his subjects, he would have been too engrossed with genetic or environmental hypotheses and might have overlooked important aspects of the human condition, *the suffering* that is often a concomitant of the illness; and if he had only seen the subjects once rather than over a lifetime, through successive generations, he might have taken a less optimistic view of illness. Let me quote a statement clearly indicating that the researcher and humanitarian need not be divorced.

> One of the most lasting impressions brought home to me by the family studies of our probands is the fact that even normal children who are successful in life can never fully free themselves of the pressures imposed on them by memories of their schizophrenic parents and their childhoods. Once one knows them more intimately, it is not rare that one perceives from the depth of their hearts a long-drawn sigh, something like: "When you've been through that . . . you can never really be happy; you can never love as others do; you always have to be ashamed of yourself and take care not to break down yourself."

Child psychiatrists of the future should keep this personal touch even in the midst of their growing scientific activities so that understanding of the child's predicament remains the core of their clinical perspective. The "little people" are child patients who have started something and cannot deal with it either by themselves or with the help of their parents. The "big people" are child psychiatrists who come along and help them not only to get over it and get along, but also to understand it. I should mention that Debbie was a subject in an ongoing research project, and so it was comparatively easy for me to keep track of her and to cultivate a longitudinal type of relationship. When she came to the Child Development Research Center, she underwent the routine physical, neurophysiological, psychiatric, anthropometric, and psychological testing that could have accounted for some of her earlier reactions to me, although the procedures were always carefully explained to the children. My total understanding of her was part of a comprehensive approach based on the Engelian biopsychosocial model of investigation. When I examined her total research dossier at any particular point in time, I would feel that my understanding was enhanced by the interdisciplinary input. I predict that the child psychiatrists of the future will develop even more refined techniques for investigating developmental psychopathologies, but I sincerely hope that they will always remember that they are dealing with a unique person.

What I have stressed chiefly in dealing with the "little people" in turmoil is the importance of seeing them as a whole, of maintaining contact with them over time, of being available during those treacherous periods during development when they especially need us, and of preparing them to become not only well-adjusted young people, but also competent parents who will help to deal more effectively with the next generation.

References

1. Bleuler, Manfred. The offspring of schizophrenics. In *The Schizophrenic Disorders* (trans. S. M. Clemens). Yale University Press, New Haven, Conn., 1978, 355–410.
2. Engel, George. *Psychological Development in Health and Disease.* Saunders, Philadelphia, 1962.
3. Freud, S. Analysis of a phobia in a five-year-old boy. *Standard Edition,* Vol. 10 (1909). The Hogarth Press, London, 1955, 5–129.
4. GAP, *Psychopathological Disorders in Childhood.* Aronson, New York, 1974.
5. Itard, J.M.G. *The Wild Boy of Aveyron* (trans. G. Humphrey and M. Humphrey). Appleton-Century Crofts, New York, 1932.

5a. Lewis, Richard (ed.) *Journeys Prose by Children of the English Speaking World.* Simon & Schuster, New York, 1969.
6. Piaget, Jean. Foreword to *Explorations in Child Psychiatry,* E. J. Anthony, Ed. Plenum, New York, 1975.
7. Sadger, J. Der psychoanalyse eines homosexuallen. *6b. sex. Zwiszhenst.,* 9, 109 (1908).
8. Yeats, W.B. Fairy and folk tales of the Irish peasantry. In Frayne, J. P., and Johnson, C., Eds. *Uncollected Prose of W.B. Yeats,* Vol. 1. Macmillan, London, 1970.

MAKING CONNECTIONS

The Formation of Maternal Filicidal Impetus from Childhood Incestuous Experiences

Christopher M. Green, M.D. (Canada)

The psychodynamic themes incorporated into maternal filicide are varied. It has been visualized as a form of extended suicide in which the mother identifies her child with herself [7]. In cases where the mothers suffer from frank psychotic illness, it has been suggested that the mother may project intolerable symptoms onto her child, the destruction of whom is a mechanism by which she attempts to gain relief [1]. Other authors have directed their attention to disturbed relationships with other family members as primary sources of the filicidal impetus. Pathological relationships with fathers [10], mothers [9], and husbands [2] have all been implicated. In these morbid relationships incest has been seen as of the primary importance. Olive [6] described a history of childhood incest in six cases of a group of 15 filicidal women. Zilboorg [11], in examining a series of depressed mothers, hypothesized that maternal filicidal impulses may arise by the mother seeing her child as a living testimony to her own incestuous past. This paper expands upon this theme. The first case describes the successful psychotherapeutic treatment of a potentially filicidal woman. In the second case, the patient, following filicide, underwent psychiatric investigation at the request of the court. Both cases provide dramatic illustration of the mechanisms that link incest and filicide.

CASE 1

Mary, a 34-year-old housewife, was admitted to the hospital in a severely distressed, depressed mental state, after strangling the family pet cat. She was unable to give an explanation for what she had done.

Mary was the second youngest in a family of seven brothers and one sister. She initially described an unremarkable childhood background but later expressed considerable hostility against her father, calling him a frightening and violent man. Following an average school career, she entered nurse training but left the course before qualifying. Shortly afterward at the age of 19 she became pregnant and obtained an abortion. A depressive breakdown followed, necessitating a period of hospitalization.

In her early twenties she met her future husband, an accountant, and married at the age of 25. The marriage proved stable, and by all accounts there had been no serious problems until she killed the family cat. At this time their daughter Julie was approaching her fifth birthday.

Mary was diagnosed as suffering from endogenous depression. With conventional antidepressive therapy her mental state gradually improved. During her stay in the hospital, however, she made oblique references to homicidal feelings against her daughter "I have swallowed a tooth and this has told me to kill my child," and, "I put one hand around Julie's neck and the other around the cat's." These remarks aroused concern for the safety of Julie. Arrangements were made to place the daughter temporarily in the care of the local authority. Mary appeared to make a good recovery from her depression. She left the hospital and was reunited with her daughter. This reunion evoked further symptoms of anxiety and depression, and she returned to the hospital. Further exploration of her psychopathology was indicated to clarify the situation. This exploration evolved into a two-and-a-half-year period of intensive psychotherapy.

Some weeks after the start of therapy Mary admitted to entertaining homicidal feelings toward her daughter. Prior to killing the cat, she had started to develop a plan in which she would give her daughter an overdose and then drive her car over a local cliff, killing them both. Along with this confession, she admitted to an incestuous relationship she had had with her father. This had started when she was five years old and terminated when she was 11 and her father attempted sexual intercourse. She expressed great hostility against him, recounting one episode of cunnilingus with special enmity. During these disclosures Mary frequently would become extremely tense, having to gain relief by smashing objects or injuring herself. This situation became repetitive, and, after much consideration, a series of pentothal abreactions were performed in an attempt to facilitate progress. A change then occurred in her descriptions of her incestuous experiences. Accompanied by intense feelings of guilt, she disclosed that they had in fact been "out of this world, a mixture of extreme excitement, happiness, and security rolled into one." Following this confession Mary appeared much happier and calmer. She went home on leave. It was arranged that she could have access to her daughter under her husband's supervision.

The leave was cut short. Mary phoned me to say that she had tried to strangle Julie with a pair of stockings. She was readmitted to the hospital. With the recommencement of therapy a new phenomenon emerged. For periods during the sessions, she would talk to me as if I were her father: "Why did you do it? You're a dirty, dirty old man. I hate you. I want to kill you." Her anger would gradually escalate, often culminating in physical attacks on me. A negative transference of almost psychotic intensity had developed. After sessions, Mary often required heavy sedation. The violence stopped with a particular event. Mary told me that she could see the devil, a black animal, whom one could interpret as representing her father. She then laughed, saying that three angels had taken him away. This episode appeared to mark a change in Mary, and for the next week she was calm.

One evening she told me she had just killed another cat in the hospital grounds. While talking about this, Mary complained of a peculiar sensation in her epigastrium. It soon became evident that this was sexual in nature. She identified these sexual feelings as the same as those she had experienced at the hands of her father. They returned repeatedly over the next sessions, becoming intense and violent in character. Between sessions her problem of self-condemnatory tension, accompanied by violent outbursts, reoccurred. The situation climaxed in a session during which she experienced sexual orgasm. Following this, her incestuous feelings and corresponding tension dissipated. It appeared that Mary had undergone a thorough catharsis of her childhood incestuous sexuality. This catharsis had a shattering effect on her mental cohesion, and she was left an insecure, pathetic figure, haunted by uncertainty. The therapeutic emphasis changed to restoration of self-confidence and coping skills. Nine months after the beginning of psychotherapy she was discharged in her husband's care. Arrangements were made for access to Julie so that she could resume her maternal role under supervision. She would return to the hospital two days a week for therapy.

One week she came with a marked change in her disposition. She was calm, composed, and confident. She informed me with *belle indefference* that her father was visiting the next day and was planning to sexually molest her daughter. She felt she had to kill Julie that night to save her from such a fate. She was sure I would understand. Her whole idea was clearly delusional. By projecting her own incestuous guilt onto Julie as a person who must be killed to be saved from paternal seduction, she was once again reerecting defenses against her own incestuous past. She was kept in the hospital. When the day of the imaginary seduction passed, Mary's idea dissipated, and so did her newly acquired self-confidence. She did, however, appear to have insight into how she had been identifying her dauther with her own childhood self. Three days after leaving the hospital, again she informed me by phone that she was being troubled by ideas of killing Julie. On her return, Mary said she had to kill Julie, not to save her from her father, but to save her from herself. Julie was just like she had been as a child, pretty, gay, and flirtatious. She would make the same mistakes and would subsequently become insane. Again, the projection and identification mechanisms that Mary was using as a defense against her own guilt were strongly challenged. Two days later Mary took a serious overdose of drugs, then made a satisfactory recovery. This was the last major traumatic event in our relationship.

Mary continued in therapy on an out-patient basis for over a year. During this period, sexual fantasies concerning her therapist emerged. A positive transference had developed with me, as therapist, assuming the role of surrogate father. Mary was able to discuss her sexual fantasies about her therapist—father in safety, without the danger of them being turned into reality. Such feelings, in this context, no longer produced intolerable guilt and therefore became acceptable. This positive transference was worked through gradually. Mary's self-confidence gradually returned, and she started to feel she could cope with life and her daughter without my support. By mutual agreement therapy was terminated.

CASE 2

In the early hours of a Saturday morning, Joan, a 29-year-old woman, killed her five-year-old daughter, Anne, by strangling her with a pair of tights. She almost immediately confessed her homicide to relatives and was then arrested by the police. In the police cells, she was in an extremely distressed state, overwhelmed by guilt for her actions. A psychiatric enquiry into the homicide was requested, and Joan was seen initially on two occasions while in police custody and then frequently over a four-week period of hospital treatment. An involved psychologist and social worker were also interviewed. Joan had been undergoing treatment from a psychologist for two years before the homicide. Her family had also received intensive investigation and support from local social services for many years.

Joan came from a large working-class family of five brothers and five sisters. Four of her siblings had received treatment for alcoholism. In her childhood, a fond relationship with her father seemed to have existed. However, in contrast to this, she possessed feelings of hostility and resentment toward her mother, who she said ridiculed her as a child. She was particularly sensitive to some taunts made about her unusually dark skin. She attended school until she was 15. She was a dull performer academically, although she claimed to have made adequate social relationships with her peers.

The most significant phenomenon of her childhood years was a gross incestuous relationship with her brothers that had developed to the point of sexual intercourse. She remembered this starting when she was nine years old and terminating at the age of 17 when she left home. Joan claimed that she had been a reluctant participant and that her brothers had forced their sexual attentions on her. In spite of this, she seemed to hold little resentment against them. This was compensated by much hostility toward her mother, who was aware of her incestuous relationship and on a number of occasions had caught her during sexual activity. She said her mother would blame her for being sexually provocative, leaving her brothers free of blame. At the age of 17, Joan was accused of seducing her brother. A violent argument ensued and she left home.

On leaving home, she established a common-law marital relationship with a man of similar age. They lived together for the next eight years, during which time she gave birth to a son and a daughter (at the time of the tragedy aged 7 and 6, respectively), and a second daughter, her victim, five years-old at the time of her death. Her common-law marital relationship was never happy. Joan found herself unable to cope with the strains of married life and having a family. Both she and her husband drank alcohol to excess. In addition, Joan would abuse tranquilizing drugs by obtaining prescriptions from seemingly numerous general practitioners. Their relationship was punctuated by violent arguments that sometimes resulted in short periods of separation. On several occasions Joan took overdoses of drugs necessitating short admissions to the local psychiatric hospital.

Two years prior to the homicide, the couple separated. At this time it was found that Joan was beating her oldest daughter excessively, and the children were placed in the care of the local social services. For the next two years Joan received constant support and counseling from the town social services department and a psychologist from the local university. During interviews with them she would often express strong feelings of guilt over her incestuous past. These appeared to be associated with a great deal of hostility and resentment against her mother. Her relationship here was markedly ambivalent. Indeed, she constantly visited her mother in an apparent search for support. It was only in privacy with her professional helpers that she was able to express her anger at her.

Four months before the homicide the children were returned to Joan's care. Things superficially appeared to progress satisfactorily. Apart from some mild signs of depression and anxiety there was no warning of the impending tragedy. Joan spent the day before the murder at her mother's home with her children. She recounted her mother making fun of Anne, calling her names, and saying that her skin was too dark, all reminiscent of the way Joan felt she herself had been treated as a child. She returned home at 11:00 p.m., feeling distressed to the point of suicide, and took an overdose of pills. Anne, who was by all accounts her favorite daughter, was, she felt, suffering as she herself had suffered as a child. The children were put to bed, Anne sleeping in the same bed as her mother. As Anne fell asleep she said, "Mommy, I love you." These words triggered a homicidal impulse. With no premeditation, Joan picked up some tights and strangled her daughter. She was arrested by the police shortly afterward, in a state of numbness and confusion over what she had done.

During the first two days of custody Joan was in a highly distressed state. She was unable to face the horror of her actions, often screaming, "My baby, my baby, I killed my baby." On the third day, at her own request, she attended her daughter's funeral. On her return, her mental state underwent a marked change. She blandly informed me that Anne was alive and well, that the date was the day before the homicide occurred, and that she was due to visit her mother that afternoon. As a hysterical defense against the horror of killing her daughter, Joan had mentally regressed to the day before the homicide. She was admitted to the hospital. Over the next four weeks, together with much mourning, she gradually returned to a realization of Anne's death. She was eventually remanded to prison to await trial.

Due to the nature of the offense, together with Joan's mental fragility, the subject of her tragedy had to be approached with delicacy. In her initial statement to the police she said she had killed her daughter to take revenge on her mother. "I shouldn't have killed my baby just to get my own back on my mom." This was followed by her stating that when she left prison she intended to kill her mother, then herself. During our initial interview she maintained that she had killed Anne as an altruistic act to save her from further suffering. While in the hospital she expanded on this theme. Anne was her favorite daughter. She looked and acted just like Joan had as a child. There were worries that Anne would be sexually abused and suffer as she had.

Discussion

These cases illustrate a number of psychodynamic themes involved in filicide. The theme of filicide as a form of extended suicide [7] is shown in Mary's fantasy of killing herself and her daughter by driving her car over a local cliff and in Joan's attempted suicide shortly before the homicide. Both cases show how disturbed relationships with other family members may be a primary source of the filicidal impetus [9,10]. In the case of Mary, it is the father who is seen as the important source of filicidal aggression, whereas in Joan filicide appears to arise in association with intense hostile feelings toward her mother.

The nucleus of both psychopathologies, however, lies in the gross guilt both patients felt over their incestuous pasts. Mary's hatred of her father arose from her sexual involvement with him. Joan's hostility was not primarily directed at her incestuous partners, her brothers, but instead at her mother, who condemned her for her seductive behavior. The cases portray filicide as a mechanism in which patients may project their own childhood incestuous sexuality onto their daughters. The act of homicide is then seen as an attempt to destroy their own incestuous guilt. Both patients identified their daughters with their own childhood selves. Each ultimately portrayed filicide as an altruistic act, to save their daughters from the same incestuous fate that had befallen them.

There are different opinions on how incest may affect the developing child. Lykionoviecz [5], in examining 26 cures of paternal incest, concluded that there were no grave psychiatric sequelae that could be related directly to the incest itself. Ferenzi [3], on the contrary, believed the incest nearly always had severe pathological consequences. Lewis and Sorrel [4] give the opinion that important factors that may determine the degree of psychological damage include the child's level of development, the quality of the parent–child relationship, the nature of the event, and whether it was an isolated or continuing experience. Rosenfeld [8] felt that in those cases where intense guilt developed, the child's enjoyment of the sexual experience was important. Both patients discussed here clearly suffered severe psychological damage and intense guilt from their incestuous relationships. A high level of sexual activity continued for many years in the context of an overall poor parent–child relationship would appear important in this context. However, it is tempting to place more emphasis on the sexual pleasure the patients obtained. This is vividly illustrated in Mary's case when the description was given of an experience that was "out of this world," consisting of a feeling of intense excitement, happiness, and security. Although Joan never admitted to enjoying her sexual involvement with her brothers, the root of her anger appeared to stem from her mother accusing her of willfully seducing them.

In summary, these cases clearly show how childhood incestuous experiences may be a possible source of filicidal impulses. Further work will determine whether this is a common source of the filicidal impetus.

References

1. Bender, L. Psychiatric mechanisms in child murderers. *J. Nerv. Ment. Dis.,* 80 (1934), 32.
2. DeVallet, J., and Sherrer, P. Un cas de psychose de degout conjugal avec reaction infanticide. *Ann. Medicopsychol.,* 97 (1939), 80.
3. Ferenczi, S. Confusion of tongues between adults and child. *Int. J. Psychoanal.,* 30/4 (1949), 225.
4. Lewis, J., and Sorrel, M. Some psychological aspects of seduction, incest and rape in childhood. *J. Am. Acad. Child Psychiat.,* 8 (1969), 609.
5. Lykionoviecz, N. Incest. *Brit. J. Psychiat.,* 120 (1972), 301.
6. Olive, R.O. Roche report, frontiers of hospital psychiatry Abstract, 4(No. 22) (1967), 3.
7. Resnick, P.J. Child murder by parents: A psychiatric review of filicide. *Am. J. Psychiat.,* 126 (1969), 73.
8. Rosenfeld, A.A., Nadelren, C.C., Krieger, M., and Boekman, J.H. Incest and sexual abuse of children. *J. Am. Acad. Child Psychiat.,* 16 (1977), 327.
9. Slater, A.K. Infanticide—Report of two cases. *Med. J. Aust.,* 48 (1961), 819.
10. Stern, E.C. The medea complex: Mother's homicidal wishes to her child. *J. Ment. Sci.,* 94 (1948), 321.
11. Zilboorg, G. Depressive reactions related to parenthood. *Am. J. Psychiat.,* 97 (1931), 927.

Yesterday's Children in Turmoil–Today's Parents

Per-Anders Rydelius, M.D. (Sweden)

It is no easy matter to foretell the long-term effects of a known situation. Indeed, in all longitudinal prospective processes, one is faced with uncertainty about the manner in which changes occurring on the social scene will affect the situation being studied. Such methodological problems are particularly pertinent in child psychiatry, a field in which it is customary to voice favorable or unfavorable predictions of a child's future on the grounds of the available data relating to the child's current symptoms and social background.

With respect to conditions in Swedish families, authors who have studied the significance of child psychiatric status have reached the conclusion that it is hardly possible to make any predictions on the grounds of the current mental status of the individual [1, 4, 7]. On the other hand, the social background and, possibly, certain symptoms and features of personality [4, 7] can be of greater importance to the prognostic assessment than the actual child psychiatric status.

As a result of a comprehensive compilation of child psychiatric literature, Rutter [5] demonstrated that so-called neurotic symptoms in children did not correspond to mental illnesses in adults, whereas other symptoms such as acting out did appear to indicate an antisocial development. In a study dealing with long-term effects on children growing up in a socially unfavorable environment with alcoholic fathers, I [6] discussed these methodological problems and concluded that although there is good reason to make prognostic assessments—at least with respect to certain social variables—it would be of greater value to perform two successive longitudinal studies, constructed along similar lines, to elucidate in definite terms the true significance of the length of the period covered by the study, both *per se* and in relation to the social changes occurring during this time.

Yesterday's Vulnerable Children in Sweden

The children considered to be the most vulnerable in Sweden in the 1950s and 1960s, that is, children from homes characterized by grave alcoholism, might constitute a less victimized group than children living under similar circumstances in Sweden today. Since adjustment problems such as asociality and drug and alcohol abuse have increased in frequency and because there has been a reduction in differences between the sexes leading to an increase in the number of women with serious adjustment problems, the children of today may well be burdened to a greater degree than the children of the 1950s in that they may have not only an alcoholic father but also an alcoholic mother. Even though some of the children growing up during the 1950s suffered both mental and physical neglect and mistreatment as a result of lamentable home conditions, the main source of their sufferings was the father in the family. The mothers of that time, although overworked and exhausted, seldom succumbed to alcoholism or drug abuse. This circumstance, which was mainly due to Sweden's policy relating to alcohol at that time, no longer applies today, with the result that there are now many women alcoholics with grave problems in the Swedish community. It may therefore be that the vulnerable children in the present population are having to meet even greater problems than those met by their predecessors and that there are other aspects of life that are worrisome today which were not at all apparent 20 to 30 years ago. It has, however, been pointed out [2] that the negative social inheritance affecting vulnerable children appears to accumulate from generation to generation, and this implies that the problems burdening certain susceptible groups will, in all probability, become greater with time.

I [7] have followed 229 of the children who grew up during the 1950s in families in which the fathers were alcoholics and generally poorly adjusted socially. These children were compared to a control group consisting of 163 matched social twins [3] and their lives as adults were investigated to discover how well, or how poorly, they had adjusted to society. As a result of the follow-up study, I was able to obtain information on how yesterday's children from deprived home environments have adjusted as today's parents. This information can be used to plan subsequent research projects designed to follow up groups that are being victimized today.

In the prospective longitudinal study in question, the original children were traced and followed up by means of blind methods, and the data were collected from various registers maintained by Swedish authorities. The main purpose of the study was to acquire, as far as possible, an objective picture of the adjustment made by the child to adult life. This part of the study covered 20 years and is now complete. A number of interesting questions remain to be studied. For example, the study did not provide answers to the following questions: Can today's adults describe how they responded emotionally to the experience of growing up? How have the experiences from those years affected their ability to form a family and their choice of husband or wife? In what way have these experiences influenced their possibilities to give their own growing children a stable home life?

Some of the factors relating to the forming of a family have been studied, however. It can be mentioned here that the boys from alcoholic homes got married at an earlier age than the boys from the control group, and they also tended to become fathers earlier. In addition, they tended to be responsible for more children born out of wedlock. Using similar statistical analyses, it was found that the girls from alcoholic homes had given birth to a larger number of children than the girls from the control group when the comparison was made at the end of the 20-year observation period. The comment can of course be made that the higher rate of adjustment problems (including difficulties in supporting the family financially, higher sickness rates, and tendencies toward substance abuse and criminality) shown by the grown-up children of alcoholic parents has obviously had an effect on their relationships to their families, but this aspect has not been elucidated in the study in question. However, a tendency toward a higher divorce rate was noted for these individuals.

Nevertheless, the data collected can supply some information about the difficulties encountered by these former children from alcoholic homes when they embark on the role of parent. To illustrate this, a number of case descriptions are given that show the background of the child in 1958 and the situation for the same individual 20 years later in the role of parent. This study has not been designed to provide any generalizations that can be said to be prevalent among those children from alcoholic homes.

Case Histories

FEMALE, AGED 31

In 1958, this girl was in poor mental condition. She was a member of one of the two families in the study group in which both the mother and father had grave problems with alcohol, the mother having been hospitalized for this reason. The girl had previously been healthy, both physically and mentally, but gave a poor emotional response at the time she was examined. Her teacher at school felt that she deviated from the rest of the class since she showed a strong tendency to withdraw. Throughout her adult life, this young woman experienced difficulties, receiving social assistance on several occasions, and being registered for criminal offenses for which she was put on probation. She was frequently ill, and during the years 1977, 1978, and 1979 she had a total of 899 sick days. She has abused both alcohol and drugs since the middle 1970s. She is unmarried. She has two children by the same man, with whom she has lived periodically and who has periodically assaulted her. The children were born in 1971 and 1973 and have at times lived with their mother, were once placed in a foster home for a period, and at times have lived with their father and his new fiancée. They have stayed periodically with their paternal grandparents, who have expressed deep concern over their condition, feeling that they were often dirty and unkempt, as well as nervous and unhappy. Efforts made to provide support and treatment through the Child Guidance Clinics failed because the mother lacked the energy to pursue the measures proposed. The Child Welfare authorities have been called to the mother's home on several occasions because a fight was going on, the boys being witness to their mother being beaten, but there is no evidence that the boys have been the victims of assault. At the end of the observation period in 1978, the Child Welfare authorities were handling an investigation of the family's situation to decide whether the mother would be permitted to retain guardianship of the children.

FEMALE, AGED 24

When she was examined as a child in 1958, her mental status was extremely poor. She was living together with her mother and father in a "summer cabin" that was in a miserable state. In winter the wind and rain blew right through the walls, and outdoor clothes had to be worn indoors. This cabin was one of several in a particular area, many of which acted as homes for male alcoholics with whom the girl associated daily. She had suffered recurrent bouts of upper respiratory infections. Reports had been received to the effect that she had often been left alone without food or attention, and when she was 5 years old, the Child Welfare authorities took charge of her for one month. During her adult life she has been in need of regular social assistance. Her sickness rate tends to be high; during the years 1977, 1978, and 1979, she was ill on eight occasions totaling 76 sick days. It is known that she has begun to abuse alcohol. She is living with a man and gave birth to a boy in 1974. After the birth she was in a distraught state and unable to cope with the baby since she was overly tired. During the baby's first year, she gave the child to her own mother to look after when she could not manage to care for him. She has been in touch with the Child Guidance Clinic for help because of problems in bringing up her child. She has left the child's father several times, only to return and move in with him again. The Child Welfare authorities have not inquired into the child's present situation.

FEMALE, AGED 28

When examined in 1959, this girl was found to be immature, shy, and unfocused. She had been hospitalized for abdominal pains and insomnia. During the observation period, she was registered for abuse of alcohol and drugs and for criminal offenses. She received probational sentences on five occasions, and was fined for 11 misdemeanors. She is in constant need of financial help. Her sickness rate is high: during the years 1977, 1978, and 1979, she had 17 periods of sick leave totaling 305 days. She is unmarried and living with a much older man who has problems with alcohol and drugs, and with whom she had a child in 1972. The man has beaten her regularly and has been sentenced to prison for the offense on several occasions. The child has not been mistreated but the mother has not looked after her properly. She has been neglected, left dirty, and not given sufficient food. The child was consequently taken from the mother by the Social Welfare authorities and placed elsewhere while inquiries were being made. After the investigation, the child was allowed to return to her mother, but her situation has not been followed up by the Child Welfare authorities.

MALE, AGED 25

When examined, the boy was found to be in a poor mental state. He had been hospitalized for psychosomatic symptoms, and he showed signs of physical neglect. In the process of growing up, he soon exhibited an antisocial behavior pattern marked by extensive burglaries and by substance abuse (sniffing solvents and excessive drinking). He was sentenced on six occasions for 18 offenses, which included assault and willful damage. He has been in regular need of social assistance and has shown a tendency toward a high rate of sickness. He was sick on 23 occasions during the years 1977, 1978, and 1979, for a total of 168 days. He has fathered two children, both girls, born in 1971 and 1975. He married the mother of the children in 1976. Because of his adjustment problems, he was not employed at the time the youngest child was born. Since he was at home anyway, he looked after the child while the mother worked. The Child Welfare authorities have not made any follow-up inquiries into the children's situation.

MALE, AGED 31

This child grew up under very difficult circumstances: his mother was mentally exhausted, and his father was a severe chronic alcoholic. He was placed in foster homes periodically and regularly displayed symptoms of ill health with abdominal pains. He also had problems in his relations with his peers. The results of a psychiatric investigation showed that he was in low spirits, that he showed signs of neglect illustrated by his poor dental status, and that his school performance deviated from that of his classmates. He had serious adjustment problems while growing up and quickly became criminalized. He became addicted to both alcohol and drugs. He was in regular need of social support. He was often ill, and was registered for 24 periods of sick leave during the years 1977, 1978, and 1979 totaling 646 days. He is unmarried but lives with a woman with whom he has a son, born in 1969. His fiancée took the child and left him during the observation period, and he no longer has any contact with his son.

MALE, AGED 30

When examined in 1958, the boy did not exhibit any adjustment problems. He showed signs of physical neglect, but there were definitely no signs of mental symptoms. During puberty, he rapidly developed an antisocial behavior pattern that included the abuse of alcohol and drugs and solvent sniffing. He has been in regular need of social help. He was sentenced nine times and received sentences of long periods of imprisonment. He is listed in the Criminal Offenses Register for more than 40 offenses. He has one child with a woman to whom he has not been married. He has no contact whatsoever with the child, and the child has not been the subject of any attention on the part of the Child Welfare authorities.

It can be seen from the foregoing case histories that many of the children from alcoholic backgrounds clearly encountered difficulties in their roles as parents. In the case of the mothers, people in their environment have often drawn attention to signs of neglect in the physical and mental care of their children, although forceful measures designed to give the children help and support have seldom been effective. In the case of the men, they obviously have often been so difficult to live with that their fiancées have taken the children and moved out. In some instances this has resulted in a complete severance of contact. The cases just described are only a very few of the original children of alcoholic parents who subsequently became parents themselves, but the situation is similar for many of the others.

The observations that have been made in the course of the study provide motivation for a continuation designed to investigate in detail the functioning of the former children of alcoholic parents from the 1950s within the situation created when they themselves build families. A further objective covered by the scope of the investigation is to describe the manner in which the social inheritance has been passed on to the next generation. It is obvious that a very large number of the children born during the 1970s have suffered from neglect in their own psychosocial care requirements, either in the form of a mother who was unable to cope or a father who was never available.

References

1. Andersson, M., Jonsson, G., and Kälvesten, A.L. *What Happened to the 1950 Stockholm Boys?* Stockholm Municipal Council Monograph series No. 38, Stockholm, 1976. (in Swedish)

2. Jonsson, G. Delinquent boys, their parents, and grandparents. *Acta Psychiat. Scand.* (suppl.) 195 (1967).
3. Nylander, I. Children of alcoholic fathers. *Acta Paediatr. Scand.*, vol. 49, suppl. 121 (1960).
4. Nylander, I. A 20-year prospective follow-up study of 2164 cases at the Child Guidance Clinics in Stockholm. *Acta Paediatr. Scand.*, suppl. 276 (1979).
5. Rutter, M. Relationship between child and adult psychiatric disorders. *Acta Psychiatr. Scand.*, 48 (1972), 3–21.
6. Rydelius, P-A. A longitudinal–prospective study of the children of alcoholic fathers. A methodological study and a description of the life situations of the children after 15 years. *Research Report from the Child Psychiatric Clinics of the Karolinska Institute, St. Göran's Hospital,* Stockholm, 1980. (in Swedish)
7. Rydelius, P-A. Children of alcoholic fathers—their social adjustment and their health status over 20 years. *Acta Paediatr. Scand.*, suppl. 286 (1981).

Infants under Stress: Tomorrow's Adults

John Cullen, M.D.
John A. Connolly, M.D. (Northern Ireland)

A search of medical data bases using the key words *stress* and *infancy* produces a very heterogeneous listing of publications in recent years. They are also surprisingly few in number (about 60) when one considers how large a literature the stress field in general has produced over recent decades. However, it is obvious that many of the major issues that have concerned researchers in child development for more than 30 years have had to do with the effects of stress in one form or another. In particular, a central role has been occupied by studies of maternal deprivation, separation and loss, and of the vicissitudes of attachment and bonding. The classic studies of Spitz and Bowlby with human subjects and those of Seay, Hansen, and Harlow [53] and of Kaufman et al. [28] in monkeys have stimulated a whole era of researchers. A keystone of this work has been the view that the disruption of mother−infant bonds occurring for a long enough time and at a critical period in the child's life usually has profound and pervasive negative effects on the child's subsequent development and future social adaptedness. It was also believed that those effects were probably irreversible.

These assumptions and the studies on which they were based have recently been reviewed by Rutter [51, 52] and also by Clarke and Clarke [10]. This valuable work has contributed a considerably more cautious approach to wide extrapolation of the earlier findings in clinical, educational, and health-care problems. It has been found that the developing organism is much more resilient than was previously claimed and that considerable restitution of function is possible [10, 26].

From these more recent studies it is clear that overt social competence and peer equivalence of intellectual attainment can be achieved or restored, albeit with increased educational and care investment. Although this resilience may be somewhat brittle, nevertheless the restitution is real and apparently can be consolidated.

Stress researchers coming from different traditions and perspectives must look at this literature with different questions in mind. They will be concerned with more psychobiological issues initially and ask if in fact their criteria for restitution have been met. For example, they will wish to know if appearances are enough. Some of the markers they use for detection of deleterious effects may be covert—biological rather than behavioral. Two biological systems have been prominent in stress studies and are used as benchmarks for rating adaptive function status. These are the endocrine pituitary–adrenal system and the cardiovascular system. Stress research also uses different constructs and paradigms for evaluating alterations in such parameters and the behavioral contexts in which they occur.

Animal studies have contributed many insights to the stress field just as they have in the more psychosocial aspects of mother–infant bonding. There is a tradition of studies on the psychobiology of development that raises important questions for health workers. Perhaps the most consistent themes in this field have been pursued by Levine and his coworkers in Stanford [32, 33, 34, 35, 36].

Beginning with rodent studies on the effects of nonspecific stimulation experiences in infancy on psychobiological adaptation [32], the work has evolved recently to encompass studies on primates of the role of the mother–infant relationship in the development of the ability to cope with stress [35].

Earlier studies [32, 36] indicated that the handling of infant rats in the sensitive period of the first seven days of postnatal life profoundly influenced their adult behavior and in particular affected in a positive direction their ability to cope with stress. This seemed to open up the possibility of experimental validation and manipulation of the issues raised by Bowlby in the clinical studies described in his monograph *Maternal Care and Mental Health* [3]. And indeed there was, over the following decade and more, an enormous range of studies that explored many dimensions of the effects of environmental manipulation in infancy and the subsequent effects on adult behavior in mammalian species. Levine [34] reviewed these developments some 15 years after his first papers, and certain highlights emerged. He now felt that accumulated evidence supported the view that the effect of handling was mediated through its effects on the mother–infant relationship, although stimulation *per se* could also have some direct effect.

Other findings also emerged. Two themes from these are still of particular significance for stress research. The first relates to a range of findings indicating that profound effects on the pituitary–adrenal system could be detected and that these endocrine effects could persist despite apparent behavioral normality in such stressful situations as the open-field test. So there seemed to be a situation in which overt coping was not accompanied by successful coping in terms of modulation of arousal in psychobiological terms. The second theme related to findings showing that mothers who had themselves been subjected to handling stress in their infancy produced offspring who showed brittle or inadequate modulation of their responses when subjected to stress in adult life. It was also found that manipulation of the mother's endocrine status by adrenalectomy before her mating led to profound effects on the responsiveness of her offspring's pituitary–adrenal system when they were required to cope with stress.

So a view had emerged that the prenatal status of the mother could have effects on the stress responsiveness of the endocrine system of the offspring and that the psychobiological response to stress was one in which behavioral and biological parameters could covary or they could be alternates given suitable environmental contingencies. These latter especially related to patterns of mother–infant relationships. Biological and behavioral dimensions do not necessarily covary in naive ways. They do remain related but in complex ways we are only beginning to discern.

This whole organism perspective was also showing new dimensions of how organisms cope with stress. It was emerging that not only was the endocrine response modulated by environmental and behavioral events but that alterations in hormones could in turn have profound effects on coping behavior [33]. These effects were to be found in perceptual processes and in learning (in particular in the learning of avoidance responses). More recently, with the explosion of knowledge in neuroendocrinology, the implication of neuropeptides and of hypothalamic factors in these processes has opened up a new era in our understanding of biobehavioral mechanisms [58].

In a recent review of the work of his own group and of others,

Levine [35] has described a whole new range of findings in subhuman primates on the stress and coping mechanisms that are modulated by the mother–infant dyadic relationship or disorganized by its disruption. These findings confirm the specificity of the attachment bonds in the dyadic relationship. Furthermore, they show that profound effects can occur in the pituitary–adrenal system if the contingencies of the mother–infant relationship are upset. It is clear that the infant manipulates the relationship by its own behavior, thus developing a cognitive map of contingencies where control, predictability, feedback and the vigor and frequency of responses all sum in the development of its coping repertoire.

There are also findings [12] that show that "aunting" by a late-pregnant conspecific does occur in squirrel monkeys. However, this aunting experience has not been found to offset all of the stress responses elicited by separation from the mother. In fact, the divergence of biological effects in the pituitary–adrenal system from behavioral ones is observed. There are persistent elevations of cortisol despite the reduction of the observable behavioral manifestations of the "protest" phase. Other studies reveal counterintuitive findings. For example, separation of infants from surrogate cloth mothers produces brisk and vigorous protest behavior, increased vocalization, and so forth, although cortisol levels may remain at basal levels. Dependency rather than attachment bonds seem to be implicated. Furthermore, separated infants maintained with familiar peers of the social group seem to show more profound depression effects than those who are isolated. Perhaps most fascinating of all is the finding that the active mother–infant relationship when the dyad is maintained in proximity is protective against novelty stress for both mother and infant. Each maintains basal level pituitary–adrenal function compared with nonpregnant conspecifics without infants exposed to the same novelty stimuli.

Much of the literature reviewed so far has been concerned with biological effects in the pituitary–adrenal system. Similar patterns of hyper- or low-arousal have been described [47] for other physiological parameters. Heart rate, body temperature, and sleep disturbances have been reported.

Cardiovascular parameters have had a significant place in developmental psychobiology, and the work of Campos [8] and Lipsitt [37] has shown how responses, especially in heart rate, are cued to developing cognitive processes. Indeed, cardiovascular processes seem to share a two-way modulating process with cerebral cortex activity not unlike the mode of the two-way processes between behavior and endocrine activity already described. Lacey and Lacey [29] had postulated effects on cortical activity deriving from alterations in levels of baroreceptor firing from the aorta with changes in blood pressure. Experimental confirmation of this postulate has gained support in a recent series of experiments by Dworkin et al. [17] in which they demonstrate effects on avoidance behavior when blood pressure is pharmacologically manipulated. Part of the experimental data we present here relate to cardiovascular responses of human infants, which for us reinforce the view that biological variables must be explored as well as behavioral ones if the effects of stress in infancy are to be evaluated fully.

Of course, a major difficulty in all of this research when considered by health professionals is to discern the relevance of the biological changes observed to the causation of disease. In fact, our models of pathogenesis are still primitive, and many of the processes involved in the genesis of the major stress diseases are poorly understood. Lennart Levi, in his work at the Laboratory for Clinical Stress Research at the Karolinska Institute, has explored many of the ways in which stress responses in the sympathomedullary and pituitary–adrenal systems may be elicited, but he has always been careful to point out that these responses may be the precursors of disease, that they are, indeed, likely to be so, but that the final elucidation of the mechanisms and of causal links has yet to be achieved [30]. Levi has contributed perhaps more than any other worker to our awareness of the importance of psychosocial factors in the multifactorial origins of disease, but much remains to be done, and our work is a contribution to this task. His own words summarize the situation much better than I could do:

In summary, we may conclude that causation of disease by psychosocial stimuli is unproven but at a high level of suspicion. The action of such stimuli on mechanisms and precursors is better understood but still rather poorly documented. There is also a high level of suspicion that interacting psychosocial factors and physical factors could prevent some mechanisms, precursors and diseases.

Before one can rationally discuss prevention, it is desirable to know more. This means research. Nevertheless there will, no doubt, be occasions when health planners may feel, in the particular circumstances of their community, that action should be taken on the basis of the existing level of suspicion (Rexed, 1971). Such action might well be in the areas of marriage (or its equivalent) counselling, handling of the baby and the young child, support at "crisis" times for the child, adolescent and adult, job satisfaction and hygiene, threat to sense of belonging in the aged (Lazarus, 1971; Roberts, 1971; Kagan and Levi, 1971; Raab, 1971). If this were to be the case, it would be important—in our opinion mandatory—to regard the action as a trial and to establish means of evaluating it for efficiency, safety and cost. This has a scientific and a social purpose. The former is to establish knowledge. The social purpose is to protect individuals from danger, and the community (and other communities) from unnecessary expense. It is also to avoid a sense of false security, to prevent delay in applying useful procedures and to provide rational support for innovative measures based on perceived cost and effect. [25]

In a more recent paper Levi [31] carries these issues much further into health-care policy formulation.

A recent search of the literature with a clinical bias has been undertaken by the present authors. Although this is by no means exhaustive, some interesting findings were noted. Some of the reports implicate disturbances of endocrine function in pathology. An interesting histological study of the adrenal glands of 41 stillbirths showed a clear stress response pattern in 28 of them. The author [16] reports a number of changes in cellular architecture, including cell change and lipid depletion, and, in the severest stress, effect cytolysis producing a cystic appearance. It is deduced that these changes indicate previous stress experiences of a nonspecific kind sustained by the fetus in utero. These changes were somewhat commoner in immature infants, but infants of low birth weight were slightly more commonly represented in the group without these stress-related changes.

Another report [43] described a single case of fatal bleeding from gastric ulceration in the first day of life. The only causative factor that could be elicited was a very high level of maternal psychosocial stress during the last trimester of pregnancy. The authors postulate a mediating role of maternal gastrin in the pathogenesis. Previously Revill and Dodge [49] had found high scores on the Life Events Inventory during pregnancy for a series of 100 mothers of infants with hypertrophic pyloric stenosis compared with a normal control group and a group of mothers whose infants had spina bifida. High anxiety levels were also found in these mothers. They also postulate a humoral agent as a mediator in causation and elsewhere suggest gastrin as the relevant factor. Gastrin is, of course, a neuropeptide with widespread CNS distribution, particularly in cerebral cortical grey matter and in the hippocampus. It is under control by somatostatin, another peptide hormone also involved in the regulation of growth hormone production under stressful stimulation. All of these factors, together with another group of growth promoting peptides collectively called somatomedins, are involved in the regulation of growth and development. Somatomedin activity in human umbilical cord plasma has been found to correlate positively with birth weight [1]. Insulin and glucose metabolism are also implicated in birth-weight regulation [23]. New data on the specialization of function in the plasma membrane of the human placenta [56] suggest different transport and receptor mechanisms, binding, and releasing, valent either for fetal or maternal humoral agents, one of which is insulin. The author [56] summarizes the situation:

> Interposed between two separate circulatory systems the placenta has a distinct polarity of its membrane specializations thus allowing different interactions at the maternal−placental compared to the fetal−placental interface. These interactions are likely to mediate placental metabolic, synthetic and transport functions.

It seems that all of these humoral activities share in very complex transactions prenatally between mother and fetus, and it is also true that these hormones show profound changes in the organism subjected to stress. Because they also relate to issues of birth weight, which is not necessarily synonymous with maturity, they represent a highly important aspect of stress in early life. Indeed, in our own data, abnormal birth weight is a feature of offspring of mothers exposed to stress during pregnancy. Psychosocial stress in pregnancy also has been associated with prematurity [41]. That abnormal birth weight is a serious health issue is indicated clearly in a recent publication of the National Institute of Child Health and Human Development [59]. It is perhaps worth noting the finding that previous heroin addicts free of narcotic use during pregnancy produce infants showing severe intrauterine growth retardation [27].

Abnormal birth weight leads to a cascade of further risk factors in separations, feeding difficulties, bonding impoverishment, and so forth. It has been implicated in later increased incidence of child abuse, although this has not been substantiated in one recent study [4]. Of course, failure to thrive in infancy also has many psychosocial dimensions both in cause and effect. For example, Pollitt, Gilmore, and Valcarcel [42] have found that infants at risk of failure to thrive are identifiable by specific behavior patterns of both mother and infant. A mismatching of behaviors occurs that training could perhaps eliminate. Cowett, Lipsitt, et al. [14] have found severely depressed sucking activity in infants who were of low birth weight and who were severely stressed in the perinatal and neonatal period. Other studies (e.g., [22]) implicate sex of infant in altering patterns of mother−infant interaction including feeding behavior.

These sex-related interaction patterns must be involved in later gender-related behaviors and sex-role factors. It is worth noting that Frankenhaeuser [17a] and her group in Stockholm have found differences in stress responsiveness in young adults related to these differences in sex and sex roles. In fact, this whole area of sex-related stress research is the subject of a large collaborative program of studies currently in progress between her department and our unit in Dublin.

Another area of considerable interest in regard to stress in infancy is the issue of breast-feeding. It should perhaps now be stated clearly that deprivation of breast-feeding in infancy is a major stress. It has both behavioral and biological implications. Rodgers [50], reporting on the findings of the National Survey of Health and Development (1946 birth cohort) in the United Kingdom, has found that "those who had been entirely bottle-fed in infancy scored significantly lower than those who had been entirely breast-fed" on a range of attainment tests after taking differences in family background into account. Biological immunity factors, which we now know are also neurally and stress-related, are a major factor in those deprivations suffered by infants deprived of breast milk and in particular of colostrum. Loss of substances contained in colostrum has been found along with stress factors to be highly significant causal factors in necrotizing enterocolitis in newborn infants [7]. So, once again we see an interaction and concomitance of somatic and behavioral variables that each need to be taken into account in elucidating mechanisms. An interesting model incorporating oligopeptides in a process of antibody-facilitated digestion and its implications for infant nutrition has been advanced by Freed and Green [18], and their model will merit close study by stress researchers, since it has many facets where interaction with neuropeptides implicated in stress could intervene. Many clinical syndromes are suggested to have links with disruption of their model. They argue that breast-feeding immunizes the gut against dietary antigens, which, they claim, cause many digestive upsets in infants of minor or major significance. Breast-feeding with colostrum is the major protecting factor.

From the psychobiological point of view, it is interesting to note that breast-feeding and suckling have an important effect on the stress responses of the lactating mother. Through increased release of prolactin, ACTH levels are reduced. This in turn reduces the perceptual world of the mother and her responses to stressful stimuli. The reduction in perceptual horizon ensures her increased availability for attachment and caring [57].

Torbjorn Åkerstedt [1a], working in Stockholm, has found depression of immunity status in subjects exposed to sleep deprivation.

Prenatal and perinatal factors have been found to influence later night waking of one-year-olds [2]. They do not find an association between parental behavior patterns and night waking. Mothers of wakers do respond more rapidly to infant crying during the daytime, but this is seen to be a separate outcome of the shared suboptimal obstetric history. Perhaps disturbed sleep patterns relate to other consequences, yet to be discerned, of altered immunity in developing infants.

Blood and cardiovascular factors have also been implicated in intrauterine growth retardation. McKillop et al. [38] have found alterations in fibrinogen–fibrin complexes in pregnant women who had babies suffering from intrauterine growth retardation. These clotting factors are believed to work through intravascular coagulation in the placenta, which has been found previously to associate with this retardation of growth in utero. They have also been found to alter with stressful environmental conditions.

Maternal blood pressure in pregnancy has also been associated with effects on the neonate and subsequent development during the first year [39, 40]. Treated hypertensive mothers had infants with more perinatal problems and with smaller head circumferences at birth and persisting in the first year. The untreated group of hypertensives had offpsring with increased incidence of serious neurological deficits, which persisted throughout the first year. An interesting study by Chisholm, Woodson, and DaCosta Woodson [9] reports an association between normal variations in maternal blood pressure during pregnancy and subsequent neonatal irritability as assessed with the Brazelton Scale. Our own findings on relationships between maternal blood pressure and that of infants raises interesting questions in connection with these data.

In summary, there seems to be ample indication from the literature that a renewed interest in stress factors in pregnancy and infancy is timely and would produce important data of immediate relevance to health-care problems. A perspective that can incorporate both biological and behavioral indices within the constructs and paradigms of stress theory could reach valuable new insights.

Experimental and Clinical Studies

The data reported in this paper represent some findings from a program of research on infancy and early child development. The studies were initiated to test the hypothesis that the basis of human adaptive function is established during pregnancy and early infancy.

The review of literature presented earlier favors two primary hypotheses: that stressors experienced by pregnant mothers are causally related to morbidity in offspring and that the mechanisms underlying adaptive functioning also may be impaired as a result of such stressors.

The main study was designed to evaluate the effects of antenatal stress on pregnancy outcome and on infant development. A variety of physical and psychosocial markers for stress were assessed in a sample of pregnant mothers, and the offspring were followed up to the age of one year to evaluate the outcome.

A sample of 200 pregnant women was obtained from outpatients attending the National Maternity Hospital, Dublin. Criteria for inclusion were that subjects be married, urban based, and less than 20 weeks pregnant. Participation was voluntary, and only three potential subjects refused to participate. The final sample represented 2.5 percent of the total hospital population in the year the study was initiated. A chi-square test for goodness of fit indicated that the sample did not differ significantly from the general population in terms of age, parity, length of gestation, and social class.

Subjects were interviewed twice during pregnancy, and data were obtained to cover two periods: the first trimester and the remainder of the pregnancy. The first interview developed a health and psychosocial background history profile on each subject. Both interviews then evaluated the presence of stressors in the areas of health and physical exertion, the quality of interpersonal relationships, life events, and environmental status. The major stress factors examined are:

Life Events Inventory
Social supports
Situational stressors
Interpersonal discord
Environmental stressors
Physical stressors

The Life Events Inventory (LEI) was based on the instrument developed by Cochrane and Robertson [11], excluding events inappropriate to a pregnant subject. The LEI rates a variety of life events and assigns a cumulative life stress score. Such scores have shown good correlations with other objective measures of anxiety, and with both the patterns and onset of illness subsequently occurring [44, 45, 46].

Situational stressor scores were based on a negative emotional and physical health profile of the subject's parents, partner, and/or children, and whether the subject had been witness to violence or accidents. Interpersonal discord was rated on the presence of marital problems, interpersonal problems with relatives or others living in or outside the family home, and whether the subject considered absconding or actually did so.

Environmental stressor measures were based on problems relating to family accommodation (lack of, change in, or sharing with others), threatened or actual loss of partner's job, and financial problems. Physical sressors included ill health and operations, employment during pregnancy and its perceived toll, and threatened abortion.

The third trimester interview repeated the stressor evaluation obtained during the first interview to assess the duration or severity of stressors arising early or late in pregnancy. Data were also gathered on the obstetric profile during labor and delivery, and on full pediatric examination carried out on the offspring during the first days of life. Further interviews were taken six weeks and 12 months postnatally. The major factors examined were:

Gestational outcome
Pediatric status
Pediatric examination conclusion
Maternal reaction to birth and baby
Type of feeding
Postpuerperal depression
Infant adaptability and temperament
Physical history and status at one year
Adaptability at one year
Psychological status at one year

Gestational outcome grouped length of gestation, labor duration, and presentation and delivery problems. Pediatric status grouped postdelivery problems with negative pediatric evaluation. Maternal reaction was based on the mother's perception of the birth experience and the baby. Infant adaptability ratings grouped feeding and sleeping patterns with temperament over the first six weeks. We grouped factors at one year of age to cover the physical history and status of the baby, the baby's adaptation to stressful experience, and the quality of the baby's relationships.

Initial Findings of the Main Study

An analysis of the correlation between grouped stress factors and individual variables in the perinatal period yielded interesting findings. A sample of significant positive correlations is presented in Table 1. Negative attitudes to pregnancy were indicated when the mother was unhappy with her pregnancy, when she disliked pregnancy in general, or when contraception had failed and resulted in the current pregnancy. As a grouped stress factor, this significantly related to congenital abnormalities of the limbs, other physical abnormalities, and dysmaturity. It also related highly with caesarean section. High life events stress in later pregnancy related to stillbirth, neonatal death, and (surprisingly) to congenital hip dislocation.

Table 1. Selected Associations Between Stress Factors and Perinatal Outcome

Stressors	Morbidity	χ^2 Significance Levels[a]
Negative attitudes to pregnancy	Cesarean section	1
	High birth weight	5
	Congenital hip dislocation	5
	Physical abnormalities	5
Situational stress	Low gestation	5
	Feeding problems	5
	Separation	5
	Low Apgar score	→5
	CDH/physical abnormalities	→5
	Postpuerperal depression	→5
Interpersonal discord	Cesarean section	5
	Feeding problems	5
	Low Apgar score	→5
	Unresponsive	→5
	High birth weight	→5
High life events stress score in early pregnancy	Jaundice	5
	Low birth weight	→5
	Puerperal depression	→5
High life events stress score in late pregnancy	Congenital hip dislocation	5
	Stillbirth and neonatal death	5

[a]Associations approaching significance (i.e., $p > .05$, $p < .08$) are indicated by an arrow.

Situational stressors relate to prematurity and infant feeding problems and predict mother–child separation in the first six weeks of life. Interpersonal discord relates to feeding difficulties and section delivery. Early life events stress relates to postpuerperal depression, and as the stress increases it parallels an increase in the severity of the depression.

Analysis was also carried out between grouped stressors and grouped outcome variables to obtain a profile of broad pattern influences on morbidity and outcome. Pearson product moment correlation coefficients and significance levels are presented in Table 2. The results outlined indicate a broad pattern of effect from a variety of pregnancy stressors on child morbidity and adaptive functioning within the first year. It is clear that pregnancy stress influences both mother and offspring postnatally.

The spectrum of effects on mothers is particularly interesting because these effects are likely to influence bonding, relationships, and the level of care available to the offspring. It is apparent from Table 1 that a negative reaction to the experience of birth itself, as well as to the baby, is related to a high level of situational and environmental stress and to the presence of problems involving interpersonal relationships in pregnancy. The general health status of the pregnant mother is also implicated in these negative reactions.

There is a significant relationship between choice of artificial feeding and the lack of social supports available to the mother. Social supports were designated as the quality of integrating with the social and cultural environment. Mothers who were not fully reared at home, whose parents were deceased, who had minimal education, or who were in trouble with the law are most likely to choose artificial feeding.

Postpuerperal depression is closely related to the presence of situational stressors and interpersonal discord in pregnancy. As life events stress increases, the severity of postpuerperal depression also tended to increase.

The immediate postnatal status of the infant is associated primarily with ill health or physical trauma suffered by the mother during pregnancy. This can be construed as a direct effect solely related to postconceptional factors.

The first marker of infant adaptability was based on the six-week postnatal interview. Feeding and sleeping patterns were grouped with temperament. It can be seen from Table 1 that poor adaptability in these terms was related to the presence of situational and physical stressors in pregnancy.

Table 2. Correlations Between Grouped Stressors and Outcome[a]

	Perinatal			Six Weeks Postnatal				One Year		
	Gestational Outcome	Pediatric Status	Pediatric Conclusion	Maternal Reaction	Feeding	Post-puerperal Depression	Infant Adaptability	Health Status	Adaptability	Psychological Status
Social supports					.1895*					
Situational stressors				.2076**		.2243**	.2045**	.1887**		
Interpersonal discord				.1486*		.1978**		.1853**		
Environmental stressors				.1417*				.2319**		.1814*
Physical stressors	.1862**	.2005**					.2211**	.1952**		

[a]Pearson product moment correlation coefficients: $p < .05$ denoted *, $p < .01$ denoted **

The general health status and health history of the offspring at one year of age shared a highly significant relationship to situational, environmental, physical, and interpersonal stressors in pregnancy. Psychological status was related to environmental stressors in pregnancy.

It can be seen that obstetric and pediatric status are affected by pregnancy stress. Early factors that indicate poor infant adaptability to the environment are also related to such stress. Such immediate effects might be expected in cases where severe pregnancy stress was present across a variety of factors. What is more significant is the apparent continuation of such effects. The general health status of the infant at the age of one year still is related to pregnancy stress. We are continuing to follow the cohort of offspring. The more subtle and no less important markers of psychobiological reactivity and adaptability are also negatively affected, which must have serious consequences in later life. This aspect was examined more closely by looking at the cardiovascular response patterns of a selected group of offspring.

Cardiovascular Studies

In one study of cardiovascular phenomena, 14 infants were selected from a main study population. The Life Events Inventory (LEI) administered to the 200 pregnant subjects in our main group gave a numerical index of life events stress loading in these mothers. Seven offspring whose mothers had LEI scores of 200 or more during both first and third trimesters were classified as the stressed group. These were matched by seven nonstressed subjects whose mothers had LEI scores of zero during both first and third trimesters. These stringent criteria were chosen for this initial study to determine boundary conditions for planning later studies.

Subjects. The stressed group on these criteria yielded seven subjects, three males and four females (mean age 15.8 months). The nonstressed group comprised seven subjects, four males and three females (mean age 14.9 months).

Measures. Four measures were recorded for each subject:

Systolic blood pressure (SBP)
Diastolic blood pressure (DBP)
Mean arterial pressure (MAP)
Heart rate in beats per minute (HR)

Subjects were assessed in their own homes. In each case the infant sat upright on the mother's knees, and the cuff was applied to the left upper arm. The parameters were recorded simultaneously at one-minute intervals for 10 consecutive measures. Subjects were awake and generally relaxed. A Dinamap Paediatric Arterial Pressure Monitor (Model no. 847) was used. This instrument uses an oscillometric technique and is of course noninvasive.

Results. The mean values obtained for the two groups are presented in Table 3. There is a consistent elevation for all values within the stressed group, although these differences did not reach statistically significant levels. Within both groups, HR displayed a consistent slight negative correlation with MAP, SBP, and DBP (MAP .27; SBP .28; DBP .4).

Sex differences were found, males displaying higher SBP and DBP than females in both stressed and nonstressed groups. Furthermore, SBP and DBP were higher in stressed than nonstressed males, and this elevation was also found in female subjects. This is illustrated in Table 4.

If we look at the patterns of successive measures of the cardiovascular responses over the period of observation, an interesting

Table 3. Arterial Pressure and Heart Rate in Stressed and Nonstressed Offspring at 15 Months of Age

	Stressed		Nonstressed	
	Mean	Standard Deviation	Mean	Standard Deviation
MAP	87.9	23.6	82.1	22.8
SBP	102.5	23.2	95.6	21.4
DBP	67.2	22.4	64	22.6
HR	132.1	16.4	130.4	16.7

Table 4. Mean Systolic and Diastolic Blood Pressure in Stressed and Nonstressed Male and Female Offspring at 15 Months of Age

	Male		Female	
	SBP	DBP	SBP	DBP
Stressed	104.7	69.8	100.9	65.2
Nonstressed	101	66	95	61.3

finding emerges. The recording procedure, the intrusion of a stranger, and the social interaction and cooperation demanded of the subjects during measurements may be regarded as stressors evoking a hemodynamic adaptive response. Looking at the data in this way, we found that the stressed group responded to the test situation at first with a marked elevation of SBP and DBP and then showed a narrower range of variance in their responses. On the other hand, the nonstressed group did not show this initial hyperreactive cardiovascular response to the same degree, but maintained a more labile response throughout the session. This phenomenon is illustrated in Figure 1.

We then looked at the possibility of finding maternal cardiovascular correlates for these phenomena. Hospital records yielded blood-pressure measures taken during pregnancy on five stressed mothers and six nonstressed mothers. We derived a blood-pressure lability measure for these mothers by computing the range between the highest and lowest scores for each subject and then obtained a group mean. When we compare these ranges for the mothers and

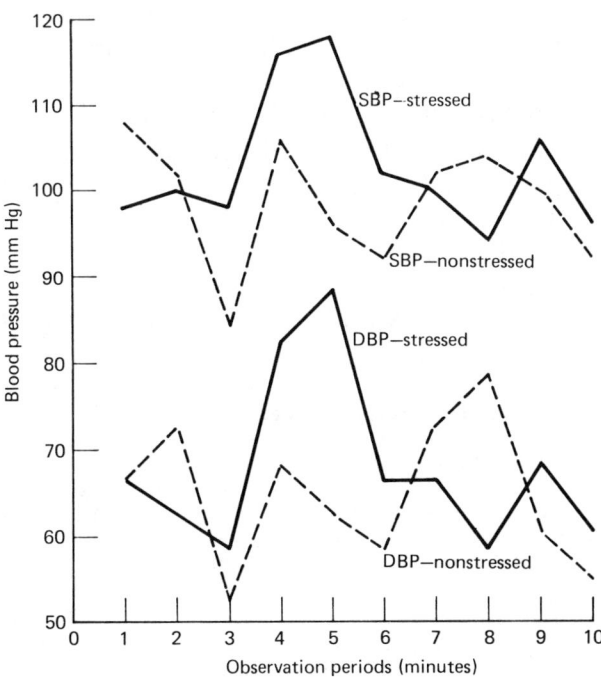

Figure 1. Mean systolic and diastolic pressures for stressed and nonstressed offspring over 10 observation periods at one-minute intervals.

their offspring as shown in Table 5, it can be seen that the nonstressed mothers display greater lability in SBP and DBP during their pregnancies; their offspring repeat this pattern for HR during labor and for SBP and DBP at 15 months of age. The major differentiating factor between the groups is the cardiovascular lability that appears to typify both nonstressed mothers and offspring. These differences, however, were not statistically significant, since the groups were small and standard deviations large, but we plan to extend our sample to find if the variance holds at significant levels with greater subject numbers.

From the clinical point of view, one finding is of particular interest. In 2-year-old children, clinical hypertension is attributed at or over the 95th percentile cutoff point, with BP reading of 112/79 measured on three separate occasions. This criterion was accepted by the Report of the Task Force on Blood Pressure Control in Children, based on various studies [48]. Two of our infants whose mothers were stressed in pregnancy can be regarded as clinically hypertensive: at 15 months they had mean BP levels of 121/78 and 117/77 over 10 consecutive observations.

These findings relate in an interesting way to an earlier normative study we had conducted. In this, blood pressure and heart rate had been measured in a group of normal, healthy, nonstressed neonates. The experiment was carried out in collaboration with James Lynch of the Medical School, University of Maryland, and the work was done in the National Maternity Hospital in Dublin. The study comprised 20 normal, fullterm infants, 10 male and 10 female, selected in order of delivery at the National Maternity Hospital, Dublin. Birth weight ranged between 3000 and 4000 grams. Examination by neonatologists excluded the presence of any illness or defect. Measures were started during the first 12 to 36 hours of

Table 5. Maternal Blood Pressure and Fetal Heart Rate[a]

	Mothers		Offspring			
	SBP	DBP	Fetal HR	SBP	DBP	(15/12)
Stressed	19	11	11.1	59	57	
Nonstressed	25	18	22	66	69	

[a]Mean systolic and diastolic range of blood pressures of stressed and nonstressed pregnant mothers; mean range of fetal heart rate during labor; mean systolic and diastolic range of blood pressures of stressed and nonstressed offspring at 15 months of age.

postnatal life, the starting point chosen to allow the immediate postnatal hemodynamic shifts to incorporate the pulmonary vascular bed and to reach equilibrium. Infants were monitored on four successive days, recording consisting of 10 successive measurements taken at one-minute intervals. Table 6 shows means and standard deviations for all subjects ($N = 20$) for all four days of sampling. Levels of blood pressure and heart rate found in this study were somewhat lower than those previously published [54, 55] with the exception of those reported by Gill and O'Brien [19]. The latter authors, however, report only on systolic blood pressure. No significant differences in HR, SBP, or DBP were found between males and females, nor were significant differences found in birth weight between males and females (Table 7). This is contrary to a finding recently reported by deSwiet et al. [54]. There was a small but not significant positive correlation (.44) between HR and birth weight (Table 7). Although the group data from the present study represent a contribution of physiological norms for the neonate in basic clinical cardiovascular parameters, the profiles of measures for the three variables HR, SBP, and DBP in individual infants throughout

Table 6. Blood Pressure and Heart Rate Values for N = 20 Neonates

	Mean	Standard Deviation
Systolic BP	70.12	6.6
Diastolic BP	37.71	5.2
Heartrate	119.2	11.8

Table 7. Birth Weights and Intercorrelations Between Blood Pressure, Heart Rate, and Birth Weight

	Birth Weight		
Males	3544 ± 284 g		
Females	3407 ± 173 g		
Correlations	DBP	HR	BWt
SBP	.9	.2	.27
DBP	—	.3	−.24
HR	—	—	.44

Table 8.

Female Infant S7, Day 1			Observation	Male Infant S18, Day 4		
HR	SBP	DBP		HR	SBP	DBP
138	77	51	1	141	83	45
115	84	46	2	136	105	57
104	106	55	3	138	99	46
129	106*	77	4	138	95	66*
144	80	62*	5	127	72	48
138	58*	39	6	127	57	32*
136	60	31*	7	108	67	33
122	65	38	8	127	71	40
120	75	33	9	133	65	33
144	60	40	10	138	75	36

a monitoring session displayed a striking lability of both SBP and DBP, especially of DBP.

Two sample profiles are given here. In Table 8, the points marked (*) indicate that changes of the order of 100 percent in DBP occurred within two minutes in one female infant (S 7) on day one and in a male infant (S 18) on day four. In the same female infant, a shift of similar magnitude occurred in SBP over the same time span but not simultaneously with the change in DBP. Overall, the profiles showed an extraordinary degree of variation in the parameters from minute to minute with no significant relationship between heart rate and blood pressure. How these changes relate to specific changes in behavior is not clear from the present study, but our observations suggest that these variables may be of considerable significance in determining patterns of response in the cardiovascular system. The clinical observations mentioned earlier give a strong impression that responsiveness to environmental stimuli and to fluctuations in internal state or behavior are well developed and that these contribute significantly to the variability found. Michael deSwiet and his coworkers have discussed some of the "within-baby" factors they discern affecting variability [54, 55].

Discussion

The findings we present in this paper represent only some salient features from a large and complex body of data. For ease of presentation in the short format available to us we have condensed both independent and dependent variables into constructs containing operationally related factors. Nevertheless, our results are interesting in that correlations are found between psychosocial stress in pregnancy and disorders of function and structure in infancy. However, these associations do not confirm causal relationships. This must await both further research and reexamination of existing literature with a view to seeking evidence in support of more sophisticated psychobiological models of pathogenesis.

A few specific issues arising from our data seem worth further comment at this stage in our research program. First, among our pregnancy stress variables, Life Events Inventory ratings are important. By and large these have stood the test of time and many diverse applications very well. It has been claimed by several workers that ratings of the individual subjective meaning and impact of these events is important, but in general adding this dimension has tended to strengthen their validity. So also the issue of the reliability of recall of life events has been discussed. Jenkins et al. [24] have researched this and have found serious discrepancies when such instruments are used retrospectively. They do not, however, find that they apply when used prospectively the way we have used them in our studies.

Another issue arising from our data concerns the differential effects of early and late pregnancy stress. If effects are exerted on the fetus, these must relate to vulnerable or sensitive periods of an embryological nature, for instance, in the case of maternal rubella and hypervitaminosis A. The mechanisms are elusive but existing literature may already contain clues. Even the apparently bizarre relationship of late pregnancy stress with congenital dislocation of the hip takes on a new aspect when the clinical literature is perused. The condition emerges as much more dynamic and resilient than its name would suggest.

Our finding of continuing lability in cardiovascular responses in nonstressed infants seems at first sight to be counterintuitive. However, if we consider the need for flexibility in the biological adaptive repertoire, this may well represent an advantage. Labile hypertension in adults is a controversial area and it has been stated that "while labile hypertension has been assumed inevitably to proceed to sustained hypertension this hypothesis has never actually been tested" [5]. Indeed, our data suggest a different pattern with increasing rigidity of response systems lying on a more pathological dimension. This approach is strengthened by a number of studies reporting these decreases in autonomic responsiveness to be a characteristic of the aging of biological systems [13]. How some of these mechanisms may be considered ontologically, with particular reference to hypertension, is elegantly discussed in a thoughtful paper by Jim Henry [21] in which he claims that "the life-long pattern of coping with disturbing events determines the mechanism and severity of hypertension."

Conclusion

We have argued for a more holistic psychobiological approach to problems of stress in infancy. This does not maintain a view that psychosocial factors are unimportant. On the contrary, we hold that our perspective ensures that these factors are seen to be truly pervasive in their effects, even to the extent of connoting profound biological changes. A paper by Goodall [20] on social factors in kwashiorkor illustrates this very well. She identifies a whole psychosocial deficiency as well as the dietary and material one in this epidemic disease of childhood in poorer societies.

The modulation of arousal and stress responses is essentially a cognitive coping process, and biological processes are at the service of cognitive functions. One of the present authors has discussed this cognitive core of the adaptive repertoire elsewhere recently in a NATO Human Factors Series volume on Coping and Health [15].

In summary, then, the consequences of stress in very early life are a serious societal issue even carrying legal implications with regard to neglect of the unborn child. These legal implications for U.S. law have been discussed recently by Bross [6]. They have concerned workers in the field for many decades. It is interesting to discover that almost 40 years ago, in 1943, the American Society for Research in Psychosomatic Problems, through its Committee on Infancy and Early Childhood, held a two-day conference at New York Hospital, on the theme, "The Psychosomatic Status of the Infant at Birth." It is therefore surprising that the First World Congress on Infant Psychiatry was not held until 1980. However, the intervening years have been far from barren. In fact, whole new fields of study have opened up, theoretical constructs have become increasingly complex, and new methodologies have uncovered subtleties of the world of the neonate that were merely a gleam in the eye of earlier workers. Some of the concerns of these earlier researchers are still with us today, but knowledge and opportunity have increased immensely, and new roles for child psychiatrists and allied professionals are opening up in caring- and prevention-oriented health-care systems.

References

1. Ashton, I.K., and Vesey, J. Somatomedin activity in human cord plasma and relationship to birth size, insulin, growth hormone, and prolactin. *Early Hum. Dev.*, 2/2 (1978), 115–122.
1a. Akerstedt, T., Gilberg, M. Effects of sleep deprivation on memory and sleep latencies in connection with repeated awakenings from sleep. *Psychophys.*, 16/1 (1979), 49–52.
2. Blurton Jones, N., Ferreira, M.C.R., Brown, M.F., and Macdonald, L. The association between perinatal factors and later night waking. *Dev. Med. Child. Neur.*, 20 (1978), 427–434.
3. Bowlby, J. *Maternal Care and Mental Health.* World Health Organization, Geneva, 1951.
4. Boyle, M., Griffen, A., and Fitzhardinge, P. The very low birthweight infant: Impact on parents during the preschool years. *Early Hum. Dev.*, 1/2 (1977), 191–201.
5. British Medical Journal. Labile hypertension *Brit. Med. J.*, 5 Jan., (1980), 4–5. (editorial review)
6. Bross, D.C. Neglect of the unborn child: an analysis based on law in the United States. *Child Abuse and Neglect,* 3 (1979), 643–650.
7. Burrington, J.D. Necrotizing enterocolitis in the newborn infant. *Clin. Perinatol.*, 5, 1 (1978), 29–43.
8. Campos, J.J. Heart rate: A sensitive tool for the study of emotional development in the infant. In Lipsitt, L.P. Ed. *Developmental Psychobiology.* John Wiley, Halstead Press, New York, 1976.
9. Chisholm, J.S., Woodson, R.H., and DaCosta Woodson, E.M. Maternal blood pressure in pregnancy and newborn irritability. *Early Hum. Dev.*, 2/2 (1978), 171–178.
10. Clarke, A.M. and Clarke, A.D.B., Eds. *Early Experience: Myth and Evidence.* Open Books, London, 1976.
11. Cochrane, R., and Robertson, A. *J. Psychosom. Res.*, 17 (1973), 135.
12. Coe, C.L., Mendoza, S.P., Smotherman, W.P., and Levine, S. Mother–infant attachment in the squirrel monkey—adrenal response to separation. *Behav. Biol.*, 22 (1978), 256.
13. Collins, K.J., Exton-Smith, A.N., James, M.H., and Oliver, D.J. Functional changes in autonomic nervous responses with aging. *Age and Aging,* 9 (1980), 17–24.
14. Cowett, R.M., Lipsitt, L.P., Vohr, B., and Oh, W. Aberrations in sucking behavior of low-birthweight infants. *Dev. Med. Child. Neur.*, 20 (1978), 701–709.
15. Cullen, J. Coping and Health—a clinician's perspective. In Levine, S., and Ursin, H., Eds. *Coping and Health.* Plenum Press, New York, 1980.
16. DeSa, D.J. Stress response and its relationship to cystic (pseudofollicular) change in the definitive cortex of the adrenal gland in stillborn infants. *Arch. Dis. Child.*, 53 (1978), 776–796.
17. Dworkin, B.R., Filewich, R.J., Miller, N.E., Craigmyle, N., and Pickering,

T.G. Baroreceptor activation reduces reactivity to noxious stimulation: Implications for hypertension. *Science,* 205 (1979), 1299–1301.

17a. Frankenhaeuser, M. Psychoendocrine sex differences in adaptation to the psycho-social environment. In Carenze, L. et. al., Eds. *Clinical Psychoneuroendocrinology in Reproduction.* Academic Press, London, 1978.

18. Freed, D.L.J., and Green, F.H.Y. Antibody-facilitated digestion and its implications for infant nutrition. *Early Hum. Dev.,* 1/1 (1977), 107–112.

19. Gill, D., and O'Brien, N.G. Systolic blood pressure in the newborn. *J. Irish Med. Assn.,* 70,14 (1977), 419.

20. Goodall, J. A social score for kwashiorkor: Explaining the look in the child's eyes. *Dev. Med. Child. Neur.,* 21 (1979), 374–384.

21. Henry, J.P. Understanding the early pathophysiology of essential hypertension. *Geriatrics,* 31, 1 (1976), 59–72.

22. Hwang, C.P. Mother–infant interaction; effects of sex of infant on feeding behavior. *Early Hum. Dev.,* 2/4 (1978), 341–349.

23. Jarai, I., Mestyan, J., Schultz, K., Lazar, A., Halasz, M., and Krassy, I. Body size and neonatal hypoglycaemia in intrauterine growth retardation. *Early Hum. Dev.,* 1/1 (1977), 25–38.

24. Jenkins, C.D., Hurst, M.W., and Rose, R.M. Life changes. Do people really remember? *Arch. Gen. Psychiat.* 36 (1979), 379–384.

25. Kagan, A. and Levi, L. Health and environment—Psychosocial stimuli: A review. In Levi, L., Ed. *Society, Stress and Disease,* Vol. 2., *Childhood and Adolescence.* Oxford University Press, London, 1975.

26. Kagan, J. Resilience and continuity in psychological development. In Clarke, A.M., and Clarke, A.D.B. Eds. *Early Experience: Myth and Evidence.* Open Books, London, 1976.

27. Kandall, S.R., Albin, S., Gartner, L.M., Lee, K., Eidelman, A., and Lowinson, J. The narcotic-dependent mother: fetal and neonatal consequences. *Early Hum. Dev.,* 1/2 (1977), 159–169.

28. Kaufman, I.C., and Rosenblum, L.A. Depression in infant monkeys separated from their mothers. *Science,* 155 (1967), 1030–1031.

29. Lacey, J.I., and Lacey, B.C. Some autonomic–central nervous system interrelationships. In Black, P., Ed. *Physiological Correlates of Emotion.* Academic Press, New York, 1970.

30. Levi, L. Stress and distress in response to psychosocial stimuli. Pergamon Press, Oxford, 1972.

31. Levi, L. Psychosocial factors in preventive medicine. In *Healthy People: The Surgeon General's Report on Health Promotion* (Background Papers, 1979). U.S. Department of Health, Education, and Welfare, DHEW (PHS) Publication No. 79–55071A, Washington, D.C., 1979.

32. Levine, S. Infantile experience and resistance to physiological stress. *Science,* 126/3270 (1957), 405.

33. Levine, S. Stress and behavior. *Sci. Am.,* 224 (1971), 26–31.

34. Levine, S. Effects of impoverished early environment—Maternal influences on adaptive function. In Cullen, J., Ed. *Experimental Behavior—A Basis for the Study of Mental Disturbance.* John Wiley, Halstead Press, New York, 1974.

35. Levine, S. A coping model of mother–infant relationships. In Levine, S., and Ursin, H., Eds. *Coping and Health.* Plenum Press, New York, 1980.
36. Levine, S., Chevalier, J.A., and Korchin, S.J. The effects of early shock and handling on later avoidance learning. *J. Pers.* 24 (1956), 475–493.
37. Lipsitt, L.P., and Jacklin, C.N. Cardiac deceleration and its stability in human newborns. *Dev. Psychol.,* 5 (1971), 535.
38. McKillop, C.A., Howie, P.W., Forbes, C.D., and Prentice, C.R.M. Soluble fibrinogen–fibrin complexes in intrauterine growth retardation. *Early Hum. Dev.,* 2/2 (1978), 139–145.
39. Mutch, L.M.M., Moar, V.A., Ounsted, M.K., and Redman, C.W.G. Hypertension during pregnancy, with and without specific hypotensive treatment. I. Perinatal factors and neonatal morbidity. *Early Hum. Dev.* 1/1 (1977a), 47–57.
40. Mutch, L.M.M., Moar, V.A., Ounsted, M.K., and Redman, C.W.G. Hypertension during pregnancy, with and without specific hypotensive treatment. II. The growth and development of the infant in the first year of life. *Early Hum. Dev.,* 1/1 (1977b), 59–67.
41. Newton, R.W., Webster, P.A.C., Binn, P.S., Maskrey, N., and Phillips, A.B. Psychosocial stress in pregnancy and its relation to the onset of premature labour. *Brit. Med. J.,* 2 (1979), 411–413.
42. Pollitt, E., Gilmore, M., and Valcarcel, M. Early mother–infant interaction and somatic growth. *Early Hum. Dev.,* 1/4 (1978), 325–336.
43. Pugh, R.J., Newton, R.W., and Piercy, D.M. Fatal bleeding from gastric ulceration during the first day of life—Possible association with social stress. *Arch. Dis. Child.,* 54, 2 (1979), 146–148.
44. Rahe, R.H., Mahan, J. and Arthur, R.J. Prediction of near-future health change from subjects' preceding life changes. *J. Psychosom. Res.,* 14 (1970), 401.
45. Rahe, R.H., McKean, J., and Arthur, R.J. A longitudinal study of life-change and illness patterns. *J. Psychosom. Res.,* 10 (1967), 355.
46. Rahe, R.H., Meyer, M., Smith, M., Kjaen, G., and Holmes, T.H. Social stress and illness onset. *J. Psychosom. Res.,* 8 (1964), 35.
47. Reite, M., Short, R., and Seiler, C. Physiological correlates of maternal separation in surrogate-reared infants: A study in altered attachment bonds. *Dev. Psychobiol.,* 11 (1978), 427.
48. Report of the Task Force on Blood Pressure Control in Children, *Paediatrics,* 59, 5 (1977), 797.
49. Revill, S.I., and Dodge, J.A. Psychological determinants of infantile pyloric stenosis. *Arch. Dis. Child.,* 53 (1978), 66–68.
50. Rodgers, B. Feeding in infancy and later ability and attainment: A longitudinal study. *Dev. Med. Child Neur.,* 20 (1978), 421–426.
51. Rutter, M. *Maternal Deprivation Reassessed.* Penguin, Harmondsworth, England, 1972.
52. Rutter, M. Maternal deprivation, 1972–1978: New findings, new concepts, new approaches. *Child Dev.,* 50 (1979), 283–305.

53. Seay, B., Hansen, E., and Harlow, H.F. Mother–infant separation in monkeys. *J. Child Psychol. Psychiat.*, 3 (1962), 123–132.
54. deSwiet, M., Earley, F., Fayers, P., and Shinebourne, E.A. In Harper, P., and Muir, J., Eds. *Advanced Medicine*, Vol. 15. Williams and Wilkins, Baltimore, 1979.
55. deSwiet, M., Faucourt, R., and Peto, J. Systolic blood pressure variation during the first six days of life. *J. Clin. Sci. Mol. Med.*, 49 (1975), 557.
56. Whitsett, J.A. Specializations in plasma membranes of the human placenta. *J. Paediat.*, 96, 3, pt. 2 (1980), 600–604.
57. Whittlestone, W.G. The physiology of early attachment in mammals: implications for human obstetric care. *Med. J. Aust.*, 1 (1978), 50–53.
58. deWied, D. Pituitary adrenal system hormones and behavior. *Acta Endocrinol.*, Suppl. 214 (1977), 9–18.
59. National Institute of Child Health and Human Development. *Little babies: Born too soon—born too small.* Department of Health, Education and Welfare, Washington, D.C., 1979. (publication 77-1079)

Children in Northern Ireland: A Lost Generation?

Liz McWhirter
Karen Trew (Northern Ireland)

Although the present ongoing social conflict in Northern Ireland, known euphemistically as the "troubles," has interested observers throughout the world since violence erupted in 1968, writings on the topic tend to be characterized more by confident assertion than by the presence of well-based knowledge. This is particularly true of many commentaries of a psychological or psychiatric nature which have considered the impact of the conflict on the children of Northern Ireland.

The flavor of some of the most prevalent views is best conveyed by a few quotations. Thus the psychiatrist Lyons asserted that "when a settlement has been brought about, those conditioned to violence, prejudice and bigotry will find it more difficult to adjust to society and will persist in their anti-social behaviour" [19]. Lyons is also quoted as believing that "in the long run we are raising a generation of bigots"[39]. Lawson's synopsis of the present period of civil strife led him to describe the young people of Northern Ireland as "part of a generation which has never known the full pleasures of life without terrorism and counter terrorism, a generation which has never been allowed to live their lives free from fear, intimidation, hate and violence" [18]. This assessment is echoed by Wilkinson: "A whole generation has grown up ... under the shadow of the gunman and the bomber constantly aware of the threat of a fresh eruption of violence" [47]. Perhaps the strongest conclusion of all is embodied in Lawson's belief that "the greatest tragedy of all" must be that "in a way [the children] are a lost generation" [18].

What the *eventual* effect on the people and community of Northern Ireland will be when—or if—the violence ends can only be a matter of speculation. The impact of the conflict in the years since 1968, though, is open to empirical test, particularly within the objective context as presented by official statistics of the violence, and by the analyses of social scientists [29].

Violence has been a characteristic feature of Northern Ireland since 1968. It has overlaid the longstanding division between Catholics and Protestants which extends beyond religious differences to encompass historical, cultural, and political diversity. Conflict and violence have also exacerbated social problems associated with some of the worst economic conditions in Europe.

Knowledge about such objective conditions is a basic prerequisite for investigating the validity of such subjective opinions as cited above. Social behavior is a vital element of socialization into conflict and violence, but this chapter is principally concerned with the complementary aspect of socialization—social awareness.

It is our belief that evidence concerning people's social awareness, perceptions, knowledge, and understanding—of religious categories, of stereotyped cues used for religious group ascription, of intergroup relations of violence and of death, for example—provides an essential *baseline* from which to examine the outcomes of the process of socialization and to approach an amelioration of some of the problems [23]. Social behavior and reactions to stress must be interpreted, at least in part, within the related context of social cognition [39]. If Northern Ireland children are "lost," it is obviously important to ask if *they* are aware of it. Until a few years ago it was not even known if the children of Northern Ireland were conscious of living in what is known to the rest of the world as a war-torn country [6]. Focusing on children's awareness of their social world—the world of adults—this paper summarizes a series of recent studies which have sampled children's knowledge and understanding of their society, with its divisions and ongoing conflict and violence.

Awareness of Sectarian Division

The divisions between Protestants and Catholics in Northern Ireland are assumed to be wide. Heskin, for example, suggested that the two groups are characterized by "separate education, versions of history, cultural activities, religious habits, residential patterns and political viewpoints" [13]. However, in order to provide a valid basis for interpreting the *development* of group awareness in Northern Ireland, it is necessary to assess the extent of separation between Protestants and Catholics as well as the nature of contact between the groups.

There is no doubt that sectarian division has been institutionalized in the religiously segregated education systems within Northern Ireland. Politics in Northern Ireland also tend to be sectarian. The vast majority of Protestants uphold the current status of Northern Ireland as an integral part of the United Kingdom, while most Catholics aspire to severing the ties with Britain in favor of a reunified Republic of Ireland [34]. Northern Ireland is, therefore, a region in which the questions of nationality and allegiance have led to lack of consensus on the basic issue of the legitimacy of the state.

Nevertheless, Catholics and Protestants have a unique shared cultural background within Northern Ireland. They speak the same language and share many social attitudes. Whyte, for example, concluded, after reviewing the available survey evidence: "One thing which emerges from these data is not the extent to which Catholics and Protestants disagree but the extent to which they are thoroughly alike on all questions, except political ones" [48].

While the existing educational systems in Northern Ireland are very largely separate [44], residential segregation is not as widespread as is often believed. It is generally confined to areas within the cities or sparsely populated rural regions. The majority of Catholics and Protestants live in integrated residential districts [2]. Furthermore, survey evidence [16], as well as anthropological research [12, 20], has indicated that within Northern Ireland there are close friendships and many personal links between Protestants and Catholics. At the same time, many commentators would agree with Beckett's suggestion that Protestants and Catholics "mingle with a consciousness of the difference between them" [1]. This view would seem to be supported by the almost universal acceptance, within Northern Ireland, of culturally determined cues for religious categorization [4, 5] and by the volume of recent psychological research on such stereotyped cues as facial characteristics [41], speech [46], and names [5]. In fact, physical differences between Catholics and Protestants in Northern Ireland are slight [38] and accents of the two communities within the same region do not differ [33].

Whether or not denominational groups *can* be distinguished is perhaps less important, to the psychologist, than the fact that people in Northern Ireland *believe* that there are real differences between the religious groups [29]. As the perceptive travel writer Dervla Murphy noted, the major problem in Northern Ireland is "the extent to which ordinary people live in an extraordinary miasma of untruth . . . the average citizen's whole personality is conditioned by myth and he is bred to live the sort of life that will reinforce the myth for transmission to future generations" [35].

It is the development of the beliefs, attitudes, and understanding of sectarian differences in the face of the contact and similarities between the groups which has provided the focus of a series of investigations carried out among young people in Northern Ireland.

Jahoda and Harrison, in one of the first studies, concentrated on children's attitudes. Using a variety of disguised tasks they demonstrated that children living in segregated areas of Belfast which are renowned for sectarian violence had developed strong negative attitudes to the outgroup by 6 years old [15]. In contrast, following a series of studies with children aged 5 to 11 years, Cairns concluded that children in Northern Ireland probably mastered discrimination between their "own" and the "other" group when they were 11 years old [5]. Cairns had, however, measured discrimination performance indirectly using a disguised recall task and stereotyped Protestant and Catholic names. He therefore had equated the knowledge of a specific cue with the ability to discriminate between groups which differ along many dimensions [28].

In contrast, we have adopted a more direct approach to investigating children's awareness of group division. Rather than examining the perceptual or affective concomitants of the child's understanding of sectarian division, we have concentrated on how children construe themselves, and their social world. In Northern Ireland, the division between Protestant and Catholic is seen to be important but the available evidence failed to reveal if this division was salient to the child.

Our research, including the work of our students, has been characterized by methods which introduce potentially sensitive topics in the context of a neutral task. McWhirter and Gamble [27], for example, examined what children in Northern Ireland, aged 6 and 9 years, understood by the terms "Protestant" and "Catholic" by embedding them into a word-definition test. Subjects ($n = 192$) came from segregated areas which had experienced sectarian conflict and two relatively peaceful integrated towns, one of which had a Protestant majority and the other a Catholic majority. Approximately half of the younger and all but a few of the older children revealed knowledge of at least one of the labels. Age, religious denomination, and majority or minority status were seen to influence the maturity of conceptualizations. Most interpretations, however, tapped the religious dimension and although the referents were often construed as different, negative allusions to intergroup hostility were infrequent.

Lawless [17] introduced the topic of religious group identity and probed children's knowledge about religious groups during an interview on a variety of related themes with 6- and 9-year-olds ($n = 96$) from integrated and segregated areas. References to intergroup hostility were again significant by their absence. Although there were differences between areas and religious groups in understanding of religious group differences, over three quarters of the 9-year-olds and half of the 6-year-olds were able to correctly identify their own religion and that of their family.

McWhirter and Duffy [26] continued the investigation of children's awareness of sectarian division by focusing on the dimensions 11- and 15-year-old Catholic girls ($n = 60$) used to describe differences between themselves and other individuals, their area and other areas, and their country and other countries. Only one of the girls spontaneously referred to religious denomination when discussing individual differences and only a small minority (3 percent) of the 11-year-olds and 40 percent of the 15-year-olds referred to denominational differences in relation to variations between areas and countries. Similarly, Trew [42, 43] found that 14 percent of 9- and 11-year-olds ($n = 609$) and only 6 percent of 18-year-olds ($n = 278$) spontaneously referred to religious denomination in response to the open-ended question "What are you?"

The investigations that have been briefly reviewed were carried out within segregated schools in which children were being taught with others from their own denomination. In order to directly examine the impact of contact between Protestant and Catholic, we [30, 31] recently carried out a study in four special schools in Northern Ireland which are *not* segregated according to religion. The study involved 452 children aged 3 years to 19 years from 35 classes in two schools for physically handicapped, one for delicate children, and a day center for maladjusted pupils. A sociometric questionnaire was administered, within each class group, by the class teacher. It included questions about actual and preferred choice of playmate, best friend, and person living nearest to the pupil. Investigating whether the number of Protestants chosen by Protestants and Catholics differed significantly from chance level within each class, it was found that in only 4 of 280 analyses did religious denomination relate to peer selection. Clearly, religious denomination was not a salient dimension for these children. Similar findings are reported in two other investigations carried out in integrated settings within Northern Ireland [5, 11].

In sum, the evidence reviewed indicates that although children are able to identify their own religious denomination and that of their family from 6 years old, denomination is not a salient dimension in self-description or in person perception. Children are aware of differences between Protestant and Catholic but concentrate on religious rather than cultural differences and do not describe the outgroup in pejorative terms. Such findings were unexpected but consistent across a number of studies carried out over a period of three years. Further research is being conducted to assess whether the findings are sustained using more direct methods. Nevertheless, it would seem that the findings to date are in accord with personal experience. Dr. Edward Daly, Roman Catholic Bishop of Derry, for example, recalling his own childhood, suggested that "our neighbours were Protestant and I spent a lot of time in their house. These are friendships I value . . . I was very much aware of being Catholic but I did not understand the distinctions between Protestants and Catholics" [10].

Awareness of Violence

In spite of appalling social conditions and deep-rooted sectarian division and conflict which is centuries old [24], Northern Ireland has been traditionally a region of relatively low levels of crime and delinquency generally, and serious crime more particularly. For example, at no time during the 1960s, prior to 1969, did the total number of murders reach double figures. Since 1969 Northern Ireland has witnessed a level of very serious crime unprecedented in its history as a result of the present period of "troubles"—the longest in eight troubled centuries in Ireland. However, while the increase in incidence of serious crime in Northern Ireland is twice that of England and Wales (120 percent compared to 60 percent increase from 1969 to 1978), the number of indictable offenses in Northern Ireland is still only two-thirds the rate in England and Wales. Although a greater proportion of juvenile offenders in Northern Ireland engage in serious offending than in England and Wales, offenses associated with political or sectarian violence constitute a relatively small proportion of all known offenses in Northern

Ireland [8]. One can therefore conclude that fears of a serious growth in antisocial behavior among the young people of Northern Ireland and the total disintegration of Northern Ireland society, compared with other areas in Great Britain and the Republic of Ireland, are largely unjustified [13, 14].

There is some evidence [3] that a number of young people would not be involved in crime were it not for the "troubles," but one cannot say that those who have become involved in arson, armed robbery, explosions, shootings, intimidation and so on, have simply drifted into a new kind of "aggro," or that they do not know what they are doing. Those who have become involved have been seen, in two small-scale studies, to differ in important psychological dimensions from conventional delinquents and from ordinary schoolboys [7, 8, 9]. Furthermore, the increased level of juvenile deviance in Northern Ireland is associated with particular urban areas exposed to extremes of both socioeconomic deprivation and civil strife [8].

Geographic analyses [37] of the violence of the last 13 years illustrate its uneven distribution. The main regions of violence have been the urban areas of Belfast and Londonderry and the rural area surrounding the border between Northern Ireland and the Republic of Ireland. The relative intensities of the violence, its form and target, vary between these regions. In Belfast, for example, the incidence of explosions from 1969 to 1977 directed at classical targets (the police and army, central and local government personnel and installations, and the infrastructure of the state) is less than expected in relation to the overall incidence, while that of economic and sectarian targets is greater than expected. Similarly, there have been fewer police and army deaths but more sectarian killings.

Much of Northern Ireland has therefore escaped direct exposure to the 'troubles'—that is, overt violence—and the measures used in an attempt to control it scarcely impinge upon day to day life. Furthermore, while the absolute statistics of the violence [36] (e.g. more than 2,000 deaths in 13 years) are hardly momentous in world terms, more people have died violently in road accidents in Northern Ireland than in incidents connected with the social conflict.

It is important to note, however, that Northern Ireland is a small landmass (approximately 13,500 square kilometers) with a population (only 1.5 million) which is composed of small, tightly knit communities. Consequently, it would appear difficult for people anywhere in Northern Ireland to totally escape the impact of the "troubles."

The first study we carried out on consciousness of violence began

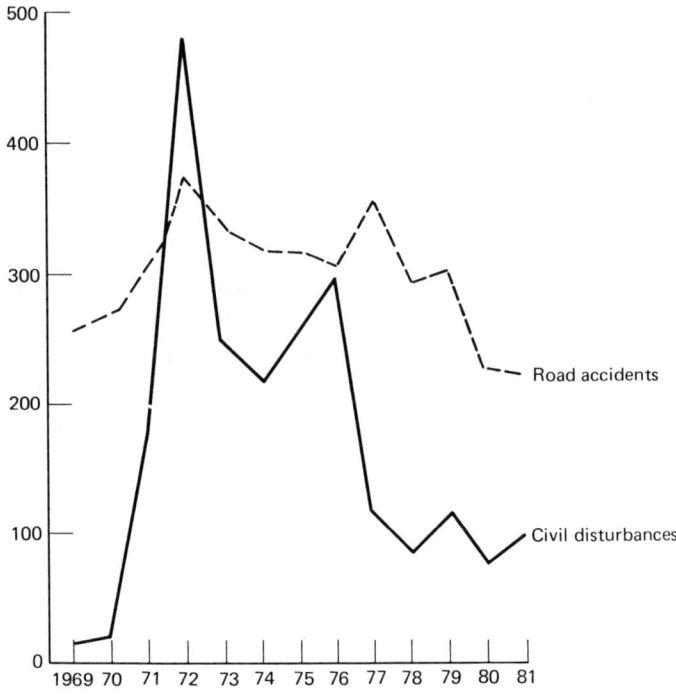

Figure 1. Deaths in Northern Ireland connected with road accidents and the security situation from 1969 to 1981. (Modified from R.U.C. Chief Constable's Report, 1978, Fig. 1A.)

toward the end of 1978 [32]. It examined awareness of violent death in children aged 3 to 16 years living in more and less violence-prone areas of Belfast. Using a disguised vocabulary test technique, supplemented by more probing questions presented casually as if incidental to the main assessment session, it was found that young preschool children living in the more "troubled" areas had a more mature understanding of the phenomenon of death than would be expected for their age. In other words, they had—at least with regard to one concept—benefited cognitively from their experience. Overall, however, the subjects ($n = 200$) attributed the causes of death more often at a general level to sickness than to accidents or violence, and at a more specific level, just as frequently to heart disease and to old age as to explosions or shootings, and more to road accidents and cancer than specific local violence. These perceptions surprisingly accurately reflect the total objective situation as given by the Registrar General's Statistics for Deaths in Northern Ireland.

Other research has investigated awareness of conflict and violence through the social reasoning scale of the British Abilities Scales [22]. Children of 5, 9, and 14 years of age, living in peaceful and troubled areas of Northern Ireland, were given the scale plus two ambiguous stories. One of these additional stories involved a stone-throwing incident and the other an unattended parcel left outside a shop. In the first of two studies less than 1 percent of the total sample ($n = 192$) interpreted the stone-throwing incident in either sectarian or political terms (e.g., stoning Protestants or Catholics, the police, or the British army) and only 26 percent perceived the parcel as a potential bomb. The second study controlled for order effects and was carried out only with Catholic children ($n = 120$) living in an area in Belfast where street rioting was more prevalent at the time of the investigation than in the previous study. This fact was reflected in the greater incidence of local interpretations given of the stoning story (45 percent) than of the parcel story (38 percent), although unlike the bomb perceptions these tended not to occur until after nondirective probing of the subjects. Not unexpectedly, there was a clear developmental trend across the three age groups in the degree to which the incidents elicited allusions to the Northern Ireland violence (stoning story: 10, 53, and 73 percent; parcel story: 0, 38 and 78 percent) but what is noteworthy is the almost total lack of such interpretations among the 5-year-olds. That so few of the youngest children saw the stoning in terms of political or sectarian rioting is perhaps encouraging. That none of them saw the potential danger of abandoned packages at shop entrances may suggest a need for increased education for survival, although whether 5-year-old children are intellectually capable of assimilating such information is open to question.

Interested more generally in environmental awareness in young people living in more and less trouble-prone districts of Belfast, McIvor [21] asked 7- and 11-year-olds ($n = 957$) to write an essay entitled either "Belfast" or "Where I Live." Clear differences that emerged in terms of area of residence reflect the fact that those areas which have suffered the highest levels of violence are urban areas also suffering severe socioeconomic deprivation. For example, approximately a quarter of the children from the troubled areas mentioned physical/social malaise and redevelopment in contrast to 4 and 17 percent, respectively, for the children from the more peaceful districts. Furthermore, while twice as many from the strife-prone areas mentioned antisocial behavior (19 percent)—vandalism, joy riding, gang fights, and so on—than from the more peaceful districts (9 percent), there was no statistically significant difference between locations in terms of incidence of "troubles"-related themes—Protestant—Catholic relations, sectarian or political violence, army, police, law and order. Essay title was, however, also important. For instance, for those living in the peaceful districts, redevelopment, physical/social malaise, and antisocial behavior were cited approximately four times more frequently in the "Where I Live" essays than in the "Belfast" essays. Themes related to the "troubles" were also more prevalent in the descriptions of Belfast (45 percent) than in the accounts of where the children lived (10 percent). Overall, only 5 percent mentioned Protestant–Catholic relations, and only 28 percent cited violence. These figures compare with 80 percent for geographical information and 83 percent for self-related material.

These data confirm the lack of salience of the violence in Belfast children's spontaneous thinking. They also suggest that the television image of Belfast colors the way the children see it and that the violence has perhaps become mentally compartmentalized so that a cue such as Belfast, with its violent media image, is needed before the door to the compartment is opened, as one of the children from a peaceful district wrote:

> I like going on holidays, but I hate going on holidays and coming from Belfast, when I was in Torquay a woman said to me "Oh, do you come from Belfast with all the bombs? Aren't you afraid?" I told her "No, you know Mrs., it's not as bad as you think, you know." That's why I don't like coming from Belfast—but only when I go on holiday. I like Belfast.

In the light of this suggestion it is interesting to note what children make of the term "violence" itself. Essays ($n = 637$) on the topic by 9- and 12-year-olds living in different areas of Northern Ireland revealed that 19 percent did not know the meaning of the word [25]. Among those which showed at least a vague idea ($n = 517$) there was a low level of awareness of sectarian conflict or hostility (5 percent) but a greater reflection of area variations in the extent and nature of the violence, similar to a temporal variation in an earlier study by Cairns, Hunter, and Herring [6]. The children from strife-prone areas in West Belfast cited more Northern Ireland type of violence—stoning, rioting, shooting, bombing, throwing petrol bombs, intimidation (71 percent)—than those living in a peaceful provincial town (58 percent). In view of the prevalence over the last few years of the struggle between the forces of the British government and Republican paramilitary groups it was not unexpected that location also interacted with religion: the Catholic children from the troubled area made more reference to Northern Ireland violence (80 percent) than the Protestant children living in a neighboring area of West Belfast (60 percent) and the Catholic children from the peaceful region (58 percent). Overall, while the children are certainly aware of the violence in Northern Ireland and its violent image (65 percent overall made reference to Northern Ireland violence), their conceptions were very global and embraced much more than the "troubles": 60 percent described general universal acts of violence which were either unspecific—bullying, kidnapping, killing—or occurred somewhere other than Ireland. However they interpreted the term, two-thirds spontaneously censured it. Two examples by 9-year-old Catholic children are illustrative. The first was written by a boy from West Belfast:

> Violence is bad. It is about smashing windows. And rooking nests. Killing birds. Violence is breaking in to some one's house and wrecking the place. Some nights cars get stolen and crashed into walls or shooting people. Wrecking seats, cutting down trees and lying in flower beds. Starting forest fires, stealing things. Throwing at saracens. Throwing petrol bombs.

The second was written by a girl from the peaceful provincial town.

> Violence is bombing and burgling and killing and whatever else. I do not know why people want to have violence in Ireland. A lot of bombings are in Northern Ireland, so I hear. People do not know what to do about it and I wish they did.

People obviously lie behind the violence, both as perpetrators and victims [24]. They take us back to the conflict and our overriding theme, intergroup relations. The causes of the violence are complex and multifaceted [29] but in our latest study [26] most of the subjects (88 percent) recognized that individual and collective acts of aggression made individuals and groups in Ireland different from other people. In spite of this comparative perspective, though, the evidence converges to suggest that relative normality prevails—within the long-rooted existing framework of conflict in Northern Ireland.

When investigating social awareness and subjective realities of the violence and conflict one must take account not only of practical ethics in terms of methodology [45] and demographic variables in terms of sampling but *also* adaptation processes in terms of interpretation. Preadolescents in Northern Ireland have never experienced any style of life other than that which has had violence at least as a backdrop. After 13 years "abnormality" has become "normality" [28]. In spite of subjective opinions and a relatively greater increase in crime in Northern Ireland than in neighboring countries, there is no evidence that the children and young people are "a lost generation."

References

1. Beckett, J.C. *A Short History of Ireland,* 6th ed. Hutchinson, London, 1979.
2. Boal, F. W., and Douglas, J. N., Eds. *Integration and Division: Geographic Aspects of the Northern Ireland Problem.* Head Press, Middlesex, 1982.
3. Boyle, K., Chesney, R., and Hadden, T. Who are the terrorists? *New Society,* 6 May 1976.
4. Burton, F. *The Politics of Legitimacy: Struggles in a Belfast Community.* Routledge, Kegan and Paul, London, 1978.
5. Cairns, E. The development of ethnic discrimination in children in Northern Ireland. In Harbison, J. and Harbison, J., Eds. *A Society Under Stress. Children and Young People in Northern Ireland.* Open Books, Somerset, 1980.
6. Cairns, E., Hunter, D., and Herring, L. Young children's awareness of violence in Northern Ireland: The influence of Northern Irish television in Scotland and Northern Ireland. *Brit. J. Soc. Clin. Psychol,* 1980, 3–6.
7. Curran, J. D. Deviant attitudes and personality of juvenile scheduled and juvenile delinquent offenders. Paper presented at Annual Conference of British Psychological Society, University of Aberdeen, April 1980.
8. Curran, J. D. Juvenile offending, civil disturbance and political terrorism—A psychological perspective. In McWhirter, L., and Trew, K., Eds. *The Northern Ireland Conflict: Myth and Reality. Social and Political Perspectives.* G. W. & A. Hesketh, Ormskirk, 1982.
9. Elliott, R., and Lockhart, W. Characteristics of scheduled offeners and juvenile delinquents. In Harbison, J., and Harbison, J., Eds. *A Society Under Stress. Children and Young People in Northern Ireland.* Open Books, Somerset, 1980.
10. Daly, E. Growing up in Northern Ireland. *Belfast Telgraph,* 3 December 1981.
11. Davies, J. Interaction within an integrated school. Paper presented at Seminar on Aspects of Community Interaction, Centre for Study of Conflict. New University of Ulster, Coleraine, January 1982.
12. Harris, R. *Prejudice and Tolerance in Ulster.* Manchester University Press, Manchester, 1972.
13. Heskin, K. Children and young people in Northern Ireland. A research review. In Harbison, J., and J. Harbison, Eds. *A Society Under Stress. Children and Young People in Northern Ireland.* Open Books, Somerset, 1980.
14. Heskin, K. Societal disintegration in Northern Ireland: Fact or fiction? *Econ. Soc. Rev,* 12, No. 2, (1981), 97–113.
15. Jahoda, M., and Harrison, S. Belfast children: Some effects of a conflict environment. *Irish J. Psychol.* 3, No. 4, (1975), 1–19.
16. Jenkins, R., and Macrae, S. *Religion, Conflict and Polarisation in Northern Ireland.* Peace Research Centre, Lancaster, 1966.
17. Lawless, H. Understanding of and identity with national and religious groups in young Northern Ireland children. The influence of conflict and contact. Unpublished B.Sc. dissertation. Queen's University, Belfast, 1981.
18. Lawson, R. Address given by General Officer in Command of British Army in Northern Ireland to Belfast Rotary Club, Europa Hotel, Belfast, 6 April 1981.

19. Lyons, H. A. The psychological effects of the civil disturbances on children. *Northern Teacher,* Winter 1973, 35–38.
20. McFarlane, G. Social life in Northern Ireland. *Soc. Sci. Res. Council Newsl.* 42 (1980), 12–13.
21. McIvor, M. Environmental understanding in Northern Ireland. Paper presented at Sixth Biennial Meeting of International Society for the Study of Behavioural Development, Toronto. August 1981.
22. McIvor, M., and McWhirter, L. Living in a troubled area in Belfast: Interpretations of potential conflict incidents. Submitted for publication.
23. McWhirter, L. Awareness of conflict. In McWhirter, L. and Trew, K., Eds. *The Northern Ireland Conflict: Myth and Reality. Social and Political Perspectives.* G. W. & A. Hesketh, Ormskirk, 1982.
24. McWhirter, L. Growing up in Northern Ireland: From "Aggression" to the "Troubles." In Goldstein, A.P., and Segall, M.H., Eds. *Aggression in Global Perspective.* Pergamon Press, New York, 1982.
25. McWhirter, L. Children's conceptions of violence in Northern Ireland: The influence of religious denomination and area of residence. Submitted for publication.
26. McWhirter, L., and Duffy, U. Interpersonal and intergroup comparisons: Perceptions of differences in a sample of young people in Northern Ireland. Submitted for publication.
27. McWhirter, L., and Gamble, R. Development of ethnic awareness in the absence of physical cues. Submitted for publication.
28. McWhirter, L., and Trew, K. Social awareness in Northern Ireland children. *Bull. Brit. Psychol. Soc.,* 34 (1981), 308–311.
29. McWhirter, L., and Trew, K., Eds. *The Northern Ireland Conflict: Myth and Reality. Social and Political Perspectives.* G.W.& A. Hesketh, Ormskirk, 1982.
30. McWhirter, L., and Trew, K. Education and social conflict in Northern Ireland: From segregation to integration? Submitted for publication.(a)
31. McWhirter, L., and Trew, K. The role of integrated education on the socialization of Northern Ireland children: An application of the contact thesis. Submitted for publication.(b)
32. McWhirter, L., Young, V., and Majury, J. Belfast children's awareness of violent death. *Brit. J. Soc. Psychol.,* 1982.
33. Milroy, J. *Regional Accents of English.* Blackstaff, Belfast, 1981.
34. Moxon-Browne, E. Northern Ireland attitude survey: An initial report. Unpublished manuscript, Queen's University of Belfast, 1979.
35. Murphy, D. *A Place Apart.* Penguin Books, Middlesex, 1978.
36. Murray, R. Patterns of violence. In McWhirter, L., and Trew, K., Eds. *The Northern Ireland Conflict: Myth and Reality. Social and Political Perspectives.* G. W. & A. Hesketh, Ormskirk, 1982.
37. Murray, R. Political violence in Northern Ireland: 1969–1977. In Boal, F. W., and Douglas J. N. H., Eds. *Integration and Division. Geographic Aspects of the Northern Ireland Problem.* Academic Press, London, 1982.
38. Potts, W. Origins of the Irish people. In McWhirter, L., and Trew, K., Eds.

The Northern Ireland Conflict: Myth and Reality. Social and Political Perspectives. G.W. & A. Hesketh, Ormskirk, 1982.
39. Rosenblatt, N. Children of war, *Time Magazine*, 11 January 1982, 16–38.
40. Rutter, M. Stress, coping and development: Some issues and some questions. *J. Child Psychol. Psychiat.*, 22, No. 4 (1981), 323–356.
41. Stringer, M., and Cairns, E. An investigation into the development of denominational attitudes in Northern Ireland. Paper presented at the Annual Conference of the British Psychological Society, University of Aberdeen, March 1980.
42. Trew, K. Social identity and group membership. Paper presented at Annual Conference of the British Psychological Society, Northern Ireland Branch, Rosapenna. May 1981.
43. Trew, K. Intergroup relations and the development of social identity in Northern Ireland. Paper presented at Sixth Biennial Meeting of International Society for the Study of Behavioural Development, Toronto, August 1981.
44. Trew, K. Education systems in Northern Ireland. In McWhirter, L., and Trew. K., Eds. *The Northern Ireland Conflict: Myth and Reality. Social and Political Perspectives.* G.W. & A. Hesketh, Ormskirk, 1982.
45. Trew, K., and McWhirter, L. Conflict in Northern Ireland: A research perspective. In Stringer, P., Ed. *Confronting Social Issues.* Volume 2. European Monographs in Social Psychology. Academic Press, London, 1982.
46. Ward, M. Evaluation reactions to four educated regional accents. Unpublished BA thesis, Queen's University of Belfast, 1980.
47. Wilkinson, P., Ed. *British Perspectives on Terrorism.* George Allen & Unwin, London, 1981.
48. Whyte, J. Interpretations of the Northern Ireland problem: An appraisal. *Econ. Soc. Rev.* 9, p. 4 (1978), 257–282.

THE GÄLLÖFSTA CONFERENCE

Introductory Remarks

Albert J. Solnit, M.D. (U.S.A.)*

In these introductory remarks I have set myself three goals. The first is to give respect to continuity and growth. The second is to reflect briefly on the need for balance between the inside life and the outside environment of the child—the clinical, diagnostic, and therapeutic approaches in the search for social, cultural, economic, and educational environments that facilitate healthy growth and development in childhood. This balance between the preventive resources and those that serve diagnostic and therapeutic needs is essential.

Each needs the other and will not be useful or effective unless the balance between the intraphysic and social environment is maintained and elaborated in a rapidly changing world. In this balance, biological considerations are vital, to some extent being indirectly expressed by intraphysic characteristics and to some extent requiring special attention vis-à-vis the relations between the body and the mind. Thus the biological and sociological sciences have the apparent seductiveness of being more concrete, measurable, objective, and lending themselves more to techniques and methods derived from the physical sciences (e.g., demographic, SES, statistical, and epidemiological factors). This perspective is incomplete but different from that of the subjective, more complex and subtle, psychological, perspective.

Each perspective needs the other to keep reasonably close to both inner and outer reality. Each is essential for understanding human

---

*Co-Chairman, International Study Group.

beings as people living in their world and at their point in the life cycle.

I wish to comment on another vital balance—that between child psychiatry and all the other crucial mental health disciplines that serve children in their families. Without clinical psychology, social work, special education, pediatrics, youth leaders, rehabilitation workers, nurses, and many others (e.g., child-care workers in hospitals and other institutions that serve children and their parents), we would be incomplete as we look backward with our multidisciplinary lenses to move forward to examine Children in turmoil: tomorrow's parents.

Summation

In summarizing the presentations and discussions of our International Study Group and in preparing for our Ninth International Congress, I again cannot forgo the opportunity to express my gratitude and that of the Executive Committee of the International Association for Child and Adolescent Psychiatry and Allied Professions to Dr. Ebba Neander, President, and Mrs. Arne Löfquist, Secretary of the Swedish Association for Child and Adolescent Psychiatry, and their many colleagues, who have provided us generously with scientific and personal hospitality to make this joint meeting of the International Study Group possible. Our Swedish colleagues and friends have tactfully and clearly opened our minds and hearts to the Swedish experience, what a distinguished American journalist, Marquis Childs, has referred to in a recent book as *Sweden: The Middle Way on Trial.** Of course, in their presentations and site visits our Swedish colleagues have concentrated on their professional and scientific experience, their research studies, and their planning and evaluation activities.

I was apprehensive that we would tend to emphasize the nonclinical studies over the clinical studies. Indeed, to a significant extent, although most of our Swedish colleagues are seasoned clinicians very much involved daily in providing expert diagnostic and therapeutic services for children and their parents, we have tended to concentrate on the facilitating or disadvantageous social environment more than on the child's inner mental life—more on

---

*Childs, Marquis. *Sweden: The Middle Way on Trial.* Yale University Press, New Haven, Conn., 1980.

epidemiological findings than on clinical problems—more on preventive than on curative experiences—more on the applied mental health areas (what we term indirect services) than on direct clinical services.

There are many reasons for this, and most of them are appropriate and understandable. First, Sweden has embarked on bold, imaginative, carefully planned and evaluated ways of improving the quality of life for children in their families and in their communities with more determination and resources per capita than any other nation in the world. It is an exciting, dedicated commitment to a better, more peaceful world for the present and future. We all need to learn from these programs and from both the positive and negative factors that such experiences reveal. And yet as Marianne Cederblad has indicated in her fascinating paper "Sweden: A Society in Turmoil?" there is much evidence of a costly transition, associated with family instability because of rapid urbanization and the threat to time-tested traditions and values, especially in regard to the continuity of affectionate relationships. There is a great deal of concern about work satisfaction, the misuse and abuse of alcohol and other addictive drugs, and the degree to which technology dominates rather than serves the need for a humanizing environment.

Such trends as the rising incidence of divorce, abortions, alcoholism, anorexia nervosa and other psychosomatic disorders, as well as "Aniara child," might indicate an emotional and ideological deprivation that is destroying or distorting the capacity of parents to provide sound psychological and emotional care for their children despite the adequacy of materialistic resources. However, such trends are indicative of a society in transition, much more open about and aware of its difficulties, and much more direct about taking on what has been uncovered in preparation for moving to a better quality of life. There is a proportionate concern about the emotional as well as the economic climate.

Here I am reminded of the great contributions of Ingmar Bergman, who concentrates on exploring the profound sorrow of human beings faced with the inevitability of mortality rather than the social ills of our times. After all, does a society shape the individual personality, or does it reflect the personalities that constitute that society?

I lean toward an optimistic emphasis, toward the need for a longer historical perspective suggesting that Sweden, an affluent society, is in transition, with the disorganizing and regressive tendencies being an index of preparation for a more stable, more humane, more child- and family-centered society.

As Colette Chiland indicates in her discussion of Dr. Cederblad's paper, Sweden is suffering from "happiness diseases" but in many respects it is apparently not as chaotic and unstable as many other countries in Western Europe. Gerald Caplan suggested that one should look for extended family support networks and what James Anthony termed personal support systems as indicators of stability and continuity.

Given these sociological perspectives, we can realize that clinical, intrapsychic perspectives are much more difficult to characterize. We need both epidemiological and clinical perspectives and indices. To some extent, in the infant studies of Peter de Chateau we found more of such a balance. De Chateau has extended the studies of Klaus and Kennel, emphasizing the critical period and its continuing impact when a mother does not have immediate and continuing physical contact with her newborn infant.

We are called on to use our expert clinical and theoretical knowledge in regard to several pressing problems that concern the everyday lives of children. We are pressed to apply our theory and the insights of our clinical knowledge because children cannot wait. Younger children need to have the best attention from parents during early infancy; they need sound day care and must have the help of teachers and schools to foster their cognitive and social development. Young children must be protected from the dangers of a world largely constructed for adults and from dangerous adult impulses.

In school and other educational settings, there should be a balance between the application of mental health principles and case finding. The former will enable teachers and principals to carry out more effectively their primary tasks of creating an environment that will facilitate children's cognitive and social development—that will strengthen the child's acquisition of symbolic learning, expression, and communication through reading, writing, and working well with numbers, and to use thinking as a trial action. It is our task to enable children to develop memory as a method for tapping the knowledge acquired through personal experience as well as that knowledge gathered over the ages and lodged in those libraries, museums, and other repositories of our cumulative historical, artistic, and philosophical understanding and expressiveness. It is a primary task for educators to establish a dynamic environment in which children's socialization can proceed according to their particular community's and culture's prevalent patterns of social expression and expectation.

Case finding in the schools should be a secondary task carried out with the assistance of mental health professionals. Thus mental health diagnostic and therapeutic services can be conducted in association with other services the schools provide or foster for children and their families, usually in the context of general health care.

Already in the first and second days, through presentations by Burt Stölhammer, Inge-Britt Stibner, Lennart Levi, Marianne Cederblad, Ulaf Brenner, and Borje Höök, in discussions by Peter Neubauer, Richard Landsdown, and Winston Richards, and in exchanges with Bengt Borjeson Ted Winther, and B. Lagerheim et al., we had the advantage of hearing how research and its applications were given high priorities in understanding and developing sound education for all children. There was also a discussion of preventive programs and intervention services concerned with child abuse.

Time limitations did not permit us to go into details about rehabilitation of abusive parents or the role of foster care and adoption for young children who have been abused. But we heard how superb the Swedish system is in exploring and describing the scope and nature of a threatening problem such as child abuse before moving too quickly into intervention and preventive programs. We also heard how daycare programs are evaluated and standards established to prevent psychological damage to young children, especially in regard to emotional and cognitive development of children under four years of age. We were impressed by the presentation of imaginative research and its applications designed to understand children's reactions to stress in daycare programs, and the effort to use behavioral and bioamine markers to define the stability of temperament and behavior in the developing child.

In our site visits to the Laboratory of Clinical Stress Research, to the Child Psychiatric Hospital in Stockholm, and to the Family Treatment Unit at SKA, we were impressed by the efforts to understand and help children and the adults who care for them, especially their parents, teachers, and case workers. We struggle to conceptualize the complexity of stress from the environment and stress from the inside—what might be termed tension discharge when the tension is derived from our drives and internal urges compared to tensions created by environmental pressures. The conflict between inner tensions and social demands is ever present.

Professor Lennart Levi introduced us to the goals, strategies, tactics, and philosophy of the Stress Research Center, by focusing on the aim of improving the quality of life for children. In his outline, he emphasized the need to keep in mind the micro and macro levels of studying and understanding children, with due respect for individual differences of vulnerability and invulnerability and of high-risk and low-risk environments. It was an elegant formulation of how to keep social engineering for a better quality of social environmental opportunities related to individual and group variations of strengths and weaknesses.

In considering the presentations and discussions of "Suicide Attempts in Sweden" by Ulf Otto, of "Alcoholism and Drug Abuse in Sweden" by Per-Anders Rydelius, and of "New and Follow-Up Research in Fostering and Adoption" by Dr. Michael Bohman, we realized how wide the net is and how repeated and interwoven are the themes. In one sense we can summarize by referring to the obstacles that stand in the way of children growing toward adulthood with the resources that will enable them to take care of their children. In that sense, what are the experiences that foster and those that pose obstacles to the child's development that will prepare them to find satisfaction and to achieve competence in their functions as parents?

As brilliantly documented by Michael Bohman's follow-up research, the psychological meaning of remaining with biological parents, of being adopted, and being in long-term foster care cannot be taken for granted. Feeling wanted permanently by parents who can provide continuity of affectionate care is best, no matter what adjective qualifies or characterizes such a family.

Many of the fascinating reports and discussions illuminate the unending and infinitely complex interactions of nature and nurture. They cannot be ignored. For example, if one studies alcoholism, the genetic factor must be taken into account. Can children's capacity to grow, identify, and extract strength from their social-emotional roots so influence their psychic functioning as to increase their capacity to be in charge of their bodies and fates, rather than to be tyrannized by their genetic inheritance?

Time limitations did not permit us to hear about and consider the mental health and developmental aspects of immigration, migratory labor, and socioeconomic class differences.

We became aware of our limited qualifications to specify what the quality of life should be. Although we have our own individual value preferences, doctors, nurses, social workers, and psychologists should realize how often we are tempted to indulge in our fantasies of omnipotence and omniscience. We should remain within our competence in assisting people—especially children and their parents—according to their life style and value preferences to reduce and prevent illness, to enhance each child's potential, and to maximize each family's integrity. In that sense, alcoholism and criminal behavior may not be best approached in terms of prevention by our professions, although we can have a great deal to say about the physical and psychological reactions to, involvement in, and contributions to alcoholism, criminal behavior, and a variety of other unhealthy human behavior patterns and preferences. This leads to issues of health education and the ways in which humans establish and protect preferred modalities of tension discharge. What is a painful stress for one child may after all be another child's joy!

Sweden—A Society in Turmoil?

Marianne Cederblad, M.D. (Sweden)

Sweden was lucky enough to be saved from the destruction during World War II which struck the rest of Europe and entered the postwar period with a strong wish for social planning and general optimism about development. The growth of economic resources during the 1950s turned the hopes into reality. Sweden took the lead among the economically high-standard societies of Europe. Dedicated social reforms distributed the growing material resources among the groups which needed them the most and the safety net of social security became more elaborate. Sweden seemed to become a model-country with increasing living standard and a social caretaking system built on solidarity.

No doubt this meant improved conditions of living for most people of the country. But the picture has shadows. The rapid socioeconomic development had to be paid. The development of the industry led to increasing environmental destruction. The efficiency of modern industry demanded more effective production which led to stress and exclusion of large groups of laborers who did not any longer meet the standard of work. The urbanization meant new cities which often became monotonous and isolating environments. The small nuclear family with two working parents gave rise to child-care problems. The old people got improved economic conditions but became more and more isolated. While serious somatic diseases were successfully conquered, psychological stress increased giving rise to mental disturbances and crisises.

This is a quotation from the former head of the Swedish National Board of Health and Social Welfare, Bror Rexed, who wrote this in a foreword to the report from a Royal Committee on Mental Health published in the autumn of 1978. He concludes that psychological problems cannot be solved by increasing the number of psychotherapists and psychiatrists, but "on the basis of a critical analysis of the society the living conditions leading to these stress situations must be changed. That is: we must investigate carefully our psycho-social environment."

If psychological problems can be used as a thermometer of the capacity of a society to maintain a high quality of life, is Sweden then a society in turmoil giving rise to a high degree of stress in its citizens? The answer of the Royal Committee was yes, based on the following examples of psychosocial problems that they think clearly indicate serious impairments of the psychological well-being of people in Sweden.

CHILDREN AND YOUTH

1. Twenty-five percent of all pregnancies are terminated by abortion.
2. Divorces with children below 15 years of age in the family increased threefold between 1963 and 1974.
3. One hundred and fifty thousand children live in single-parent homes.
4. Psychological problems are found in 30 percent of 4-year-old preschool children.
5. More than one-third of boys and one-fourth of girls in grade 9 (16 years of age) drink alcohol in intoxicating amounts.
6. One-fifth of those taking the medical examination for military service show neurosis or pathological personality.
7. During military service, 30 percent of the service people show major personal problems.
8. Thirty percent of students have psychological disturbances and three times as high a frequency of suicide as comparable groups.

WORKING LIFE

1. Thirty percent of workers experience work as psychologically stressful.
2. Two-thirds feel pressed for time.
3. One-seventh are psychologically exhausted at the end of the working day.

OLD AGE

1. Twenty percent of the old people of Stockholm have nervous problems.

2. Of the 70-year-old people in Gothenburg, one-eighth of the men and 25 percent of the woman need psychiatric treatment.
3. Of women 65 to 74 years of age, 25 percent use sleeping pills and 15 percent use tranquilizers.

GENERAL

1. Impaired psychological well-being is reported by 30 percent of the population.
2. Ten percent of all men suffer from alcoholism.
3. Seven hundred fifty million tablets of psychopharmacological drugs are sold each year (Sweden has 8 million inhabitants).
4. Four times as many crimes are reported compared with 20 years ago.
5. Nearly 2000 suicides per year, a rise of 20 percent during the last 15 years, are reported. This increase is especially high among women and younger persons.
6. Twenty thousand suicide attempts per year are reported.

Certain factors in a modern, urbanized, industrialized society like Sweden may account for the exasperating fact that a rising social, material, and economic standard of living has not led to improved mental health, although it has improved the somatic health as well as given rise to excellent conditions in general.

Why are Swedish children and young people, who are perhaps the healthiest, best fed, best dressed, most educated and intellectually stimulated, and least authoritarian repressed of all young people in the world not also the happiest, most harmonious, and least neurotic? And why do they not grow up to become harmonious, responsible adults, free of anxiety and depression? My analysis covers three areas:

Changes in the family structure.
Changes in the upbringing conditions of children outside the family.
Values and "meaning of life" transmitted to young people.

Changes in the Family Structure

Size. During the twentieth century, family size has gradually diminished. In 1910 the most common size was five persons or more

(33 percent), whereas in 1975, one or two persons per household are the most common (about 30 percent each). In Sweden during the 1970s a couple has on average 1.8 children whereas a single parent has 1.4 children.

During the twentieth century the divorce rate also has increased tremendously. In 1910 the number of divorces was less than one thirtieth of the number in 1978. The percentage of divorces involving children under the age of 15 has been approximately the same: two-thirds. During the last half of the 1970s, approximately 15,000 marriages with small children are dissolved each year. This is of course a major crisis in the lives of the children involved.

Out of single-parent families, the largest group consists of divorced women (31 percent). Forty-six percent are unmarried women, but 40 percent of these live with somebody. Many divorced mothers marry again or live more or less steadily with a man. The percentage of marriages in which one or both spouses have been married before has also increased from 11 percent in 1901 to 19 percent in 1978. The reason that it has not increased more is probably that the total number of marriages has decreased (halved) since 1944, although the population has increased, which is due to the fact that many people prefer to live together without being formally married. Since many of these "conscience marriages" probably also dissolve each year, the true number of divorces with separation traumas for children is probably much larger. Some children experience several such separations from successive new fathers and sometimes half-siblings during their growth.

Roles. Industrialization has meant changing roles of parents. Lopata investigated 600 housewives in Chicago who stated that they saw their own most important role as mothers and considered their husbands mainly as breadwinners. The husbands themselves also saw their main role as breadwinners. Other investigations have shown that the self-esteem of the husbands is based to a large extent on a successful fulfillment of the role of breadwinner. The modern nuclear family thus often can be seen as a "mother" married to a "breadwinner." This role specialization easily leads to intense relations between a mother and her dependent children and a distant, emotionally underinvolved father. Or, according to Brendon (also describing the United States), leads to a father who is often away from home, a mother who feels alone in her parenting role, and feelings of helplessness as authorities in both. They abdicate as parents, the children and their gang of age mates take over. We get a distortion of a child-centered culture in which the youngsters are in power and the parents look to them for guidance.

A Swedish sociologist, Rita Liljeström, is of the opinion that this holds true for Sweden as well and that it is the consequences of socioeconomic factors that have isolated the family, taken the work of the father away from the home, and created similar families consisting of a single breadwinner and a housewife.

In Swedish society, however, only around 35 percent of preschool children have mothers who are full-time housewives and mothers. In the homes where the mothers work part-time or full-time, there are other consequences for the children. The quality of the child-care arrangements while the mothers work is of course important. The strain of the resulting "double work" is especially hard on single-parent families. Divorced women have the highest frequency of employment (80 percent), yet their income is less than half that of a family with two parents). Their risk of requiring social aid is four to five times as great as that of women without children or couples with children. In these overburdened families, the quality of parent–child relationships easily might be affected in a negative way. Studies have shown that Swedish women work approximately 40 hours per week in the household, although they work outside the home whether they are married or alone. Even in Sweden, the husbands don't help much in the household in the majority of families!

Mobility. Whereas in 1910, 75 percent of the population lived in rural areas, in 1980, 80 percent live in towns and cities. This change has been noticed especially during the last 20 years. Political decisions increased the high mobility. The so-called moving-van policy of the 1960s involved decisions to move the labor force to certain regional centers where it was considered most profitable to concentrate industry. Still ½ million Swedes move across parish borders each year, and ¼ million move within the parishes; that is, 10 percent of the entire population moves each year. Mobility is the greatest for young people and for families with two or more children. The result is uprootedness and loss of contact with relatives and childhood friends, who could constitute an important psychological network for the family at moments of stress. The children have to change daycare centers and schools and find new friends. As Liljeström puts it, "The people of the farms in the 19th century lived within a frame of lasting human relations. Modern man lives without a safety-net of relationships."

Changes in the Upbringing Conditions of Children Outside the Family

Out of all Swedish preschool children, approximately one-third are at home with their mothers, 15 percent are in daycare centers, 15 percent are at family day-homes, and the rest have various private arrangements (a young girl as baby sitter, a privately arranged family day-home, a grandmother, etc.).

All these child-care models can add positive factors to the environment of the child, but they can also mean additional stress. We have already discussed the changes in the situation of the family in modern society. The small size and the frequent moves with loss of contact with relatives and old friends can lead to a feeling of isolation and emptiness of the housewife−mother, who also loses her role when her children are grown. Studies in England have shown high frequencies of depression (around 30 percent) in home-working mothers with small children. This probably holds true for Sweden as well. The risk for the children of this group is few relations outside the home leading to overinvolved mother−child relations.

Those children who are in daycare centers, and also sometimes those being taken care of by day mothers or young baby sitters instead run the risk of too many, frequently disrupted relationships. The staffs of the centers consist mostly of young women and many have their own children. They are therefore often on pregnancy leaves or home with their children in addition to taking sickness absences and ordinary vacations, so that the parent substitutes often are different persons each time. Day mothers work in that position for three years on average, which means that many children change day mothers during their preschool years. Young baby sitters often work only for a year and then continue their education. Someone has calculated that a child who spends all of his or her preschool years in daycare centers may be taken care of by up to 200 nurses during those 6 years!

For those children who have private day-homes, the quality of care varies. Some are good, but others try to make more money by taking too many children, who are sometimes neglected. Young baby sitters are often too immature to take sole responsibility for small children for long hours and don't know enough about the psychological needs of children. Grandmothers are of course dedicated and more experienced, but they may be ailing, tired, or too indulgent. Often the shared responsibility of mothering awakens the autonomy struggles of adolescence between mother and grandmother as the younger generation becomes more dependent on the older again.

School children. Out of Swedish school children 7 to 10 years of age, 30 percent have their mothers at home full-time. Twenty-five percent go to a recreation center (that is, a daycare center for school children) or a family day-home (half at each). About 50 percent have private arrangements. Out of the latter group there are some children who must take care of themselves, "key children" or "banana-in-plastic-bag children." These children often spend their time at the department stores of the suburbs or at the public library with very little constructive contact with adults. I must point out, however, that 55 percent of the women in Sweden who work and who have children under the age of 17, work part-time. Since schools function for 20 hours per week during the first grade and 30 hours per week during the third, most children only have to take care of themselves for a few hours each day, except during vacations. This is still a problem for many children, and there are plans to solve it by arranging after-school activities with various youth organizations.

In summary, children in Sweden experience a childhood either characterized by too few, overinvolved relations in a very small, isolated nuclear family with little variation of role models to identify with, or their childhood is characterized by a large number of broken relations of various depths but of short duration. The only lasting relation, that with their mother (and maybe father), is often handicapped by the parent being exhausted when the family is together.

Apart from those with women in child-caretaking positions, the children seldom have intimate contacts with adults in working situations and therefore are alienated from a very important sector of adult life.

In clinical child psychiatric practice in Sweden, we have noticed an increasing number of two psychiatric disorders, which may be extreme reactions to these upbringing conditions: anorexia nervosa and what has been called "the Aniara child"—named after the Swedish Nobel Prize winner Harry Martinsson's spaceship poem "Aniara." Anorexia nervosa is increasing in clinical praxis. Modern treatment has focused on autonomy problems activated during adolescence but based on very early disturbances of symbiosis and individuation. The previously described conditions of the modern nuclear family easily can be seen as aggravating these problems in vulnerable individuals.

The Aniara child is characterized by a weak ego and a shallow capacity for contact. Such children are restless, impulse-driven, and with a short attention span and low level of frustration, which gives rise to school problems. When growing up, these people develop into narcissistic, pleasure-seeking individuals whose relations are superficial and manipulative. They have many superficial and exchangeable contacts but few lasting and committed relations. This personality type may develop in vulnerable persons as a result of the repeated separations that characterize the growing up of many Swedish children.

In *The Culture of Narcissism* [3], the American psychologist Christopher Lasch relates borderline personality disorders and the descriptions of similar conditions in contemporary novels and plays to certain crucial phenomena in postindustrial society. He sees these conditions as the extremes of more general character traits which are the results of various factors.

The weakening of parental authority, due to the alienation of working away from the home and the rapidly changing society, makes the life experience of the parents irrelevant as a guide for the children. Since the 1930s, experts have made parents insecure in their parenting role through continuously changing advice: on the-clock-feeding (1930); permissiveness (1950s); stress on authenticity of feeling; for instance, in parent effectiveness training (1960s).

As a result, the inhibiting, controlling, and guiding function of the superego, which largely merges with the ego, is weakened through the weakness of the parents. Society reinforces this pattern through indulgent education in the schools and this fails to train the ego. Through advertising and the mass media, a hedonistic cult of consumption is encouraged. By surrounding the consumer with images of the good life, the mass culture encourages the ordinary person to cultivate extraordinary tastes, to identify with the privileged minority against the rest, and to fantasize life of exquisite comfort and sensual refinement. This simultaneously makes the person unhappy with his or her lot. By fostering grandiose aspirations, it also fosters self-denigration and self-contempt. This focus on personal gratification is increased by a loss of historical continuity: the sense of belonging to a succession of generations originating in the past and stretching into the future.

Values and "Meaning of Life" Transmitted to Young People

During the twentieth century, religion has lost its meaning for increasing numbers of people in Sweden. We still have a state religion, the Lutheran (protestant) faith. However, in the goal descriptions of the Swedish preschools and at school in general, it is explicitly stated that the teachers will be objective and not influence the values of the pupils except for basic democratic values: cooperation, respect for others, tolerance, solidarity, and so forth. Ninety-six percent of Swedes belong to the state church, but the number leaving the church per year has doubled from 1970 to 1979. The numbers of baptisms and funerals have remained the same during the last decade, but the proportion of church marriages has diminished. In 1910, 7 percent of all marriages were outside the church, in 1978, 38 percent were outside it. I think it is true to say that most Swedes have an uninvolved, disengaged attitude toward religious questions. They may go to church on major Christian holy days like Christmas and Easter, and they often baptize their children and bury their dead within the church, but this is more a sign of abiding by tradition than taking a personal stand. Maybe this situation is due to our 44 years of social-democratic rule, which has stressed materialistic values, maybe it is a *Zeitgeist* in Western European industrialized societies that has focused on concrete, material goals rather than on spiritual development. We have not replaced religion by any other ideologies like Marxism. Instead, an ideological vacuum has been created, filled only with general democratic values and without any answers to the existential questions of why and for what do we live. Much of the aimless, listless attitudes that we meet in the youth of today seem to be the result of upbringing by adults who don't advocate strong personal belief in values beyond an individual existence. Devoid of the spiritual aspects of life, people regress to an egocentric, pleasure-seeking attitude, which doesn't seem to give any lasting satisfaction and, in fact, provides a low quality of life.

The theme here is stress: turmoil or mastery? How can the turmoil of the present society be turned into mastery? This question is discussed in a new book by Jan Grönholm, published by the Swedish Secretariat for Future Studies. Grönholm states that economic and technical development has reached its limits and that development now has to enter another direction focused on human consciousness. He stresses the central beliefs of many religions as well as theories of modern physics, which all describe the holistic aspect of the universe and the human mind and the inseparable interdependency of the part and the whole.

The English professor of physics David Bohm has put forward a theory of the world as a hologram. In the hologram, the whole is represented in every part. One example of the hologram character of reality is the DNA molecule, in which all the information needed to build a whole body is stored. The view of the world as a hologram is not new, however. People have experienced the world in this way in altered states of consciousness. The American physicist Fritiof Capra [1], in his book *The Tao of Physics*, has described the parallels of Eastern wisdom and modern physics. "The more we enter the sub-microscopic world the more we understand how the modern physicist like the eastern mystic has come to see the world as a system of inseparable interchanging components in constant flow and with man as an integrated part of this system." The insight into this, he argues, is the consciousness—the development of which is the next step in the development of mankind.

Sociologists claim that each society has a central project. In our society this is material growth. The new central project that could give our society a meaningful direction that he and future-researchers advocate is human development. The goal should be the self-actualizing person described by Abraham Maslow. A person who is independent, creative, spontaneous, integrated, open, and cooperative. This person has a strong feeling of self-worth and is focused on the well-being of the totality. Her or his actions are guided by a wish for development and by love and care for others. She or he lives in the present but at the same time sees her or his life in a greater perspective, feeling responsible not only to the family but to society and humankind. To create such a personality, society must be organized to give the individual a possibility to take responsibility, to be creative, and to deepen the feelings of togetherness with others.

This is not possible in the present society. A change has to be made toward what has been called the B-society: a small-scale, ecologically adjusted, decentralized society focused on togetherness and personal development. The Norwegian peace researcher Johan Galtung [2] describes this society: A micro-industrial society consisting of villages of about 1000 inhabitants where 75–80 % of the population lives. Farming and industry are organized as co-operatives. More handicraft and subsidance households. The small scale gives more possibilities for participation in democratic decisions. The material standard will be less than in the present large-scale, centralized A-society but the quality of life will be increased.

This may sound utopian, but there seems to be a tendency in Swedish society to become more open to these ideas. At a public vote in 1980 on nuclear power plants, nearly 40 percent of the population voted against nuclear power, which is also a symbol for the continuation of the postindustrial A-society. They voted for a society with alternative forms of energy, which means development toward a B-society along the lines described by Galtung.

References

1. Capra, F. *The Tao of Physics*. Random House, New York, 1975.
2. Galtung, J. *Members of Two Worlds: A Developmental Study of Three Villages in Western Society*. Columbia University Press, New York, 1971.
3. Lasch, C. *The Culture of Narcissism*. Norton, New York, 1978.

Long-Term Effects on Mother—Infant Behavior of Extra Contact During the First Hour Postpartum

IV. Study Design and Methods

Britt Wiberg
Peter de Château, M.D. (Sweden)

The main purpose of this article is to present the research design and methods used in a longitudinal study aimed at testing the hypothesis that early postnatal interaction between mothers and infants can influence the development of their relationship. In most studies on the same subject, many different investigative methods have been used [4, 5, 10, 15, 16, 17, 24, 25, 26, 28, 30, 40, 41, 42, 44, 47, 51]. The experimental designs in many studies also differ greatly, which makes direct comparison impossible. Furthermore, the selection of the subjects and their allocation to these studies is not at all uniform, adding another problem to the already existing ones. The statistical methods differ, and so do the evaluation and interpretation of the results.

The conclusions drawn from these studies and their impact on day-to-day perinatal care has been impressive. However, this in itself includes a dangerous development. If a routine is to be replaced by a new one, great sensitivity in practical application is needed. No such change should be made in too rigorous a way, even if there is evidence of implications for perinatal care. Infants differ greatly from each other right from the start. Their families have different capacities and backgrounds. Flexibility regarding individual requirements of each and every family is therefore needed. It is most regrettable that certain modes of early stimulation and soothing are considered universally beneficial, regardless of a given infant's particular needs [10, 13].

The danger of too much generalization from contemporary research on mother–infant relations has recently been pointed out (47). We fully share this opinion and would also add that detailed information about research projects is often difficult to obtain. This makes the judgment and interpretation of these studies less than adequate. This paper, therefore, must be considered an endeavor to fill the gap, especially since some parts of our studies have been replicated by others [8, 28, 35].

Study Design

MATERIAL

This longitudinal, prospective study was started in December 1974 and aimed to examine the effect that extra contact—limited to 15 to 20 minutes—immediately following delivery might have on the behavior of mother and infant and on the development of their relationship [10, 15, 16]. A general outline of the times of various follow-up studies, the methods used, and the participating experimenters are given in Figure 1.

The basic conditions for participation in the study were that mothers and infants were healthy and lived in our hospital catchment area, and that pregnancy and delivery were normal and the neonatal period uncomplicated. The study was carried out in a university hospital and included 42 mother–infant pairs divided into two groups:

1. *P group* (n = 20): Primiparous women given routine care with newborn infants.

2. *P+ group* (n = 22): Primiparous women given extra contact (an extra skin-to-skin and suckling contact with their newborn infants) followed by routine care.

SELECTION CRITERIA

The medical criteria that all mother–infant pairs had to meet (Table 1) were a were a maternal age of 20–29 years, no history of previous abortions or miscarriages, length of pregnancy 38–42 weeks, no use

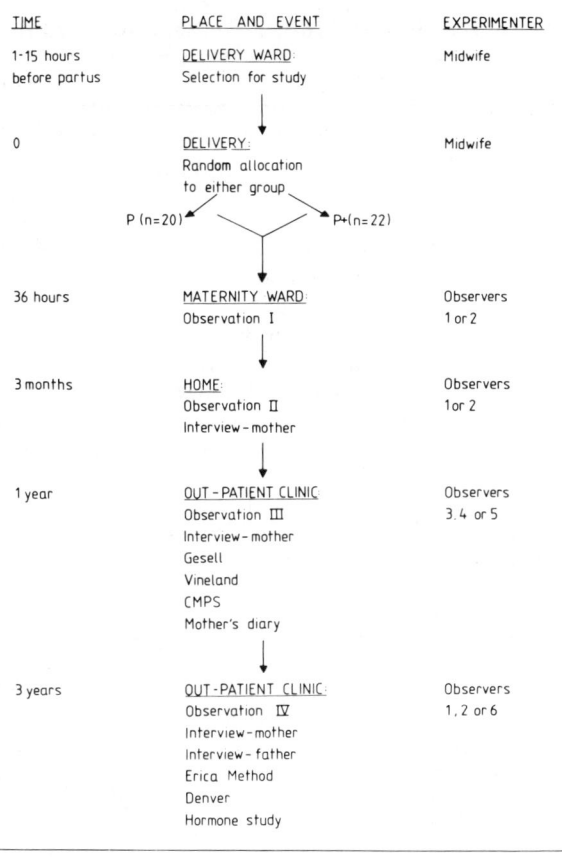

Figure 1. General outline of study design and methods used at different times in follow-up studies.

of drugs except iron medication and vitamins during pregnancy, normal weight gain [37], normal blood pressure and Hb percentage, and no proteinuria [36]. The mother must have started labor spontaneously at full term. All infants must have been born in vertex presentation, have a birth weight of between 3000 and 4000 grams, and have no signs of intra- or extrauterine asphyxia. There must have been no signs or symptoms of congenital malformation or disease at physical examination one day and six days postpartum. Many of these criteria have been described as optimal obstetrical conditions [38, 48]. The number of mother–infant pairs participating in the different parts of the study at different occasions is given in Table 2.

Table 1. Medical Criteria That All Mother–Infant Pairs Had to Meet

	Mother	Infant
Age	20–29 years	Single child (no twins)
Parity	0	Apgar Score: ≥7 1 minute postpartum
Pregnancy	I—normal	
Length of pregnancy	38–42 weeks	Weight: 3000–4000 grams
Delivery	Spontaneous labor ≤ 24 hours	No malformations
	Vertex presentation	
	≤ 200 mg pethidin (or equivalent) 1–6 hours before parturition	

Table 2. Number of Mother–Infant Pairs Participating in Different Parts of the Study

Time	P group	P+ group	Total
Selection	24	26	50
Delivery	20	22	42
36 hours postpartum	20	22	42
3 months postpartum	19	21	40
1 year postpartum	15	18	33
3 years postpartum	18	20	38

SELECTION PROCEDURE

When the mother arrived at the hospital for delivery, the midwife made a preliminary selection based on previous obstetric history, present pregnancy, and place of residence. The records of these mothers were marked "study" and numbered in order of arrival. Fifty mothers were selected for the study. General care, observation, and preparation for delivery were carried out according to standard routine procedures. The mothers were delivered by the midwife on duty; due to the duration of labor, this was very often not the same midwife who was present at admission. Immediately after delivery, the midwife or nursing aid helping her compared the number on the mother's record with a coincidence table. According to this table—placed in a locker in an office outside the delivery room—mothers were assigned randomly to either the routine care group (P) or the extra-contact group (P+). Eight mother–infant pairs who did not fulfill the established criteria concerning residence, delivery, infant, or neonatal period were excluded (Table 3). The final groups thus comprised 42 mother–infant pairs.

The groups were comparable in mean maternal age, civil status, socioeconomic status, education, mean number of visits to the antenatal clinic, maternal weight gain during pregnancy, and mean gestational age (Table 4). An equal proportion of fathers was present at delivery, and the mean duration of labor and amount of analgesia used were comparable in the two groups [10].

ROUTINE CARE IMMEDIATELY FOLLOWING DELIVERY (P GROUP)

After delivery, the baby lies on the delivery table, between the legs of the mother. Mouth and upper airways are rinsed and the stomach emptied. Face, trunk, and legs are wiped dry with a towel. The mother is then given a brief view of the infant but usually she does not touch it. Numbered bracelets are put around the wrist of both mother and infant. After cord clamping, two to six minutes postpartum, the baby is taken to another part of the delivery room for weighing, measuring, bathing, physical examination, Credé prophylaxis, and dressing. This takes approximately 30 minutes. In the meantime, the mother is helped to deliver the placenta, is washed, and cleaned. The baby—with clothes on—is put in a crib and covered with a blanket. The crib is placed beside the mother's bed so that she can watch her baby and touch its face. In some instances the baby, dressed and wrapped in a blanket, is placed in the mother's bed. The mother, the infant, and the father (if present) stay together in the delivery room for approximately two hours after the actual birth, at which time the mother and the infant are transferred to the maternity ward.

Table 3. Mother–Infant Pairs ($n = 8$) Excluded from the Study After Preliminary Selection in the Delivery Ward

P Group ($n = 4$)[a] Reason for Exclusion	P+ Group ($n = 4$)[b] Reason for Exclusion
Bleeding postpartum	Ablatio placentae
Hyperbilirubinemia neonatorum	Hyperbilirubinemia neonatorum
Not living in our catchment area	Not living in our catchment area
Wrong observation time	Wrong observation time

[a]P = primiparous mothers with routine care after delivery.
[b]P+ = primiparous mothers with extra contact following delivery.

Table 4. Data on Mother–Infant Pairs in the Two Observational Groups

	P ($n = 20$)[b]	P+ ($n = 22$)[c]
Mean maternal age (years)	25.5	25.0
Mean age of fathers (years)	26.3	25.6
Married and regularly living together	19	20
Socioeconomic status I/II/III[a]	3/9/8	5/7/10
Mean number of visits to antenatal clinics	13	13
Mean of mothers' weight gain (as a percentage of weight at delivery)	16.5	17.3
Mean gestational age (weeks)	40.4	40.1
Fathers present at delivery	17	19
Analgesia		
$\quad$ N$_2$O	19	20
$\quad$ Pethidin chlorid	12	11
$\quad$ Pethidin in mg (mean)	85	90
$\quad$ Time before delivery (range)	2–8 hours	2–12 hours
$\quad$ Diazepam	5	5
$\quad$ Time before delivery (range)	2–8 hours	3.5–12 hours
$\quad$ Pudendal blockage	19	19
$\quad$ Time before delivery	15 min.–3 hours	15 min.–2 hours
Mean duration of delivery (hours and minutes)	7.40	7.43
Range of duration of delivery (hours and minutes)	1.48–15.32	2.38–14.34
Sex of infant (males/females)	13/7	12/10
Mean birth weight (grams)	3386	3532
Mean apgar score at 1 and 10 minutes	9/9	9/9

[a] Socioeconomic status: I = highest; II = middle; III = lowest.
[b] P = Primiparous mothers and infants with routine care after delivery.
[c] P = Primiparous mothers and infants with extra contact following delivery.

EXTRA CONTACT IMMEDIATELY FOLLOWING DELIVERY (P+ GROUP)

Mouth and upper airways are rinsed, the stomach is emptied, the body dried with a towel, and a numbered bracelet is fastened around the wrists of infant and mother as in routine care. The midwife puts the naked baby onto the mother's abdomen after clamping the cord. This skin-to-skin contact begins approximately 10 minutes postpartum (Figure 2). About five minutes later the midwife moves the baby up onto the mother's chest and helps it suckle from the mother's breast. This extra contact lasts for about 15 to 20 minutes. After this period, when the baby is about 25 to 30 minutes old, the routine procedure described above is continued.

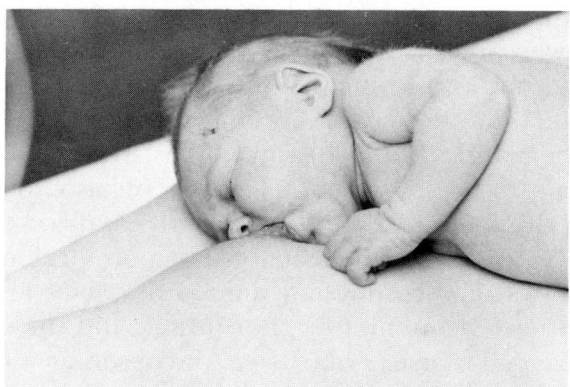

Figure 2. The extra skin-to-skin contact immediately following delivery (P+ group only).

ROUTINE CARE IN THE MATERNITY WARD FROM ABOUT TWO HOURS AFTER DELIVERY UNTIL DISCHARGE FROM THE HOSPITAL SIX TO EIGHT DAYS LATER (P AND P+ GROUPS)

For the first three days after delivery, the mother sees and nurses her infant every four hours during the day. During the night, and for most of the day, the infant stays in a separate nursery. During the second half of the postpartum week, the infant stays in the mother's room in the daytime. The mother takes a more active part in the care of her infant, bathing it, changing nappies and clothes, and so on. During the night, most infants remain in the nursery. Most of the rooms in the maternity ward accommodate four mothers and their infants.

Methods at 36 Hours

Before leaving the delivery floor, the mothers were asked to participate with their newborn infants in an ongoing study on breast-feeding and child development and were told that they were to be observed later on in the maternity ward. None of the mothers refused, probably because the approach was made through the midwives, who by that time were well known to and trusted by the mothers.

OBSERVATION OF MOTHER–INFANT BEHAVIOR AT 36 HOURS

All subjects were observed about 36 hours after delivery (range 32 to 40 hours) in the mother's room during breast-feeding. All mothers were in four-bed wards. Two observers participated in the study, and the subjects were randomly assigned to one of them. They did not know to which group the mother–infant pairs belonged. Only one observer was present at each observation. The mothers were told that we did not know much about normal behavior during the neonatal period and that we were interested in the interaction between mother and infant during breast-feeding. They were encouraged to proceed as usual. They were also told that only normal and healthy mothers and their healthy and full-term infants were to be observed. During the observation period the other mothers in the ward were nursing their own babies as usual. The respective positions of the mother, her infant, and the observer are shown in Figure 3. To be less obtrusive, the observer was present in the room for a few minutes before the infant's crib was brought in. Before actual observation during breast-feeding, notes were made about how the mother picked the baby up from the crib and the way she carried it to her bed or chair for breast-feeding [10]. No conversation between mother and observer was allowed during the observation period. Thirty-five different behavioral items, 29 maternal and 6 infant, were scored and noted on a checklist.. Most of the observational items are self-explanatory; full details and definitions are given elsewhere [10].

DURATION AND TECHNIQUE OF OBSERVATION AT 36 HOURS

The observation period was 15 minutes, divided into 20 periods of 15 seconds for actual observation and 20 periods of 30 seconds for writing the observations on the checklist. A small taperecorder provided signals through an earphone to indicate the observation and writing periods. This apparatus was shown to the mothers and

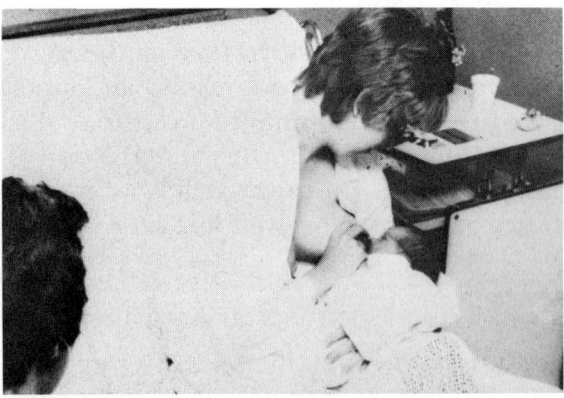

Figure 3. The position of the mother, the infant, and the observer during the observation session 36 hours postpartum. [10]

its use explained before the actual observation was started. Behavior that occurred during the observation period [10] was scored as 1. After the observation, the score for each item of behavior was added up, and the total was used as a measure of the frequency of the particular behavior during the observation period. The maximum score for any item was therefore 20. Items of behavior not included in our observation list sometimes occurred but could not be used for data analysis.

INTEROBSERVER RELIABILITY AT 36 HOURS

The two observers were compared before and after the study proper. Each of these reliability studies comprised eight mother–infant pairs. The observation was performed during ordinary breastfeeding. These mothers and infants did not meet any specific criteria other than that pregnancy, delivery, and the first postpartum days had been normal. The mothers had agreed to the presence of two observers. The correlation coefficient r was above .90 for all of the 35 behavioral items both before and after the study.

After completing the observation at 36 hours in the maternity ward, the observer talked to the mother and answered her questions. On a specially designed form the observer registered the name, address, age, and civil and socioeconomic status of both mother and father. During this conversation we asked if we could contact the mother again for a follow-up study when the infant was three months old. All mothers agreed to this.

Methods at Three Months

The follow-up study was carried out during a home visit and included observation of mother–infant free play and a personal interview with the mothers.

OBSERVATION OF MOTHER-INFANT BEHAVIOR AT THREE MONTHS

The same two earlier observers participated in this study. The appointment for the home visit was made by a secretary. The mother–infant pairs were assigned randomly to one of the two observers, neither of them being aware of which group (P or P+) to which the mother–infant pairs belonged. All home visits were made at 1 p.m. At this time most infants were asleep. After an initial interview, mother–infant free play approximately 2 to 2½ hours after the last feeding was observed. This is a good time for observation [2], since the infant is usually alert and cooperative. The mother and infant were asked to place themselves on a carpet on the floor. The observer also sat on the floor, approximately one meter away from them (Figure 4). Before the observation started, the mother was told by the observer that we wanted to watch her and her infant together during 10 minutes of free play. The mother was given a bell, a dangling ring, and a rattle bag similar to those used in Gesell Developmental Schedules [20]. The mother could use the toys in whatever way and sequence she liked. Sixty-one different behavioral items (33 maternal, 28 infant), most of which were very descriptive of what was observed, were scored and noted on a checklist [10].

DURATION AND TECHNIQUE OF OBSERVATION AT THREE MONTHS

During a pilot study, we had discovered that infants very soon became tired during observation. The mean frequency for crying during observation for eight infants was 0.25 during the first five minute period and 1.40 during the second. The mothers used a dummy more frequently during the second half of the observation time than during the first half. The observation periods were therefore kept to 10 minutes, and good cooperation was obtained from all mother-infant pairs. This observation period of 10 minutes was divided into 10 periods of 15 seconds for actual observation and 10 periods of 45 seconds for writing the observation down. The number of items observed made it necessary to have a longer writing

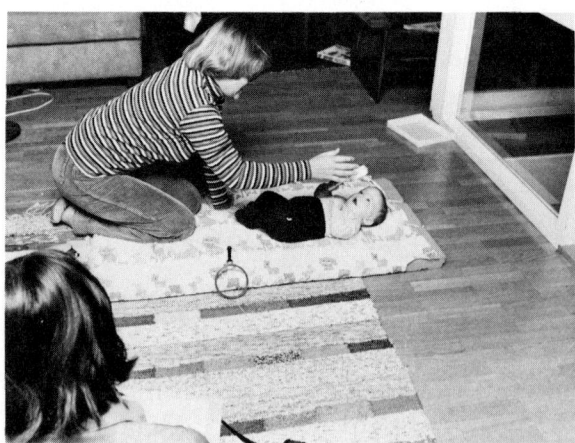

Figure 4. The position of the mother, the infant, and the observer during the observation 3 months postpartum.

period than at 36 hours. The same small tape recorder provided signals through an earphone to indicate the observation and writing periods. The use of this apparatus was known to the mothers from our first observation at the maternity ward, and, if necessary, was reexplained to the mothers before the observation period started. Behavior that occurred during this period was scored as 1. After observation, the score for each item of behavior was added up, and the total was used as a measure of the frequency of that particular behavior item during the observation period. The maximum score for any item was therefore 10. As on the previous occasion, behavior not included in our observation list sometimes occurred but could not be used for data analysis.

INTEROBSERVER RELIABILITY AT THREE MONTHS

For reliability purposes, a study was made of 11 mother–infant pairs during a routine three-month checkup at the Child Health Center in our hospital before the study proper started. These mothers and infants did not meet any specific criteria other than that pregnancy, delivery, the first postnatal week at the maternity ward, and the first three months at home had been normal. They also agreed to participate in the reliability study and to the presence of two observers. The correlation coefficient r was not lower than .92 for any of the 61 items used during the observation.

PERSONAL INTERVIEW WITH THE MOTHERS AT THREE MONTHS

A structured but unstandardized personal interview was also held with the mothers during the home visit. The interview took place before the actual observation of mother–infant behavior during free play started and consisted of questions grouped into four main categories:

1. Mother's preparation for and perception of pregnancy, delivery and neonatal week.
2. Coming home and the first three months at home.
3. Current situation.
4. Duration of breast-feeding.

Methods at One Year

The design of the one-year follow-up study is given in Table 5.

Table 5. Design of the One-Year Follow-Up Study of Control and Extra Contact Groups in the Out-Patient Clinic

Methods of Examination	Observers	Participant(s)[a]
Arrival of mother and infant		M and C
Observation of mother and infant behavior during a physical examination of the infant	(1 + 2 or 3)	M and C
Personal interview with the mother	(1)	M
Gesell Developmental Schedules	(2 or 3)	C
Vineland Social Maturity Scale	(2 or 3)	M
Cesarec-Marke Personality Scale	(2 or 3)	M
Mother's diary of infant's feeding and sleeping habits	(2 or 3)	M and C
Duration of breast-feeding, final discussion	(2 or 3)	M and C

[a] M = mother; C = child; (1) = pediatrician; (2 and 3) = psychologists.

OBSERVATION OF MOTHER AND INFANT BEHAVIOR DURING A PHYSICAL EXAMINATION OF THE INFANT AT ONE YEAR

Observation of maternal and infant behavior followed a standard pattern. The subjects were randomly assigned to one of the two new observers. Only one observer was present at each observation period. All observation took place in the same examination room of the clinic during a routine physical examination of the infant by a pediatrician. The approximate positions of mother, infant, doctor, and observer and the placement of the furniture in the examination room are shown in Figure 5. The same doctor conducted all the examinations. The observer in chair A was present when mother, infant, and doctor entered the examination room. The observation period started after an initial talk and after the mother had undressed her infant. This period was divided into two parts: one of 7 minutes and 30 seconds while the infant was seated in its mother's lap on chair C and a second part of the same duration while the infant was lying on the examination table D. In both parts of the observation, a routine and standardized physical examination was made by a doctor, who was at E for the first part (26 items, 19 maternal and 7 infant) at F for the second part (25 items, 18 maternal and 7 infant) of the observation period. No conversation between the observer and the other persons in the room was allowed during the actual observation period. Of course mother, infant, and doctor could communicate freely among themselves during the whole period. Maternal and infant behavior was scored according to two separate checklists [17].

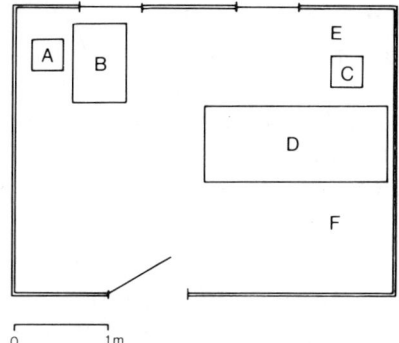

Figure 5. The approximate position of the mother (at C) and the infant (at C or D), the doctor (at E or F) and the observer (at A) during observation of a physical examination of the infant at one year. A = chair (psychologist's position); B = table; C = chair; D = examination table; E and F = doctor's positions. [13]

DURATION AND TECHNIQUE OF OBSERVATION AT ONE YEAR

The total observation period was two times 7 minutes 30 seconds; each period was divided into 10 periods of 15 seconds for actual observation and 10 periods of 30 seconds for writing the observations down on the checklist. As in the earlier studies, the same small, portable tape recorder was used, providing signals through an earphone to indicate the observation and writing periods. Behavior that occurred during the observation time was scored as 1. After the observation period, the score for each item of behavior was added up, and the total was used as a measure of the frequency of that particular behavior during the observation. The maximum score for any item during one of the two periods was therefore 10, and for the total period, 20. As on the previous occasions, behavior not included in our observation list sometimes occurred but could not be used for data analysis.

INTEROBSERVER RELIABILITY AT ONE YEAR

For reliability purposes, a study was made of eight mother–infant pairs during a routine checkup at the Child Health Center before and after the study. These mother–infant pairs met some basic criteria such as normal pregnancy, delivery, development, and absence of illness. For none of the 51 items used during observation was the correlation coefficient r lower than .90 [22].

PERSONAL INTERVIEW WITH THE MOTHERS AT ONE YEAR

A short, semistructured interview covering socioeconomic and occupational circumstances, health, some child-rearing practices, and the father's participation in the daily care ofsthe children was held at the beginning of the one-year follow-up study. This interview contained a total of 15 questions.

GESELL DEVELOPMENTAL SCHEDULES AT ONE YEAR

All the children were given the Gesell Developmental Schedules, which consists of five major categories: gross-motor, fine-motor, adaptive, linguistic, and personal-social development [20, 21]. Each child was examined individually by one of the two psychologists with the mother present during the examination.

VINELAND SOCIAL MATURITY SCALE AT ONE YEAR

The Vineland Social Maturity Scale was developed by Doll [18] at the Vineland Training School. The scale measures social development and maturity in children. A Swedish version has been used since 1960 [31]. The greatest value and strength of this method lies in its indirect, through-the-mother approach to the subjects. The mothers were assigned randomly to one of the two psychologists, who interviewed them.

CESAREC-MARKE PERSONALITY SCHEME AT ONE YEAR

Cesarec and Marke [6] constructed a personality scheme (CMPS) based on Murray's theories of psychogenic needs [34]. This inventory might be regarded as one of the most comprehensive multidimensional personality inventories available and standardized in Swedish. The factors measured are achievement, affiliation, aggression, defense of status, guilt feelings, dominance, exhibition, autonomy, nurturance, order, and succurance. In addition to these factors, there is also an "acquiescence" scale measuring a tendency to answer yes no matter what the question is. Five factor indices based on factor analysis were calculated: (a) neurotic self assertion; (2) dominance: a nonneurotic need to dominate; (3) aggressive nonconfirmity; (4) passive dependency; and (5) sociability. The personality questionnaire was administered individually to each mother by one of the two psychologists.

MOTHER'S DIARY OF INFANT'S FEEDING AND SLEEPING HABITS AT ONE YEAR

During the week before the follow-up at the hospital, all the mothers were asked to keep a diary, using a standard form, concerning infant feeding (two days) and sleeping habits (one week). Most mothers kept these diaries very thoroughly.

DURATION OF BREAST-FEEDING AT ONE YEAR

The data were collected during the personal interview with the mothers at three months and at one year and checked against the Child Health Center records.

Methods at Three Years

After three years, a total of 38 mother–infant pairs were studied (Table 2). Some of the pairs missing at one year did agree to come this time. The general outline of the three-year follow-up is given in Figure 1, a more detailed schedule in Table 6.

MORNING SESSION AT THREE YEARS

Upon arrival at the clinic at approximately 9:30 a.m., the family was given a short introduction by experimenters 1 and 2. After this introduction, the parents and the child were separated. The parents were interviewed by a doctor (experimenter 1) and answered a questionnaire. Both parents completed the questionnaire during the same period of time but independent of each other. The questionnaire covered some of the routines during the neonatal period,

Table 6. Design of the Three-Year Follow-Up Study of Families with Extra Contact and with Routine Care After Parturition

Time	Method of Examination	Observers	Participant(s)[a]
9:30 a.m.	Arrival of family	(1, 2)	M, F, and C
10:00 a.m.	Observation (interview)	(1, 2)	C (M and F)
11:00 a.m.	Denver Test	(3)	C
	Interview continued	(1)	M and F
12:00	Luncheon		M, F, and C
1:00 p.m.	Videotape recording	(1)	M and C
2:00 p.m.	Observation (2)	(2)	C
3:30 p.m.	Final discussion	(1)	M and F

[a] M = mother; F = father; C = child; (1), (2), and (3) = experimenters 1, 2, and 3.

general child development, and attitudes toward child-rearing practices. The actual social, economic, and family structure situation were also covered, as well as some questions about reproductive behavior and family planning. When the questionnaires were completed, a discussion about the ongoing study took place, and individual questions of concern to the actual couple were discussed. During this time the child went with a psychologist (experimenter 2) into a separate room for a structured and standardized observation of play in accordance with the Erica method, a worldwide technique for psychodiagnosis of children [9].

While the parents were still with experimenter 1, the child was taken to the next activity, a Denver Developmental Screening Test [19] carried out by a psychologist (experimenter 3). The DDST consists of four major parts: personal-social, fine-motor—adaptation, linguistic, and gross-motor development. The same psychologist examined all the children individually.

AFTERNOON SESSION AT THREE YEARS

At noon the family gathered again to have lunch in a private room at the clinic, and some time was also scheduled for rest. At about 1 p.m., mother and child were invited to play with dolls representing their own family in a doll's house. The mother and child were given the following instruction: "I want you to play what happens on an ordinary day in your family." A videotape recording of this session was made (30 minutes). In the meantime, the father was asked to wait outside. As soon as the recording had been completed, the whole family was asked to watch a playback with experimenter 1. This was done to give the parents an opportunity to see what had actually been recorded and also to get their opinions about the recording. When the playback was completed, its content was discussed, and the parents were asked if they felt that the recording was natural and like an ordinary interaction between mother and child. If not, the tape was to be destroyed. None of the parents expressed doubts and thus all the tapes were used for analysis. This analysis consists of three different parts and is still not complete:

1. *Quantitative analysis:* 22 different items are included, 12 on maternal and 10 on child behavior. Many of the items are identical to those used in earlier parts of this study, for instance, contact, touching, and body contact. All tapes were analyzed by two new independent (and blind) observers. Reliability between observers was obtained before the actual analysis of the tapes was carried out and was checked again afterwards.

2. *Qualitative analysis:* A new method was developed to enable a qualitative analysis of mother–child interactional play [50]. In contrast to earlier analysis, mostly dealing with frequencies of behavior, special sequences of interaction were evaluated. The total content of all tapes could not be used, since this contained far too much information. Therefore, certain appropriate aspects were chosen: the emotional climate, maternal behavior (such as comforting, supporting, and encouraging), the child's reactions (passive, active, destructive, constructive), mother–child communication, development of conflicts, and conflict solution. Three new, blind observers were used and interobserver reliability was tested and maintained during analysis.

3. *Mother to child speech/conversation:* All tapes were transcribed, and a method was developed for analysis of conversation [46]. Aspects of language development and understanding as well as of speech interaction between mother and child were included.

At the end of the day, child play was again observed (observation 2, Table 6) while the parents had a final discussion with experimenter 1 about what had been studied during the day.

HORMONAL STUDIES AT THREE YEARS

Urine samples were collected during different periods at the hospital and, to obtain base lines, after night rest and daytime activities during different periods of a day at home. The samples were used for analysis of urinary catecholamines and cortisol. Free adrenaline and noradrenaline were analyzed by fluorimetric method [1, 52], and cortisol was analyzed by means of a radioimmunoassay [43]. Samples were obtained at the following times in the hospital: (1) at 10 a.m., on arrival; (2) at noon during tests and interviews; (3) at 1 p.m., during lunch; (4) at 3 p.m., during mother–child play. These periods included differences in stress and rest, creating different conditions appropriate for the measurement of the hormones at different levels. On a separate day at home (Saturday), under minimal activity conditions, urine samples were obtained at 7 a.m. (night urine), 10 a.m., noon, and 2 p.m.

Short Summary of Results

The results of this longitudinal study have been reported extensively elsewhere [10, 11, 12, 13, 15, 16, 17]. Here a very brief and simplified summary is given in Table 7. At 36 hours postpartum,

Table 7. Influence of Early Postnatal Contact at Different Times Postpartum[a]

	36 Hours	3 Months	1 Year	3 Years
Maternal behavior	+	+	+	?
Infant behavior		+	+	?
Interview		+	+	+
Child development			?	−
Vineland test			−	
Mother's diary			−	
Breast-feeding		+	+	
Adrenalin excretion				+

[a] + = positive relation; − = no relation; ? = tendencies

mothers with extra contact showed significantly more holding, encompassing*, and close body contact with their infants than mothers with routine care. At three months after delivery, mothers with extra contact spent significantly more time looking at and kissing their infants, and their infants laughed and smiled more often and cried less frequently. At one year, mothers with extra contact more often held their infants with positive empathy, and they also exhibited more ATL† and more often talked positively to their children than mothers with routine care. At three years there were no longer any clear-cut, statistically significant differences in maternal and child behavior, but tendencies pointed to more close body contact and touching for extra-contact mothers. The interview at one year revealed a number of differences between the two groups: mothers tended to return to gainful employment and to start toilet training their children later in the extra-contact group. There were twice as many siblings born during the three-year follow-up period in extra-contact families. In four out of five parts of the Gesell Developmental Schedules, children with extra contact immediately after delivery were ahead of the children in the control group. The results of the Vineland Social Maturity Scale, the Denver Developmental Screening Test, and maternal diaries on infants' sleeping and feeding habits, (except breast-feeding) revealed no major intergroup differences. The mean duration of breast-feeding was 175 days in the extra-contact group as opposed to 103 days in the control group. At three years, adrenaline and noradrenaline

---

*Encompassing is defined as the mother's upper arm, lower arm, and hand around the infant's body.
†ATL means affectionate touch love and is defined as any extra touching of infant or infant's clothing by mother's fingers, not in connection with feeding or caretaking.

excretions were somewhat higher in mother–child pairs with early extra skin-to-skin and suckling contact. The differences between the two groups were more pronounced for boy–mother dyads than for girl–mother dyads in almost all measurements at all four occasions of follow-up.

Discussion

In studies concerning the possible long-term effect of early mother–infant interaction on the development of their relationship, many different methods have been used at different intervals. Experimental conditions also differ greatly, and it is not always clear whether the groups studied are fully comparable in other respects. It is therefore very difficult to make a direct comparison of results obtained in these studies. The fallacies in the methods used in studies of this kind are still incompletely explored.

Direct observation is a very suitable method for studying mother–infant relations [32, 39]. The most obvious advantage of observation is that one can see what is happening without having to rely on poorly established techniques. Therefore, in the early parts, direct observation was preferred to filming and videotape recording, techniques that may be experienced as less natural. The camera lens, moreover, covers a restricted area [7], and analysis becomes excessively time consuming and expensive. During direct observation, on the other hand, one must be selective about what is to be observed and recorded. There is always the risk that valuable information will be missed. It is obviously an advantage if a limited number of behavioral items to be observed can be chosen from the start.

Clear-cut definitions of behavioral items were made in advance and agreement on their occurrence settled. The presence of an observer may be disconcerting [29], but mothers during their stay in the maternity ward are used to contact with the hospital staff and did not show any signs of discomfort during the observation. For the newborn infant and its mother, the maternity ward is a "natural" environment in our culture, since there are no longer any home deliveries. During our observation in the maternity ward, a great number of observational items were used. Some of these items were chosen from the literature [3, 27, 29, 39, 49] and others from our own experience. A high interobserver reliability was obtained, thus reducing the bias of each observer. In the follow-up studies at three months and one year, the same methods were used as in the maternity ward. By that time, the home had become the dyad's natural environment and may therefore be considered the most suitable setting for studies of mother−infant relations. At three years, our interest was focused on sequences of behavior and interactions, thus the videotape technique was preferred.

Indirect procedures for studying mother−infant relationships, such as interviews, questionnaires, and diaries, have limitations [32]. Mothers may have a limited memory about things that have happened in the past, and they may give a distorted report of their relationship with their children, being influenced by what is believed to be culturally acceptable mother−infant behavior. Therefore, retrospective reports have been limited. The value of interviews and questionnaires is greater if they are combined with other methods of study.

Since a mother often has difficulty in recalling data exactly from the recent and more distant past, both for herself and her child [23], other ways of collecting data have been used. To obtain more reliable data on breast-feeding, the children's health records were collected and used when calculating the duration of breast-feeding. Data concerning the mother's pregnancy, delivery, and earlier obstetrical history were collected from her records, from antenatal clinics, and from the maternity ward. To evaluate the postnatal adaptation and state of health during the neonatal period, objective criteria like birth weight, laboratory investigations, and duration of hospital stay were taken from the infant's records at the maternity and neonatal wards. By using objective data from existing records made by third persons unaware of our interest in particular facts, circumstances, or measurements, some of the disadvantages of interviews and questionnaires possibly have been compensated for.

Our department has a large body of experience in the Gesell Developmental Schedules and the Denver Developmental Screening Test. This is one of the main reasons that these tests were used in the longitudinal study. In our opinion, it is of great importance to use methods that are familiar to the experimenters from their routine practical work with children. The child's development is expressed in the same major ways, and the child was examined individually by a psychologist in both tests. To obtain information about the mother's perception of the child's social behavior and social environment, a structured and standardized interview using the Vineland Social Maturity Scale was held with all mothers. The opportunity to relate the Gesell Developmental Schedules to the Vineland Social Maturity Scale was also taken.

The samples in our studies were random from the start. A large number of relevant and accessible background factors were comparable in both groups. Nevertheless, an unknown bias could have slipped into the investigation. The validity and value of the results of these and other studies have been questioned fairly. To meet some of these criticisms and to enable us to be more confident about the results, a checkup on the psychogenic needs of the mothers was made one year after delivery. For this checkup the Cesarec-Marke Personality Scheme [6], based on Murray's dynamic theory [34], was used. The CMPS is considered one of the most useful and accessible of the multidimensional personality questionnaires standardized for Swedish conditions and has proved to be stable over time when used on the same subjects [45]. The CMPS measures the mother's perception of herself and obtains a systematic description of psychogenic needs. The two groups were fully comparable in psychogenic needs such as achievement, defense of status, dominance, exhibition, autonomy, nurturance, order, and succurance. It is therefore unlikely that these factors can account for the differences found in other parts of our study.

Problems of methodology in the study of the parent—infant relationships and their development are many and are far from solved today [14]. Many different investigative methods have been used without any of them being completely satisfactory. Combinations of methods have been employed to try to overcome the disadvantages of each used alone, but looking at the subject from a variety of angles has not always reduced the inaccuracies.

Acknowledgments

Parts of this study were supported by the Swedish Medical Research Council (project no. 5443), the Swedish Save the Children Federation, the Karolinska Institute, the March of Dimes Foundation, New York, and the Medical Faculty, University of Umeå.

References

1. Andersson, B., Hovmöller, S., Karlsson, C.G., and Svensson, S. Analysis of urinary catecholamines. An improved autoanalyzer fluorescence method. *Clin. Chim. Acta,* 51 (1974), 13—28.
2. Beintema, D.J., and Prechtl, H.F.R. *A Neurological Study of Newborn Infants.* Spastic International Society Publications, London, 1968, 24, 30.
3. Bowlby, J. *Attachment and Loss,* vol. I. Hogarth Press, London, 1969.
4. Carlsson, S.G., Fagerberg, H., Hornman, G., Hwang, P., Larsson, K., Rödholm, M., Schaller, J., Danielsson, B., and Gundewall, C. Effects of

various amounts of contact between mother and child on the mother's nursing behavior. *Dev. Psychobiol.*, 11 (1978), 143–150.

5. Carlsson, S.G., Fagerberg, H., Hornman, G., Hwang, P., Larsson, K., Rödholm, M., Schaller, J., Danielsson, B., and Gundewall, C. Effects of various amounts of contact between mother and child on the mother's nursing behavior. A follow-up study. *Infant Behav. Dev.* 2 (1979), 209–214.

6. Cesarec, Z., and Marke, S. *CMPS Manual.* Skandinaviska Testförlaget AB, Stockholm, 1968.

7. Cooper, E.S., Costella, A.J., Douglas, J.W.B., Ingleby, J.D., and Turner, R.K. Direct observations. *Bull. Brit. Psychol. Soc.* 27 (1974), 3–7.

8. Curry, M.A. Contact during the first hour with the wrapped or naked newborn: effect on maternal attachment behaviors at 36 hours and three months. *Birth Fam. J.*, 6 (1979), 227–235.

9. Danielsson, A. *Ericametoden.* Psykologiförlaget AB, Stockholm, 1965.

10. de Château, P. *Neonatal Care Routines: Influences on Maternal and Infant Behaviour and on Breast Feeding.* Umeå University Medical Dissertation, New Series: 20, 1976.

11. de Château, P. Long-term effect of early post partum contact: one-year follow-up. In *Emotion and Reproduction,* 20B, (1979a), 1185–1190.

12. de Château, P. Effects of hospital practices on synchrony in the development of the infant–parent relationship. *Semin. Perinatol.,* III (1) (1979b), 45–61.

13. de Château, P. Early post-partum contact and later attitudes. *Int. J. Behav. Dev.* 3 (1980a), 273–286.

14. de Château, P. Parent–neonate interaction and its long-term effects. In Simmel, E.C., Ed. *Early Experiences and Early Behavior: Implications for Social Development.* Academic Press, New-York 1980a, 109–179.

15. de Château, P., and Wiberg, B. Long-term effect on mother–infant behavior of extra contact during the first hour post partum. I. First observations at 36 hours. *Acta Paediat. Scand.* 66 (1977a), 137–144.

16. de Château, P., and Wiberg, B. Long-term effect on mother–infant behavior of extra contact during the first hour post partum. II. A follow-up at three months. *Acta Paediat. Scand.* 66 (1977b), 145–151.

17. de Château, P., and Wiberg, B. Long-term effect on mother–infant behavior of extra contact during the first hour post partum. III. A follow-up at one year.

18. Doll, E.A. *The Vineland Social Maturity Scale.* Revised, condensed publication of the Training School at Vineland, Department of Research No 3, New Jersey, 1936.

19. Frankenberg, W.K., and Dodds, J.B. The Denver Developmental Screening Test. *J. Pediatrics,* 71 (1967), 181–189.

20. Gesell, A., and Amatruda, C.S. *Developmental Diagnosis. Normal and Abnormal Child Development,* 2nd ed. Harper & Row, New York, 1947.

21. Gesell, A. *General Instructions to Accompany the Gesell Developmental Schedules.* The Psychological Corporation, New York, 1949.

22. Guilford, J.P. *Fundamental Statistics in Psychology and Education,* 4th Ed. McGraw-Hill, New York, 1956.

23. Jarrow, M.R. Problems of methods in parent–child research. *Child Dev.* 34 (1963), 215–226.
24. Kennell, J.H., Jerauld, R., Wolfe, H., Chesler, D., Kreger, N., McAlpine, W., Steffa, M., and Klaus, M.H. Maternal behavior one year after early and extended post partum contact. *Dev. Med. Child Neur.* 16 (1974), 172–179.
25. Kennell, J.H., Trause, M.A., and Klaus, M.H. Evidence for a sensitive period in the human mother. In *Parent–Infant Interaction,* Ciba Foundation Symposium 33. Elsevier, Amsterdam, 1975, 87–101.
26. Klaus, M. H., Jerauld, R., Kreger, N., McAlpine, W., Steffa, M., and Kennell, J. H. Maternal attachment—Importance of the first partum days. *New England. J. Med.* 286 (1972), 460–463.
27. Klaus, M. H., and Kennell, J. H. Mothers separated from their newborn infants. *Pediatr. Clin. N. Am.* 17 (1970), 1015–1035.
28. Kontos, D. A study of the effects of extended mother–infant contact on maternal behavior at one and three months. *Birth Fam. J.,* 5 (1978), 133–140.
29. Lewis, M. State as an infant–environment interaction: an analysis of mother-–infant interaction as a function of sex. *Merrill-Palmer Q.,* 18 (1972), 95–121.
30. Lozoff, B., Brittenhamn, G. M., Trause, M. A., Kennell, J. H., and Klaus, M. H. The mother–newborn relationship: Limits of adaptability. *J. Pediat.,* 91, 1 (1977), 1–12.
31. Magne, O., and Wahlberg, G. *Vinelandmetoden Manual,* 3rd Ed. Skandinaviska Testförlaget AB, Stockholm, 1961.
32. Moss, H. A. Methodological issues in studying mother–infant interaction. *Am. J. Orthospychiat.* 35 (1965), 482–486.
33. Moss, H. A. Sex, age and state as determinants of mother–infant interaction. *Merrill-Palmer Q.* 3 (1967), 19–36.
34. Murray, H. A. *Explorations in Personality* Oxford University Press, New York, 1959.
35. Nagel, M., and Wimmer-Puchinger, B. 6th International Congress of Psychosomatic Obstetrics and Gynecology. Abstract 27, 1980.
36. Pasamanick, B., Rogers, M. E., and Lilienfeld, A. M. Pregnancy experience and the development of behavior disorder in children. *Am. J. Psychiat.,* 112 (1956), 613–618.
37. Pitkin, R. M., Kaminetzky, H. A., Newton, M., and Pritchard, J. A. Maternal nutrition: A selective review of clinical topics. *Obstet. Gynecol.,* 40 (1972), 773–785.
38. Prechtl, H. F. R. Neurological findings in newborn infants after pre- and postnatal complications. In Jonxis, J., Ed. *Nutricia Symposium: Aspects of praematurity and dysmaturity.* Stenfert Kroese, Leiden, 1968, 303.
39. Rheingold, H. L. The measurements of maternal care. *Child Dev.* 31 (1960), 565–575.
40. Ringler, N. M., Kennell, J. H., Jarvelle, R., Navojosky, B. J., and Klaus, M. H. Mother to child speech at two years—Effect of early postnatal contact. *J. Pediat.,* 86 (1975), 141–144.
41. Ringler, N. M., Trause, M. A., and Klaus, M. H. Mother's speech to her two-year-old, its effect on speech and language comprehension at 5 years. *Pediat. Res.,* 10 (1976), 307–312.

42. Ringler, N. M., Trause, M. A., Klaus, M. H., and Kennell, J. H. The effects of extra post partum contact and maternal speech patterns on children's IQ, speech and language comprehension at five. *Child. Dev.* 49 (1978), 862–865.
43. Ruder, H. J., Guy, R. L., and Lipsett, M. B. A radioimmunoassay for cortisol in plasma and urine. *J. Clin. Endocrinol. Metabol.* 35 (1972), 219–224.
44. Sosa, R., Kennell, J. H., Klaus, M. H., and Urrutia, J. J. The effect of early mother–infant contact on breast feeding, infection and growth. In *Breast Feeding and the Mother,* Ciba Foundation Symposium 45 (new series). Elsevier, Amsterdam, 1976, 179–193.
45. Strandman, E. Depressive disorders: Genetic, clinical and diagnostic concepts. *Umeå University Medical Dissertations,* New Series 29 (1977).
46. Strömqvist, S. *Lindguistic Effects at Three Years of Age of Extra Contact during the First Hour Post Partum. I. On Communication and Transcription.* Child Language Research Institute, Stockholm, 1979.
47. Svejda, J., Campos, J. J., and Emde, R. N. Mother–infant "bonding": Failure to generalize. *Child Dev.* 51 (1980), 775–779.
48. Thoman, E. B., Leiderman, P. H., and Olson, J. P. Neonate–mother interaction during breast feeding. *Dev. Psychol.,* 6 (1972), 110–118.
49. Thoman, E. B., Turner, A. M., Leiderman, P. H., and Barnett, C. R. Neonate–mother interaction: Effects of parity on feeding behavior. *Child Dev.,* 41 (1970), 1103–1111.
50. Wiberg, B., Kuoppa, S. M., Nilsson, A., Widmark, S., and de Chāteau, P. A qualitative analysis of maternal–child interaction during free play. BLF, 21–22 March 1980 in Umeå.
51. Winberg, J., Wahlberg, V., and de Chāteau, P. Breast-feeding–early initiation and duration, an epidimiological study. In (Freier, S., and Eidelman, A. I., Eds.), *Human Milk. Its Biological and Social Value.* Excerpta Medica, Amsterdam, 1980, 283–286.
52. von Euler, U.S., and Lishajko, F. Improved technique for the fluorometric estimation of catecholamines. *Acta Physiol. Scand.* 51 (1961), 348–355.

Daycare for Three-Year-Olds

AN INTERDISCIPLINARY EXPERIMENTAL STUDY

Marianne Cederblad, M.D.
Börje Höök (Sweden)

In 1974, a broad interdisciplinary experimental study was made of the density of personnel (teacher–child ratio) at 10 daycare centers in Stockholm. One hundred three-year-olds were followed for 18 weeks with daily observations and physiological measurements. The results have been presented in a series of articles in Swedish of which this report provides a summary. An increased density of personnel was associated with a reduced incidence of behavioral disorders, fewer conflicts, higher satisfaction, and lower urine levels of the hormones adrenaline and noradrenaline in the children. Absence due to sickness of the personnel decreased notably. On the whole, the results show that an increased density of personnel resulted in clear improvements for both the children and the nurses. In correlation studies we found that children in small groups had fewer behavioral disorders and lower hormone excretion levels. The relation to the time spent daily in the nursery was less clear. The density of personnel and the group size seem to have been of special importance for anxious and inhibited children. In 1977, a follow-up study was carried out on 69 of the children by means of interviews with preschool personnel. It was found that behavioral disorders at age six were highly predictable from the information on behavioral disorders and home environment at age three.

This project was supported by the Swedish Medical Research Council and the Swedish National Board for Health and Welfare.

Background

The institution of the day nursery underwent a tremendous expansion in Sweden during the 1970s. More and more children of preschool age spend a good deal of their waking time in day nurseries or in part-time groups ("playschools"). In 1978, more than 100,000 children were enrolled in day nurseries, with an equally large number enrolled in part-time groups.

How a day nursery should best be organized is currently the subject of lively debate. The factors most discussed are density of personnel, group size, and the number of hours per day a child spends at a daycare center. Scientific research on day nurseries has, however, been limited for the most part to pedagogical questions. Very little is known about the effects of various factors in the daycare milieu on the health and well-being of the children and the personnel. On the other hand, it is known that the home environment has a very strong influence on a child's development and behavior [2, 4, 6, 7]. Many children spend 8 to 10 hours in a day nursery every day. The influence of the daycare milieu and various factors within it on a child therefore can be just as important as conditions in the home environment.

Purpose

The aim of this investigation was first and foremost to study experimentally the effects of changes in personnel density. One hypothesis was that an increased teacher−child ratio should entail an improved psychosocial environment for both the children and the nurses. For the children, this presumably would result in positive changes in behavior as well as a reduced physiological stress level and lower morbidity. Positive changes of attitude could be expected in parents and personnel, with a concommittant reduction in sickness absence among the personnel. Second, the investigation proposed to study the significance of the group size and the length of time spent daily in the nursery. This part of the investigation, however, was carried out solely on the basis of correlation studies rather than experimentally. The investigation subsequently acquired a third purpose, namely to establish a basis for a longitudinal study.

The Study Itself

Stockholm was divided into the inner city, the older suburbs and the new suburbs. From these, a total of eight daycare centers was selected at random. At two of the centers, two classes were included. During the first half year, 1974, a total of 107 full-time children were in the day nursery classes. Seven of the children were excluded from the investigation because they left the daycare center or because they were unable to leave a urine sample. Thus the investigation in the end comprised 100 children, 47 boys and 53 girls. On January 1, 1974, the youngest child was 2½ years old and the oldest was 4½.

The experiment lasted 18 weeks. During the first nine weeks, half of the classes were provided with additional nurses to increase the density of personnel from the figure of one nurse per five children (1:5) recommended by the Social Welfare Board to one nurse per three children (1:3). Halfway through the investigation, the extra personnel were shifted to the other classes for the same length of time. This crossover design meant that every child was studied under two different trial conditions. Thus a child's behavior at a normal density of personnel was compared with behavior at an increased density of personnel. During both of the nine-week periods, the first four weeks constituted an adaptation period and were not taken into account in drawing up the results of the experiment. The extra personnel consisted of temporary employed youth who lacked formal training. A few of them, however, had worked in day nurseries before.

Every day during the experiment two urine samples were collected from each child, the first after two hours of noon rest, and the other after two hours of free play. Each day the nursery personnel recorded the time a child arrived and the time it left the nursery, the reasons for any absences, how many children and how many of the personnel were present, and the occurrence of any symptoms of illness or aberrant behavior in each child. A child's behavior during the free play period was observed daily by assistants in the project. For one week each month, a child psychologist systematically observed occurring conflicts and interactions in the child groups during play, for two hours in the morning and two hours in the afternoon.

Every month, the parents reported current stress factors in the child's home environment (life changes occurring in the family during the preceding month) in a mail questionnaire. At the beginning, middle, and end of the study, the parents and the nursery personnel were interviewed about the child's behavior in 25 different respects (25 different variables or symptoms). In the first parent interview, information on the family background was also gathered. This information was later used to determine, by the method developed by Kälvesten and Meldahl [8], the degree of constant psychosocial stress factors in the home environment (family disturbances). Three times during the study, the parents and the personnel evaluated the child's level of contentment and their own satisfaction with various factors in the daycare milieu, in mail questionnaires. At the end of the study, further interviews were made with parents and nurses to round out the information gathered.

In the spring of 1977, a follow-up interview was made with preschool personnel concerning the behavior of 69 of the children who were still attending preschool institutions in the Stockholm area. Information on the sickness absence of the children during the intervening period (1974 to 1977) was also gathered.

The First Results of the Experiment

Four of the day nursery classes were excluded from the experimental analyses because the intended increase in density of personnel was not achieved. In two of these the number of nurses was not increased, and in the two others the increase was canceled out by a simultaneous increase in the number of children. The effect of the experiment was therefore evaluated on the basis of 62 children and 15 nurses.

The density of personnel each day in each class was calculated by dividing the number of working days for the nurses taking direct care of the children by the number of children present. On the average, the density of personnel in the six classes increased from about 1:4.5 to about 1:2.5. However, variations from day to day were appreciable, mainly because of variations in the number of child absences. Days with fewer than three children per adult also occurred during the period with a "normal" density of personnel.

The increase in density of personnel did not influence the incidence of illness among the children. On the other hand, the children's behavior in the nurseries was affected. An increased density of personnel reduced the incidence of serious behavioral disorders. For example, the number of children exhibiting strong outbursts of aggressiveness decreased from eight to four, and the number of children with signs of severe anxiety fell from seven to four. The children also became more active, had more contact with one another, and got along better. The first analyses of urine samples also indicated that the excretion of the stress hormones adrenaline and noradrenaline had decreased in the children.

Table 1. Effect of Changing Density of Personnel (Teacher–Child Ratio) from Low (1:5) to High (1:3)

	Density of Personnel		
Dependent Variable	Low	High	Level of Significance[a]
Children			
sickness absence[b]	15.7	16.5	—
adrenaline rest[c]	12.2	11.2	*
noradrenaline rest[c]	63.7	61.4	o
adrenaline play[c]	25.6	25.2	—
noradrenaline play[c]	84.7	84.5	—
overall symptomload[d]	164.8	131.1	*
aggression-hyperactivity[d]	38.6	29.5	—
anxiety-inhibition[d]	88.5	67.1	*
psychosomatic reaction[d]	5.5	5.6	—
conflicts[e]	0.82	0.64	*
satisfaction[f]	4.25	4.40	**
activity[g]	3.14	3.28	*
interaction[g]	2.96	3.06	o
Personnel			
sickness absence[b]	12.5	6.1	*
attitudes to parents[h]	4.03	4.26	**
Parents			
attitudes to day nursery[h]	4.30	4.49	o
attitudes to personnel[h]	4.18	4.32	o

[a]Level of significance (*t*-test for correlated observations): o = $p<.10$, * = $p<.05$, ** = $p<.01$
[b]Days of sickness absence, in percent of days of presence plus days of sickness absence.
[c]Picomols/minute.
[d]Summation of points for individual symptoms (behavioral disorders) according to interviews with the nursery personnel.
[e]Average number of conflicts started during two hours, according to child psychologist observations.
[f]Child contentment, according to ratings by the nurses from 1 (low) to 5 (high).
[g]Ratings by the project assistants from 1 (low) to 5 (high).
[h]Ratings from 1 (negative) to 5 (positive).

The higher density of personnel also had a positive influence on the nurses. Absence due to illness decreased sharply, on the average by more than 50 percent. Nurse attitudes to parents also became more positive, and so did the attitudes of parents to the day nursery and its personnel.

Behavior Disorders of the Children

The interviews with the parents and the personnel about 25 behavior variables of the children (e.g., anxiety, aggressiveness, depressive mood, self-esteem, contact with peers, sensitivity) were based on the list of symptoms constructed by MacFarlane [12] and adapted to Swedish by Jonsson and Kälvesten [7]. In the first published results of the experiment, our measure of behavioral disorders was merely how many symptoms the children had out of the possible 25. Later, the interview material was gone over more thoroughly. All the symptoms, as well as the degree to which they were manifest, were evaluated relative to one another, and rated on a point scale from 0 to 100. In this way we were able to take into account that a symptom could be present to various degrees of severity, and that some symptoms were more serious than others. The overall measure of a child's symptom load was thus the sum of the point ratings for the individual symptoms. Summations were also made for different subgroups of behavioral disorders. The points for symptoms like aggressiveness, hyperactivity, and defiance were summed up as aggression-hyperactivity; the points for anxiety, shyness, inhibited aggression, and so forth were summed up as anxiety-inhibition; and the points for nervous stomach, enuresis, and so forth were summed up as psychosomatic reaction.

The interviews with the nursery personnel, thus systematized, show clearly that the increase in *density of personnel* in the experiment had a favorable influence on the incidence of behavioral disorders in the children. The overall degree of symptom load diminished. Above all, the children became less anxious and inhibited and less aggressive and disorderly. The incidence of psychosomatic symptoms, however, was not affected. The positive effects were most pronounced in children who came from good homes and in older children. They were also more pronounced for boys than for girls.

Behavioral disorders also varied with *the size of the group*. Children in the large nursery classes (15 enrolled children) displayed anxiety-inhibition type symptoms more often than children in the smaller classes (10 to 12 enrolled children). This difference was at least as distinct in the follow-up three years later. Children who previously had been in the large classes were more dependent on their mothers, less active, more anxious, and more sensitive to praise and criticism in 1977 than were children who had been in the smaller classes.

Behavioral disorders also varied with the *time spent in the nursery each day*. Children who spent a relatively short time per day at the center (less than seven hours) had more symptoms of the anxiety-inhibition type (i.e., inhibited aggression, shyness, and poor self-esteem) than the other children. Children who spent a long period each day (more than nine hours), displayed more acting out and psychosomatic symptoms. For example, they were more often aggressive, ate too much, and wet themselves. Children spending a moderate amount of time each day (seven to nine hours) displayed the lowest incidence of symptoms.

Behavior Disorders in Relation to the Psychosocial Home Environment

Behavioral disorders varied with the *life changes* of the family. An increased incidence of temporary psychosocial stress factors was accompanied by a greater number of behavioral disorders in the children. Above all, symptoms of the aggression-hyperactivity type became more common.

The incidence of behavioral disorders in the children also varied with the more constant psychosocial stress factors in the home environment. The correlations between *family disturbances* in 1974 and behavioral disorders at the same time were relatively weak (about $r = .25$), but the correlation with behavioral disorders three years later was much stronger ($r = .57$). Children with severe stress in the home environment in 1974 often had behavioral disorders in preschool institutions in 1977. It may be that disturbances in the family have a cumulative effect and therefore have more pronounced repercussions at a later time in the child's life. Another possibility is that the families that had problems in 1974 had even worse problems in 1977.

Conflict Behavior of the Children

The two child psychologists observed a total of 934 conflicts in the day nursery classes. Eighty percent of them were between two children, 15 were started by an adult with a child, and five by a child with an adult. Almost all the children both had started and had been involved in conflicts. Conflicts started by adults or by children with adults were almost always conflicts of ideas; that is, they had to do with the content of activities such as listening to a story instead of playing fire engine. Between children, conflicts over things were most common. For example, a child would attempt to take a toy that another child had; the other child would resist, and the personnel would intervene to divert attention, conciliate, console, and give help. Another common type of conflict, aggressions, occurred, in which a child for no apparent reason would physically attack another. The nurses often intervened in this type of conflict, especially when the attacked child began to cry. Sometimes the personnel would intervene negatively, for example, by scolding or even grabbing and shaking the child, shouting and threatening.

The children's conflict behavior was correlated with neither group size nor the time spent each day in the nursery; it was, however, influenced by the density of personnel. The children started fewer conflicts on days with a high teacher–child ratio than on days with a low ratio. The difference was most marked for boys from disturbed homes. The nature of the conflicts also changed. Physical aggressions became less common, and children who came into conflicts more often resisted and less frequently ran away.

Conflict behavior was strongly related to the sex of the children. Boys started three times as many conflicts as girls. Family background also bore a relation to conflict behavior. Children from families with considerable problems started more conflicts and got into more conflicts than other children. The nature of the conflicts also differed. Boys from disturbed homes more often started aggressions.

We also studied the behavior of the nurses. At a high density of personnel, entered into conflicts somewhat more often, but the way in which they did so was not noticeably changed. Positive behavior such as diversionary or conciliatory efforts did not occur more often than at a low density of personnel. On the other hand, there were differences in this respect among the different categories of personnel. Preschool teachers entered into conflicts in a positive way more often than the rest of the personnel. Similar differences were found between nurses in small and in large classes. In the small nursery classes, the personnel more often intervened positively in the children's conflicts. These two results were related to one another, since the large classes often lacked preschool teachers. There was also a clear relation between the children's conflict behavior and the nurses' evaluations of the children. The personnel liked children who started many conflicts less. It is perhaps a natural reaction to think that "disorderly children are a bother," but it is unfortunate, since it is just such children who often come from disturbed homes and who therefore have an especially great need for a good relationship with the personnel.

Adrenaline and Noradrenaline Excretion of the Children

An individual's psychological stress level can be measured by the level of the hormones adrenaline and noradrenaline excreted in the urine [11]. Various types of stress result in an increased excretion, especially of adrenaline [5]. There have been many studies of this factor in adults, but so far none on children in a nursery environment. Our results are based on about 6000 urine samples. For most children, samples from the noonday rest and from the following play period were available for 30 to 40 different days. The estimation of adrenaline and noradrenaline in urine was made by a fluorimetric method [1].

The experimental increase in *density of personnel* had the effect of reducing adrenaline and noradrenaline excretion during the midday rest. The greatest decrease in hormone excretion was found in anxious and inhibited children, older children, and boys. Adrenaline excretion during play also decreased somewhat. Covariations between changes in density of personnel from day to day and the children's hormone excretion were also studied. We were able to include children from all 10 nursery classes by not taking into account whether the changes in density of personnel were due to the experiment. The results showed very good agreement with those from the experiment.

Covariations between hormone excretion and group size were also studied. Children in the large day nursery classes had a higher level of hormone excretion during rest than children in the small classes. The difference was most marked in noradrenaline excretion in girls. Anxious and inhibited children had distinctly higher adrenaline urine levels during rest if they belonged to large classes than if they belonged to small ones. On the other hand, there was no clear relation to the time spent in the nursery each day. Children who spent a short time each day had a higher adrenaline excretion level during the midday rest than children spending a moderate to long time, whereas children spending a long time each day perhaps had a somewhat higher noradrenaline level.

Hormone excretion in the children was clearly related to sex. Boys excreted markedly more adrenaline and noradrenaline per kilogram of body weight than girls, both during the rest and during the play period. On the other hand, there was no clear correlation between hormone excretion in the children and their home background.

Covariations between hormone excretion and illness were also studied. The findings show that sickness absence among the children was preceded by changes in behavior and an increased adrenaline excretion.

Attitudes and Beliefs of Parents and Personnel

In an interview toward the end of the study, 25 of the personnel and parents of 71 of the children gave their opinions about various aspects of the day nursery. Both parents and nurses considered three children per adult to be the ideal density of personnel, 10 children in a class to be the ideal number of children, and six hours to be the ideal amount of time spent per day in the nursery. The parents' evaluations of the day nurseries and their personnel were clearly related to these ideal notions. The further the actual group size and density of personnel diverged from the levels the parents considered ideal, the poorer were their assessments of the nursery and its personnel.

The parents were also asked whether they would choose some other form of child care than a day nursery if they had the opportunity. Practically all answered no. When asked what was best in their nursery, the parents answered, for example, that the staff was good, that the children showed that they were contented, and that the day nursery was close to their home. Some negative judgments concerning the nurseries were poor contact with the nurses, too many changes of personnel, crowded quarters, and a dreary outdoor playground. The nurses' judgments about the nursery mostly concerned relations within the group of personnel. The most common positive judgment concerned companionship and the good sense of community. On the other hand, at some of the day nurseries the personnel spoke frankly of antagonism within the group.

Follow-up Study

Up to now, just one longitudinal child psychiatric study has been done in Sweden [9]. There is a dearth of such studies in other countries as well. Often, only the stability (constancy) of individual symptoms has been studied, with the finding that the type and degree of behavioral disorders change as a child develops [3, 9, 10, 12]. This sometimes has invited the conclusion that behavioral disorders in small children are not so serious, that "the children grow out of them with time." Even if individual symptoms are not stable, it is nevertheless fully possible that the child's overall load of symptoms and other combinations of behavioral disorders are more constant and predictable. The purpose of the follow-up interview in 1977 was therefore first and foremost to determine whether it was possible to predict the children's total load of symptoms at the age of six on the basis of information concerning behavioral disorders, home situation, and so forth at age three. If a child's behavior over time can be predicted, children exposed to a high risk of emotional and social maladjustment can be detected and various preventive measures can be taken.

It was found that the total load of symptoms at age six was highly predictable from behavioral disorders and family disturbances at the age of three ($r = .68$). Children who displayed major behavioral disorders at age six also had had problems in regard to family background and/or behavioral disorders at age three. Hyperactivity and aggressiveness at age three were symptoms having clear relations to the total load of symptoms at age six (about $r = .50$).

Combinations of behavioral disorders displayed a much higher stability between the ages of three and six than individual symptoms. Only a few symptoms (especially hyperactivity) approached the level of constancy of total symptom load, aggression-hyperactivity, and anxiety-inhibition (approximately $r = .60$). It was also noteworthy that anxiety-inhibition showed as high a stability as aggression-hyperactivity, since a number of earlier studies had shown that social behavioral disorders are more stable than introverted neurotic symptoms [13]. This is probably not the case in the preschool age.

Eighty-four of the children were studied once again in the spring of 1980. Behavioral disorders, hormone excretion, and home background were studied in relation to one another and to the information from the 1974 and 1977 studies.

Discussion and Conclusions

Most studies in child psychiatry are of the observation type; that is, the incidence of various disorders in different environments is studied, after which an attempt is made to draw conclusions from the covariations. In contrast to this, our study of density of personnel was designed as an experiment. This means that we will be able to draw conclusions concerning cause and effect. The increase in density of personnel had the following effects:

1. The excretion of the hormones adrenaline and noradrenaline with the urine decreased in the children.

2. The interviews with the day nursery personnel showed that the incidence of behavioral disorders in the children decreased. The children became less aggressive and disorderly, as well as less anxious and inhibited.

3. The observations of the psychologists showed that the number of conflicts within the child group decreased. Behavior in conflicts also changed; for instance, physical aggression became less common.

4. The evaluations of the personnel showed that the children were more contented at the nurseries.

5. The observations of the project assistants showed that the children became more active and had more contact with one another.

6. Nurse attitudes to parents became more positive, and the parents' evaluations showed that they in turn were more satisfied with the day nursery and its personnel.

7. The sickness absence of the nurses decreased sharply. This may be seen as a reflection of the stressful work situation with which the personnel must normally cope. The effect is thus very important from the standpoint of work environment. The children are also influenced indirectly in a positive way, since it is not necessary to employ so many temporary substitutes.

The upshot of the findings is that we obtained all the effects we expected from an increase in density of personnel with the exception that the morbidity among the children was not changed. The data, gathered in many different ways, all point in the same direction. All in all, they show that an increase in density of personnel does indeed bring about tangible improvements for the children. Moreover, these are not effects bearing merely on parent and nurse expectations, since the children's physiological reactions were also affected; furthermore, changes in their behavior were observed by the child psychologist. The findings presumably would be reproduced in the converse case as well; that is, a reduction in density of personnel would result in manifestly poorer conditions for the children.

The effects of the experiment concern children and personnel at only six of the day nursery classes. However, there is no evidence that the exclusion of four classes had any influence on the results. The omitted change in density of personnel was not due to sickness absence of the nurses. The covariations between hormone excretion in the children and changes in density of personnel from day to day, calculated by employing data for children from all of the day nursery classes, show the same result as the experimental study.

The significance of the size of the children's group was not studied experimentally. The children in three relatively large day nursery classes were compared with the children in seven relatively small classes. This means that factors other than group size may have been responsible for the differences among the children. On the other hand, it is also possible that the effect of group size may be even more marked than indicated here, since such an effect may have been concealed by the fact that the children were also influenced by changes in density of personnel and other factors. Thus the interpretations of these results are more speculative than for density of personnel. The findings do, however, point in the same direction. The children in the large classes tended both to have a higher urine hormone level and to be more anxious and inhibited than children in the smaller classes. The latter finding may be interpreted as a reflection of a better relationship between the personnel and the children in the small classes. This interpretation is further supported by the fact that the personnel of the smaller classes intervened in a more positive way in the conflicts. It is also noteworthy that differences between children from large and small classes persisted three years later, despite the fact that the children were in other day nursery classes. Moreover, the size of the group is of course closely related to personnel density. Increasing the group size without adding nurses at the same time also means a decrease in personnel density, and thus may be expected to have negative effects. To shed more light on the significance of group size for the behavior of day nursery children, a long-term experimental study is necessary.

The assessment of the effect of time spent each day in the nursery also requires an experimental study in which, for example, a six-hour working day would be introduced for the parents. In this respect our study is only a covariation study, since the variations actually existing among the children in the spring of 1974 were used to divide them up into three groups which were then compared with one another. Children spending a relatively short time per day in the nursery were more shy and inhibited than the other children, and also had a higher adrenaline excretion during the midday rest. A possible explanation is that the relation is spurious. The difference in adrenaline level may be due to the fact that the children spending only a short time were less tired and therefore slept less during the rest than the other children. Another explanation is that the children's disturbances were the reason for the short time spent in the nursery and not vice versa. Some of the parents may have been able to shorten their working day or organize their time differently so that the children did not need to be so long in the nursery if they were discontented there.

The children spending a long period each day in the nursery also differed somewhat from the other children. They tended to have more psychosomatic symptoms and symptoms of the aggression-hyperactivity type, and perhaps also a somewhat higher noradrenaline excretion. However, the differences were markedly small. A possible explanation is that the long nursery day was offset by the fact that the group of children is small early in the morning and late in the evening, and that the personnel density is therefore higher at these times. It is important to point this out since the charge is sometimes heard that day nurseries are not 100 percent used the entire time they are open. Since children spending the longest time per day in the nursery often come from the most stressful psychosocial environments (single mothers, parents of low socioeconomic status) it is an asset for the daycare milieu to be as good as possible at the beginning and at the end of the day. These children then get some of the compensation they need so much.

Sensitivity to factors in the day nursery milieu varies from child to child. Density of personnel and group size seem to play an especially significant role for anxious and inhibited children. The increase in personnel density resulted in a marked reduction in the incidence of symptoms of the anxiety-inhibition type. The reduction in hormone excretion was also especially marked for anxious and inhibited children. Children in the large nursery classes more often had symptoms of the anxiety-inhibition type than children in the small classes, and of these anxious and inhibited children, those in large day nursery classes had a higher adrenaline excretion than those in small classes. The positive effects of the increased density of personnel were also particularly marked for older children and boys. These groups are very possibly those children who are easy to forget about when the personnel density is low and the nurses must devote most of their attention to the smallest children, who require more care and attention, and to the restless and extroverted children.

Children from psychosocially disturbed families were especially benefited by changes in density of personnel regarding conflict behavior (according to observations), probably due for the most part to the climate in the children's group. However, their behavioral disorders (according to the interviews) were affected much less, perhaps because they have to do with more long-term stresses. The relatively brief experimental intervention was unable to offset the pronounced disturbances in their home environments. On the whole, however, the findings indicate that these children as well were favorably affected by the increased density of personnel. Since day nursery placement is used as a supportive measure for children from problem families, it is important to point out that the mental hygiene effect of such a measure probably depends a great deal on how the daycare milieu is shaped.

The experimental increase in personnel density had many clearly positive effects, despite the fact that it lasted only two months. Children attend day nurseries for long periods, up to six years. The long-term effects of various factors in the daycare milieu may therefore be many many times greater. A daycare center can be a valuable complement to the home, but then the qualitative features of the center must be accorded a great significance. One of the most important qualitative factors is probably personnel density, since it is a prerequisite for the quality of the contact that develops between the adults and the children in the nursery.

References

1. Andersson, B., Hovmöller, S., Karlsson, C.-G., and Svensson, S. Analysis of urinary catecholamines: an improved auto-analyzer fluorescence method. *Clin. Chim. Acta,* 51, (1974), 13–28.
2. Bellman, M. Studies on Encopresis. *Acta Pediatr. Scand.,* Suppl. 170, (1966).
3. Chamberlin, R.W. Can We Identify a Group of Children at Age 2 Who are at High Risk for the Development of Behavior or Emotional Problems in Kindergarten and First Grade? Department of Pediatrics, University of Rochester School of Medicine, Rochester, New York 1977.
4. Expert Committee on Child Mental Health & Psychosocial Development, Geneva, 1976.
5. Frankenhaeuser, M. Behavior and circulating catecholamines, *Brain. Res.,* 31, (1971), 241–262.
6. Jonsson, G. Delinquent boys, their parents and grandparents. *Acta Psych. Scand.,* Suppl. 195 (1967).
7. Jonsson, G., and Kälvesten, A.-L. *222 Stockholmspojkar.* Almqvist & Wiksell, Stockholm, 1964.
8. Kälvesten, A.-L., and Meldahl, G. 217 Stockholmsfamiljer. Tiden, Stockholm, 1972.

9. Klackenberg, G. A Prospective Longitudinal Study of Children. *Acta Pediatr. Scand.*, 224:71, 1971.
10. Lapouse, R. The epidemiology of behavior disorders in children. *Am. J. Dis. Child*, 111, 594, 1966.
11. Levi, L., Ed. Stress and distress in response to psychosocial stimuli. *Acta Med. Scand.* Suppl. 528, 1972.
12. MacFarlane, J. W., Allen, L., and Honzik, M. P. *A Developmental Study of the Behavior Problems of Normal Children between 21 Months and Fourteen Years.* University of California Press, Berkeley, 1954.
13. Robins, L.N. *Deviant Children Grown Up,* Williams & Wilkins, Baltimore, 1966.

Reports from the Project

Cederblad, M., and Höök, B. Beteenderubbningar och katekolaminutsöndring hos treåriga daghemsbarn i Stockholm. *Läkartidningen* 77:3366-3368 1980.

In the Reports Series from the Laboratory for clinical stress research:

Cederblad M., Höök B., Kagan, A. R., Levi, L., Borg, A., Falk, K., Karlsson, C. G., and Lind, E. Daghemsvård för treåringar: Inverkan av personaltäthet—en tvärvetenskaplig, experimentell studie. No. 46, 1976.

Kagan, A. R., Cederblad, M., Höök, B., Levi, L. Evaluation of the effect of increasing the number of nurses on health and behavior of 3 year old children in day care, satisfaction of their parents and health and satisfaction of their nurses. No. 89, 1978.

Cederblad, M., and Höök, B. Daghemsvård för treåringar—en tvärvetenskaplig, experimentell studie. III. Attityder och åsikter hos föräldrar och personal. No. 55, 1977.

Cederblad, M., and Höök, B. Daghemsvård för treåringar—en tvärvetenskaplig, experimentell studie. IV. Inverkan av faktorer i daghemsmiljön på barnens beteenderubbningar. No. 78, 1978.

Cederblad, M., and Höök, B. Daghemsvård för treåringar—en tvärvetenskaplig, experimentell studie. V. Inverkan av faktorer i hemmiljön på barnens beteenderubbningar. No. 79, 1978.

Cederblad, M., and Höök, B. Daghemsvård för treåringar—en tvårvetenskaplig, experimentell studie. VI. *Konfliktbeteende,* No. 80 (1978).

Cederblad, M., and Höök, B. Daghemsvård för treåringar—en tvåretenskaplig, experimentell studie. VII. Inverkan av faktorer i daghemsmiljön på barnens utsöndring av adrenalin och noradrenalin. No. 118, in press 1981.

Cederblad, M. Daghemsvård för treåringar—en tvärvetenskaplig, experimentell studie. VIII. *Interaktionsbeteende,* No. 119 (1981).

Cederblad, M., and Höök B. Daghemsvård för treåringar—en tvårvetenskaplig, experimentell studie. IX. Barnens sjukfranvaro under experimentperioden samt under ytterligare tre år. No. 120, 1981.

Cederblad, M., and Höök, B. Daghemsvård för treåringar—en tvärvetenskaplig, experimentell studie. X. *Sammanfattning,* No. 121 (1980).

Cederblad, M., and Höök, B. Beteenderubbningar hos förskolebarn: stabilitet och predicerbarhet från tre till sex års ålder. No. 81, 1978.

Psychosocial Risk Factors in Children

Ragnar Jonsell, M.D. (Sweden)

The number of young people with serious psychological complaints and social maladjustment has become a major problem for the community in Sweden and for many other countries. Pediatricians and other physicians see many children with symptoms (e.g., abdominal pains, headache, poor eating) for which no organic explanation can be found. Are some of the patients who are brought to a pediatrician with symptoms lacking a somatic background identical with those who much later pose intractable problems for psychiatrists and social authorities? If so, can early diagnosis and adequate measures by the pediatrician prevent a serious psychiatric or social maldevelopment in certain cases?

The material for this study was collected at the pediatric outpatient clinic of Umeå in northern Sweden. Families with a very low economic standard or poor housing were uncommon. Because of the public system of security in Sweden, economic factors cannot be considered to have had a selective effect on the persons who attended the pediatric clinic. In the year from July 1, 1970 to June 30, 1971, a record was made of all visits to pediatricians at the Umeå Hospital. Patients making an initial visit (defined as one that was not a follow-up visit) numbered 4152, of whom 37.6 percent had an appointment. The rest were emergency cases. At each visit the examining physician judged whether psychological factors had an essential bearing on the child's symptoms, using three alternatives: yes (5.2 percent), doubtful (8.3 percent), and no (86.5 percent). The distribution by age is reproduced in Figure 1. The term psychological factors is used here in a wide sense, that is, the fundamental cause might be the child's constitution, emotional or social environment, or endogenous psychological disorders. Two groups of subjects were formed from all the cases and were judged yes (PY) or doubtful (PD). In addition, a control group was obtained from a sample of the (PN) cases and matched for the variables sex, age, and place of residence.

For the most common complaints in which a psychological factor was probable or suspected, a breakdown by age is given in Figure 2. In some instances it was only after several contacts with the health service that the background of the patient's symptoms became clear. In 19.7 percent of the PY group the patients received a referral to the child psychiatry clinic, were recommended to renew an existing contact, or asked to make use of a referral issued earlier. Many parents either declined a proposed referral straight away or else let it lapse, even though an appointment had been arranged within a week. In such cases the pediatrician often seemed to believe that the patient was being looked after, and there was therefore no form of follow-up arranged at the pediatric clinic.

A considerable proportion of the patients presented indefinite

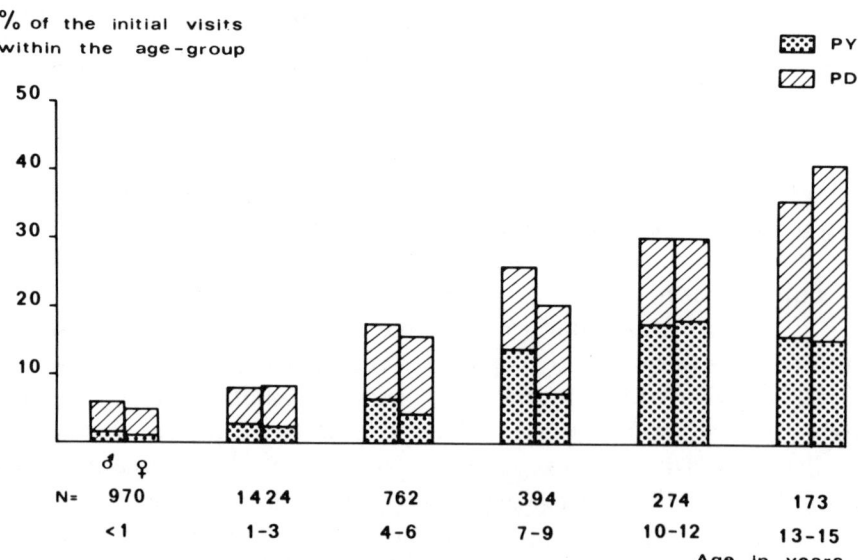

Figure 1. Proportion of PY and PD cases among the total number of initial visits, according to sex and age group. Age in completed years.

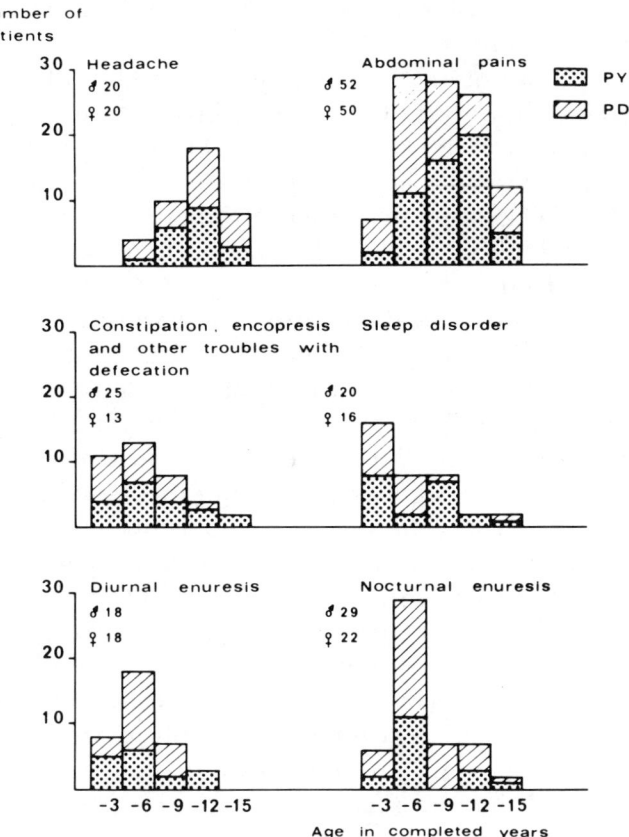

Figure 2. Actual visit. Distribution of some common psychogenic complaints (suspected and probable) in different age groups.

somatic symptoms, and the frequency of both respiratory and other virus infections was relatively high, even in the PY group. This may reflect a reduced tolerance to the child's symptoms by parents who are under stress for other reasons. It is also conceivable that somatic symptoms are used more or less unconsciously as a "passport" for discussing very different problems with a physician. Many of the PY cases were left without an active pediatric follow-up or a referral elsewhere. Since very few patients refuse medical measures and referral when their children are ill, it is surprising how many refuse a referral to a child psychiatrist. This attitude, which is often reinforced by relatives and neighbors, probably rests on preconceptions about child psychiatry and the concept of psychiatric disorder. Several studies suggest that many of the patients who are not followed up return to health services later on with the same or other indefinite symptoms.

The group did not differ statistically in number of previous initial visits or emergency visits. There were, however, many patients who had made several visits with different symptoms and problems. At previous initial visits or admissions many of the children, particularly in the PY group, presented problems that were judged to involve psychological factors. This was particularly common among the older children.

Broken homes due to divorce or death were considerably more common in the PY group (12.6 percent) than in the PN group (4.6 percent), $p < .001$. Mothers who had been less than 20 years old when the patient was born were more common in the PY than in the PN group, 12.3 percent and 4.8 percent respectively ($p < .001$). The groups did not differ significantly in family income, occupation, or socioeconomic group. The number of parents who had been registered sick for nervous complaints or disorders at some time during the child's lifetime was significantly higher in the PY than in the PN group. The differences were marked for the parents of children aged 4 to 12 years, whereas the frequencies were similar for those aged 13 to 15 years (Figure 3). The families in the PY group featured in the social register considerably more frequently than those in the PN group. The families that had been broken up by divorce or death had an increased incidence of registered sickness for nervous disorders among both the fathers and the mothers, and these families were overrepresented in the social register. Families with a record of nervous disorders featured more frequently in the social register. The fathers with a record of nervous disorder were overrepresented in the temperance register and the mothers were overrepresented in the social assistance register.

The material collected for this study covers practically all the contacts patients have had with pediatricians or child psychiatrists in the area served by the hospital. One can assume that the physician made a note of psychogenic complaints in the pediatric records if he or she considered them important, but no doubt there were problems that escaped detection due to lack of doctor's time, the presence of more prominent complaints, or lack of contact with the patients. The attendance figures and the size of the population served by the hospital suggest that 15 to 20 percent of all children aged 0 to 15 years made one or several initial visits to the pediatric clinic. There is thus a large need for help, which parents and various bodies interpret as medical. It is questionable whether the communi-

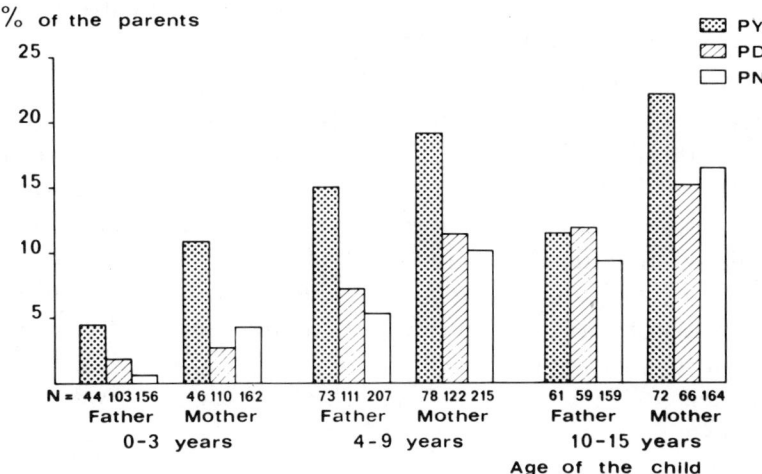

Figure 3. Parents who had reported sick for mental or nervous complaints or disorders during the child's lifetime.

ty's resources for health services and social welfare are correctly structured to meet the real needs of many of these families. Studies have pointed out that the somatically inclined pediatrician may neglect to obtain important information about the patient's behavior and situation, information that may be crucial for an understanding of the illness or symptoms. The training of medical students in these matters is poor, and during their training they loose a good deal of their original ability to establish contact with parents, apparently because the training is excessively concerned with technical aspects.

There is no laboratory procedure that can help the doctor detect the patients at risk. But I think there are some signals that the doctor can observe.

1. The anxiety of the parent(s) is out of proportion to the condition of the child.
2. There are recurrent visits to an outpatient clinic with different symptoms.
3. Patients fail to appear at appointed visits but claim to have priority as emergency cases.
4. Patients want tranquillizers but will not offer a thorough anamnesis.
5. Parent(s) have depressive, agitated, or deviating behavior.
6. Parent, brother, or sister has a serious or protracted illness.
7. There is serious conflict between the parents.

8. Parenthood is described in an exclusively negative way ("always troubles with the child").

There is always some likelihood that the presenting symptoms have a somatic background, and large resources are often invested—in the form of laboratory tests, x-ray examinations, and consultations—in ruling out an organic cause. These efforts cannot be dismissed in general as unnecessary, but there are cases that show that many investigations could be cut down substantially if a more thorough history were obtained and further personal contact provided at a second visit.

Consider some simple advice, which I try to give to young colleagues:

1. Reduce the immediate somatic investigation to the minimum required to exclude an imminent urgent disease, and give an appointment within one to two weeks with time to take a good anamnesis.
2. Shut off the telephone, and do not admit sudden trespassers (e.g., students, nurses) except for emergencies.
3. Try to speak individually with parents and older children.
4. If parents admit to them, contact other doctors who treat family members.

Another advantage would be access to child guidance specialists (psychologist, social worker, and, if possible, child psychiatrist) within the same locality as the pediatric out-patient clinic. The patient could then be referred on a simple door-to-door basis and the parents would not have to admit that they had been to see a psychiatrist. In time, such an integration would eliminate the prejudice against child psychiatry and the continuous contact between pediatric and psychiatric specialists would provide further training on a practical basis as well as further mutual understanding. Although these measures may appear time consuming, they would certainly save the health service from many unnecessary new visits (often out of hours, when costs are higher) and large investigations. One could also prevent certain cases from developing into serious psychiatric and social problems. Efforts should be made to benefit from a situation in which the parents express a need for help.

References

1. Apley, J., and McKeith, R. *The Child and His Symptoms*. Oxford, 1968.
2. Goodall, J. Clinical clues to emotional disturbances in children. *Clin. Pediatr.*, 12 (1973), 178.
3. Green, M. A developmental approach to symptoms based on age groups. *Ped. Clin. N. Am.*, 22 (1975), 571.
4. Jonsell, R. Patients at a Pediatric Out-patient Clinic. *Acta Pediatr. Scand,* 66 (1977), 723–734.
5. Korsch, B.M., and Aley, E.F. Pediatric interviewing techniques. *Curr. Probl. Pediatr.*, 3, 7 (1973).
6. Simmons, J.E. The pediatric clinician's job. In Green, M., and Haggerty, R.J., Eds. *Ambulatory Pediatrics*. Saunders, Philadelphia, 1968, 110.
7. Wolff, S. *Children Under Stress*. Lane, London, 1969.

Drug Abuse and Alcoholism Among Children and Youth in Sweden

Per-Anders Rydelius, M.D. (Sweden)

Since the end of World War II, alcohol consumption has steadily gone up in Sweden. Parallel with this general rise in consumption we have seen evidence of alcoholism among teenagers. In addition, a new problem has been apparent since the middle of the 1960s: the use and abuse of narcotic drugs. The serious abuse of alcohol and other drugs among children and youth is a rather new problem in Sweden, and the clinical importance of this has become greater and greater during the 1970s.

School children have been investigated annually since 1971 as to their habits of use and abuse of alcohol, narcotics, tobacco, and so forth. These students are, on each occasion, 13 and 16 years old. The results from the investigations of 1978 are available [7, 8]. In the spring of 1980, the Swedish government released a study on the heavy addiction of narcotic drugs. This study, using data collected from the fall of 1978 to the spring of 1979, is an update of the actual situation of heavy addiction in Sweden and is called the UNO-investigation [28]. This paper concerns these investigations and others carried out at the Department of Child and Youth Psychiatry, Karolinska Institute, St. Görans Hospital in Stockholm.

Abuse of Narcotic Drugs

In the UNO-investigation, the case-finding study revealed that approximately 20,000 persons (78 percent men, 22 percent women) use drugs. Of these drug addicts, 3 percent were 10 to 17 years old, and 7 percent were 18 to 19. Sweden has a population of 8,316,000 persons (4,121,000 men and 4,195,000 women). This means that about 0.38 percent of the men and 0.11 percent of the women are known as drug addicts. In the 10- to 17-year-old age group, only 0.06 percent of the youngsters were known as addicts. The corresponding figure in the 18- to 19-year-old age-group was 0.65 percent. The three dominating drugs were, in order of magnitude, the cannabis group, the amphetamine group, and the opiate group. Other drugs were rare and of less importance. Many addicts used more than one drug. Fifty-one percent of the cannabis addicts used or had used another drug. The corresponding figure for the amphetamine users was 71 percent and for the opiate users, 74 percent.

The number of heavy abusers in the study (defined as using "daily injections," "regular injections," "daily use," and "injections") was approximately 8000, 41 percent of the total. The mean age was 27 years. In this group of heavy abusers, 1 percent corresponded to the 10- to 17-year-old age group and another 5 percent corresponded to the 18- to 19-year-old age group. From this you could say the only 0.01 percent of Swedish youth aged 10 to 17 were heavy addicts compared to 0.18 percent of 18- to 19-year-olds. This figure could be higher, since the estimate of error in the investigation points to a total of 10,000–14,000 heavy abusers in the country as a whole. Eighty percent of the most serious addicts in this group were concentrated in the three big cities in Sweden: Stockholm, Gothenburg, and Malmoe. Small communities with less than 10,000 inhabitants corresponded to about 1 percent of the total known users. Thus heavy abuse of narcotic drugs in Sweden seems to be almost only a big city problem.

The group of heavy addicts was dominated by men (76 percent of the total) who have used drugs for a long time, often more than five years. The greater part was unemployed, and 53 percent had been condemned to prison because of delinquency. Almost half of this group (46 percent) was also known as alcoholics.

From the school investigations it is clear that there have been differences from 1971 to 1978 in the narcotic habits of the youth. The predominating drug is cannabis, and has been all the time.

However, there are less and less students using or having used narcotic drugs. The same tendency has been seen in tobacco smoking and solution sniffing. However, there are indications that the group using narcotic drugs is a multiproblem group, experienced in sniffing solutions, drinking alcohol and showing disciplinary problems in general. Alcohol consumption is higher among teenagers as a whole.

From these studies you could conclude that abuse of narcotic drugs among children and youths is of minor importance in child psychiatric practice. There is however, evidence that this group of teenagers and young adults who show problems with delinquency and serious abuse of narcotic drugs and alcohol needs extensive support from an early age, when child psychiatrists could do much.

Curman and Nylander [4] and Nylander [16] have followed patients who had been treated at the Child Guidance Clinics (CGC) in Stockholm from 1953, 1954, and 1955. This prospective study, which has run for 20 years, has shown that 7 percent of the boys and 3 percent of the girls developed serious abuse (two-fifths became alcoholics, two-fifths became drug addicts, and one-fifth abuses both alcohol and drugs). The group of future addicts did not differ from the general CGC group in age or sex distribution. The average age of this group at the time of CGC contact was 9 years, and one-quarter had been in contact with the CGC before school age. Compared with the rest of the CGC group, the future addicts more often came from badly disturbed homes with alcoholic fathers or mothers, mentally sick parents, or parents who had divorced. Both boys and girls often showed symptoms of acting out (hyperactivity, lack of concentration, aggressiveness). Half of the boys and one-third of the girls had already shown antisocial symptoms (pilfering, theft, absconding). The child psychiatric diagnosis did not differ significantly between the future addicts and the CGC group in total.

One of the biggest problems with this group at the time of CGC contact was for the CGC staff to collaborate with the families. Therapy often came to an abrupt end. Only 10 percent of the boys and 17 percent of the girls had received any form of real therapy. Furthermore, 60 percent of this group also became criminals with heavy records. These dimensions present a challenge to child psychiatrists to find ways of helping this group of children.

For the group of established teenage drug addicts, there have been many attempts to give effective treatment. During the 1970s, a treatment chain was developed for this group in Stockholm. The social authorities in the city have the Maria-policlinic, which deals exclusively with young addicts of all types. The clinic also supports a chain of treatment homes, called the *Hasselakollektiven,* where the teenagers are treated during a three-year period in a program including school education. The results of this program are promising, but a long-term follow-up is not yet done.

Alcohol Abuse

Alcoholism among children and youth has been known since the 1800s. At that time, in Sweden and in most other countries in Europe and North America, alcoholism was a serious problem. It was seen among men, women, youth, and children. Even the syndrome of alcoholfetopatia was known among physicians. The threat that alcohol presented to the well-being of people at that time was met with worldwide restrictions and movements against the drug. As a result of this, the problem of alcoholism decreased in clinical importance, and in Sweden it became a problem almost exclusively among men. Abuse among women, youth, and children became extremely rare. Probably as a consequence of this, much knowledge about the pathogenesis of alcoholism and the threats this drug poses to human health also disappeared.

In an interesting paper on the historical aspect of the effects of drinking on offspring [29], the authors conclude that today's generation has discovered "news" that was already discovered in the nineteenth century. In 1896, the Swedish Medical Association had a committee studying the problem of alcoholism in youth, which concluded that "alcoholism came earlier if a child started to drink than if an adult did so" [25].

From the beginning of the twentieth century until 1977 it was a crime to be drunk in Sweden. Publicly drunken adults were taken into custody, and drunken children usually were brought to their homes, but both categories were registered in a central alcohol register. In the local place, offenders were registered with the local temperance boards and child welfare committees. These registrations, together with statistics on alcohol consumption, reveal that after World War II there has been a rise in registrations of drunkenness as well as a rise in the consumption of alcohol [3, 22]. The consumption has almost doubled since 1945 and in 1974 the level equalled the average from 1860 to 1900.

From 1945 to the 1970s, these drunkenness registration Figures have increased steadily. The biggest rise is for men, and especially noteworthy is the fact that, between 1971 and 1976, every eighth man registered was a boy 19 years old or younger. In women, the biggest rise has been among younger women, and every fourth was a girl aged 19 or younger between 1971 and 1976. These figures also show that the risk of relapse into drunkenness is high. After three known occasions, this risk is almost 100 percent [2].

At the St. Görans Hospital in Stockholm there has been a special interest in the problem of alcohol abuse among children and youth. The result of this interest has been three separate studies, of which two are longitudinal prospective ones. In a retrospective study [5], all boys who had been known to the Child Welfare Committee in Stockholm between 1958 and 1959 for uncomplicated public drunkenness and who were not known earlier for drunkenness or delinquency were investigated for relapse during a five-year period. This study showed that relapse groups were more often psychosociologically handicapped than nonrelapse groups.

This study was followed by two prospective studies. The first [18] was an intensive study of first-time drunkards not older than 18 and without previous records of delinquency. The study showed that boys in this situation often had an alcoholic or mentally ill father and had themselves shown symptoms of psychic deficiency and disciplinary problems in school. During a five-year period relapses were recorded. In comparing a nonrelapse group with a group with three or more relapses, it was found that the relapse group more often had alcoholic or mentally ill fathers, had more often reported symptoms of psychiatric deficiencies, had more often shown disciplinary problems in school, or was judged to be psychiatrically deficient when examined. The relapse group also showed personality disorder by not reacting with anxiety at the time of the first arrest.

The second study [19, 23] aimed at early recognition and early child psychiatric intervention with this group of young drunkards to prohibit a proceeding into alcohol abuse. This study took place in Umeå from 1967 to 1972. Every child and teenager up to 17 years of age found drunk was taken directly to the Department of Child and Youth Psychiatry at the University Hospital. Umeå, a university city in northern Sweden, had at that time a population of about 50,000, of which approximately 10 percent were in the actual age interval for the study. During the five years from 1967 to 1972, 149 children with a mean age of 15 years 5 months (range: 10 years, 0 months to 16 years, 12 months) were arrested for public drunkenness.

These youngsters were, from a psychosociological point of view, heavily burdened. To a large extent, they came from broken or unsatisfactory homes. Their mothers were often single parents, usually worn out from hard work. Their fathers were often alcoholics. In many cases these children had shown symptoms of maladjustment at home or at school from an early age. Approximately one child in five had previously been in contact with the Child and Youth Psychiatric Department. Of the total youth population of this age group they represented a small proportion (approximately six per thousand). Of 149 youngsters, 92 were admitted to the hospital 99 times, and 57 were not available for examination at the department because they had been detained by the police (in most cases because of suspicion of involvement in crimes other than drunkenness, but in some cases because of refusal from the child in question to have any contact with the department at all).

The 92 children admitted to the hospital had treatment and support according to their status and needs. In some cases this meant only an overnight stay at the department and a judgment of status and psychosociological situation, but in other cases a clinic treatment was undertaken, and some cases were treated as inpatients at the department for more than one month.

During a five-year period from the first drunken offense, relapses into drunkenness were then recorded. This showed that approximately every fifth child, mostly boys, became serious misusers and abusers of alcohol. This group often became delinquent as well, sometimes including criminal acts of serious nature. The relapse group had need of social welfare and used the sickness insurance more often than was normal for these age groups. There were no differences between the group detained by the police and the group admitted to the hospital in these aspects. The future high-risk group of those admitted to the hospital had indeed been recognized at the first drunken occasion and had had treatment and support.

The high-risk group was composed of children heavily psychosociologically burdened in the way described above, and often had been found drunken on weekdays. The low-risk group often had been found drunk on special occasions or weekends.

Nylander [15] presented a study on children of alcoholic fathers showing that boys and girls in such families were psychiatrically deficient, had problems in school, and often suffered from headaches or stomachaches. Compared with the controls, the children from the alcoholic fathers often sought advice at pediatric clinics. The pediatrician, however, did not understand the psychosociological aspects of the child's somatic complaints and often made extensive investigations of the child without reaching a somatic diagnosis. The conclusions of this study were that children who live under severe emotional stress, as these children of alcoholics did, tend to show symptoms of conversion type, and if they seek help, they often come to pediatric or pediatric surgery departments, and hardly ever to child psychiatrists.

In a prospective longitudinal study of the same material [26], it has been shown that boys from alcoholic fathers have alcohol-problems more often than controls do, and are prone to delinquency and need support from social welfare.

From these studies, one may conclude that the serious abuse of alcohol among children and youth in Sweden is restricted to a small, heavily psychosociologically burdened group that is also prone to delinquency. Findings similar to those mentioned above are reported from many other studies [1, 6, 9, 13, 14]. This fits with Winokour's opinion on "primary alcoholics" having an early debue in both alcoholism and delinquency [30].

Jonsson [10, 11] is of the opinion that children growing up under the conditions mentioned above actually are suffering from a social inheritance, which accumulates from generation to generation, producing more and more symptoms of social deviance in offspring. Therefore, young alcoholics and drug addicts could, as parents, be a great risk to their own children's well-being and good social outcome. That this could be true at least for boys has actually been shown by Nylander [15], who investigated children of alcoholic fathers, and Rydelius [26, 27], who has followed these children for 15 and 20 years. The great risk for alcoholic mothers is that children can be born with mental retardation and deformations. Such mothers often have problems in rearing children as well.

Some studies [12, 21, 23] point to the fact that these groups of youngsters are very difficult to treat. This could be because treatment is not very effective when it starts several years after the pathogenic environmental factors have had their most deleterious effects. These children should be detected very early and given support and treatment from the beginning [17, 20].

It is probable that some young people start to drink in a socially acceptable way, thereby grounding habits that will in the future give rise to an alcoholism probably without delinquency, but with more medically orientated symptoms. This group of "learned alcoholics" are different from primary alcoholics and probably could be rescued by receiving proper information and limitations on their alcohol habits in time.

Conclusions

Alcohol consumption has risen in Sweden since the end of World War II. Since 1974, the consumption has once again reached the average for the period 1860 to 1900, when alcoholism among men, women, youth, and children was common. From investigations of the alcohol habits of school children, it is clear that both boys and girls drink more alcohol today than at the beginning of the 1970s. This could mean a risk of more alcoholism in the future population. Serious abuse of alcohol among teenagers today is restricted to a psychosociologically heavily burdened group, which often is delinquent as well. The same group is also prone to the abuse of narcotic drugs, but in the teenage groups these addicts still are small in number. The average "heavy addicted narcoman" in Sweden is a 27-year-old man, living in one of the big cities, who is known for bad social adjustment, delinquency, and alcohol abuse. In my opinion, his situation is grounded in his childhood, due to psychosociological environmental factors and probably hereditary factors as well, and preventing a bad outcome for him and for his future children is a great challenge to child psychiatrists.

References

1. Blacker, E., Demone, H., and Freeman, H. Drinking behavior of delinquent boys. *Q.J. Stud. Alcohol.*, 26 (1965), 233.
2. Collet, J., Om risken för återfall i fylleri. *Alkoholfrågan* 57 (1963), 210.
3. Collet, J. Konsumtion och missbruk av alkohol under första halvåret. *Alkohol och Narkotika*, 5 (1978), 20.
4. Curman, H., and Nylander, I. A 10-year follow-up of 2268 cases at the CGC-clinics in Stockholm. *Acta Pediatr. Scand.*, Suppl. 260 (1976).
5. Eklund, L., and Nylander, I. Risken för åfterfall i fylleri bland Stockholmspojkar. *Soc. Med. Tidskr.*, 42 (1965), 210.
6. Helgason, T., and Asmundsson, G. Behavior and social characteristics of young asocial alcohol abusers. *Neuropsychobiology*, 1 (1975), 109.
7. Hibell, B. Några utvecklingstendenser i den nordiska ungdomens alkoholvanor. *Nord. Med.*, 95 (1980), 173.
8. Hibell, B., and Jonsson. E. Skolungdomens alkohol-, narkotika-, tobaks- och sniffningsvanor 1978. *Alkohol och Narkotika*, 8 (1979), 19.
9. Jessor, R., Collings, M., and Jessor, S. On becoming a drinker: sociopsychological aspects of an adolescent transition. *Ann. N.Y. Acad. Sci.*, 197 (1972), 189.
10. Jonsson, G. Delinquent boys, their parents and grandparents. *Acta Psychiatr. Scand.*, Suppl 195 (1967).
11. Jonsson, G. *Breaking Up the Social Inheritance*. Tiden/Folksam, Stockholm, 1973. (in Swedish)
12. McCord, J., and McCord, W. A follow-up report on the Cambridge Somerville Youth study. *Annals. Am. Acad. Pol. Soc. Sci.*, 322 (1959), 89.
13. MacKay, J. R., Murray A., Hagerty, T. I., and Collins, L. Juvenile delinquency and drinking behavior. *J. Health Hum. Behav.*, 4 (1963), 276.

References

14. Mader, R. Alcoholism in adolescent criminals. *Acta Paedopsychiatr.* 32:2 (1972).
15. Nylander, I. Children of alcoholic fathers. *Acta Pediatr. Scand.*, 121 (1960).
16. Nylander, I. A 20-year prospective follow-up of 2164 cases at the CGC-clinics in Stockholm. *Acta Pediatr. Scand.*, Suppl. 276 (1979a).
17. Nylander, I. Asocialitetsutveckling av barn. *Läkartidningen*, 76 (1979b), 2396.
18. Nylander, I., and Rydelius, P.-A. The relapse of drunkenness in non-asocial teen-age boys. *Acta Psychiatr. Scand.*, 49 (1973), 435.
19. Nylander, I., and Rydelius, P.-A. *Int. J. Ment. Health*, 7:3−4 (1979), 117.
20. Nylander, I., and Zetterström, R. Uppfödningssvårigheter hos späda barn- ett psykosocialt problem. *Läkartidningen* 74 (1977), 4199.
21. Powers, E., and Witmers, H.L. An *Experiment in the Prevention of Delinquency* Oxford: Columbia University Press 1951.
22. Rapport 73, 74, 75, 76, 77, 78, 79. Alkohol och Narkotikafakta och debatt. Stockholm. Centralförbundet för alkohol- och narkotikaupplysning 1973, 1974, 1975, 1976, 1977, 1978, 1979.
23. Rydelius, P.-A. Barnpsykiatriskt omhändertagande av unga fyllerister. *Läkartidningen*, 75 (1978a), 1607.
24. Rydelius, P.-A. Methanol intoxication—a differential diagnosis also of current interest in child psychiatric practice. *Acta Paedopsychiatr.*, 43, (1978b), 261.
25. Rydelius, P.-A. Alkoholmissbruk hos barn och ungdom. *Läkartidningen*, 76 (1979), 2399.
26. Rydelius, P.-A. A longitudinal-prospective study of the children of alcoholic fathers. A methodological study and a description of the life situations for the children after 15 years. Research report from the Child Psychiatric Clinics of the Karolinska Institute, St. Görans's Hospital, Stockholm, 1980 (in Swedish).
27. Rydelius, P.-A. Children of alcoholic fathers. Their situation 20 years later. (*Acta Pediatr. Scand.*, suppl. To be published).
28. UNO-undersökningen: Tungt Narkotikamissbruk—en totalundersökning 1979. Liber, Stockholm, 1980.
29. Warner, R., and Rosett, H.L. The effects of drinking on offspring. An historical survey of the American and British literature. *J. Stud. Alcohol.* 36 (1975), 1395.
30. Winokour, G., Rimmer, J., and Reich, Th. Alcoholism IV: Is there more than one type of alcoholism? *Br. J. Psychiatr.* 118 (1971), 525.

Suicidal Behavior in Childhood and Adolescence

Ulf Otto, M.D. (Sweden)

Nearly everything already ought to have been said about youngsters and suicidal acts. Does anything remain to say after the words of Schopenhauer: "The suicidant wants to live, he is only dissatisfied with the conditions in which he lives"? Or what John Syms said in 1637: "Suicide cannot be prevented so much through argument against the act itself as by the discovery and the removal of the causes and the motives"?

Let us begin by defining briefly what we mean by the concept of suicidal acts. Many have tried, but we use the definition of Stengel [5], who is of the opinion that suicide is an act that individuals consciously commit to damage themselves and that this damage leads to death. Attempted suicide is also an act that individuals consciously commit to damage themselves, but in this case the damage does not lead to death. Many doubtless feel that, in spite of the fact that so much has been written about this subject, it still seems to be difficult to sum up the suicide problem generally. Perhaps, at least where children and adolescents are concerned, there has been more talking than investigation. Or, as Kreitman [1] says: "Those of us working in the area, however, might say without undue cynicism that we know everything about suicidal behavior except why people engage in it and why some forms of it are increasing." The fact that we find it difficult to put the finger on self-destructive behavior is not a particularly unique situation when dealing with problems of such complicated character. The concept contains too many factors, all too many specialists become involved, and it is difficult to get a concrete grip on the problem in its entirety.

Personality, inheritance, childhood conditions, current environment, and current situation—these involve geneticists, physiologists, physicians, psychiatrists, psychologists, sociologists, educators, clergymen, and others.

According to WHO [6], suicide is among the first 10 causes of death in most Western countries. The greatest increase has been in the middle and late adolescent groups. For these groups the rate has doubled in the last 20 years, and it is currently listed as the world's fifth leading cause of death in the 15- to 19-year age group. A large number of adolescent suicides go unreported. Accidents are a leading cause of death in adolescence, and many of them are probably suicides that are not certified as such in an attempt to avoid the cultural stigma associated with it.

In Sweden we had a comparatively stable suicide frequency for several years of about 1500 victims annually, of whom more than 1000 were men and just under 500 were women. But during the 1970s, this frequency has increased to nearly 2000 victims annually. The increase occurs almost exclusively within the younger age groups. Let us, as an example, have a look at 1976. In this year in Sweden:

342 children and youngsters died in accidents, of which 234 were in traffic accidents.

15 children were maltreated to death or murdered.

56 children committed suicide and another 23 attempted suicide.

At least once a week one child committed suicide.

At least once a day one child attempted suicide.

Figure 1 represents the official death statistics up to 19 years of age in the years 1960 to 1977, showing the mean rise of suicides from the period from 1960–1969 to 1970–1977.

In my study, of the 1727 young people and children who made suicide attempts in the years 1955 to 1959, 80 percent were girls. During the last decade there has been a tendency to an equalization between the sexes. The common reasons are unhappy homes, conflict with parents, school problems, loss of confidence, feelings of inferiority, identity problems, and problems of sexual adjustment. We often found the loss of an important person during early childhood.

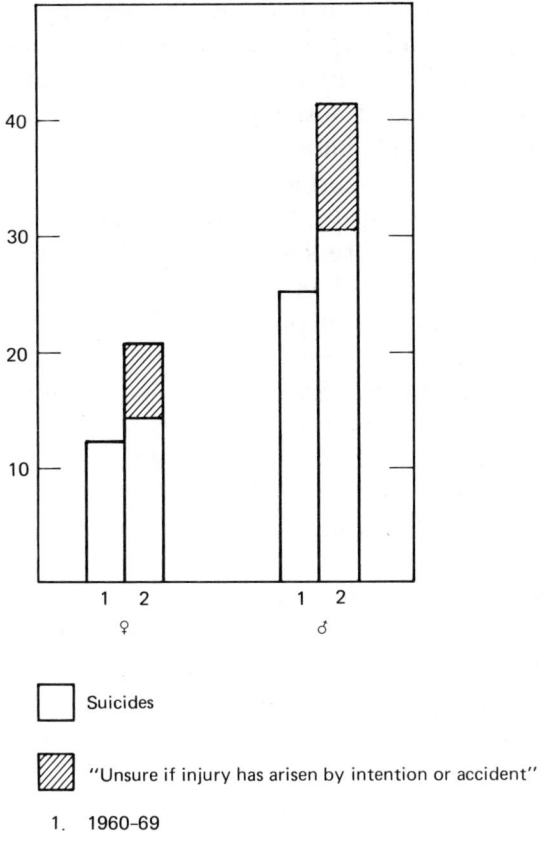

Figure 1. Average number of suicides in Sweden for children aged 0 to 17 during the years 1960–1969 (1) and 1970–1977 (2) according to official statistics.

But why the rise today? Is the reason perhaps the rapidly increasing change in economic, social, and moral circumstances in Western societies? In a society, the connections between different social institutions can be seen as a wheel, where the hub is the family and the spokes are the various institutions with which the individual comes into contact. They might be educational, religious, economic, and political institutions, for example. If the wheel turns slowly, the balance between the institutions can be suspended, but if the wheel turns too quickly, we see how the spokes melt into one another and become indistinguishable. Boundaries are obliterated, different institutions force their way into each other's domain. This has happened often during the last 20 years, and we have seen economic and political institutions increasingly intrude upon the family unit.

Family stability has been broken down both on the social and the emotional plane and has found it increasingly difficult to answer for the psychic stability of its members. And today, at least in Sweden, many children and adolescents grow up in a turmoil of emotional, social, and economic chaos.

Soubrier [4] once asked a very important question: "Are we about to be confronted with the birth of a suicidogenic society?"

In June 1981 a congress was held by the Nordic Council for Arctic Medical Research in Uleåborg in northern Finland to discuss suicides. In the northern part of Finland there has been a tremendous rise in suicides. They are attributed to the rapidly changing situation when people leave the sparsely populated areas to the old people and increase their alcohol consumption. During this century, the Eskimoes of Greenland have experienced an enormous revolution by entering Western civilization in a very old, traditional country. In 1954, alcohol became available for sale, and now the consumption is over 20 liters per person over 15 years of age (counted as 100 percent pure alcohol. In Sweden the consumption is about 9 liters per year. They now have 50 suicides per 100,000 inhabitants. Finland also has a tragic record of 26 suicides per 100,000 inhabitants. In northern Finland it is 38. In rapidly changing Alaska it is 35, but on the very slowly changing Färöarna it is 2.7 suicides per 100,000 inhabitants. In North America it was 17 per 100,000 in 1973, but only 6.7 in 1954.

There are not many scientific studies on this topic in Sweden. Since my thesis in 1971, very little has been done. This seems to be a question either of taboo or of circumstances too complicated to deal with.

My follow-up [3] study of 1727 attempted suicides by children and young people shows that 3 percent of all girls and not fewer than 10 percent of all boys died as a result of renewed suicidal acts committed after a rather short period—less than 10 years. The danger of successful suicide was greatest for three high-risk groups: boys in general, girls who used active methods, and young people whose suicide attempt was part of the development of a psychosis.

This same study showed that, seen as a group, the young people who attempted suicide later as adults differed from a control group in certain characteristic ways. The boys more often have been exempted from military service because of psychic disturbance. Both sexes are more often unmarried. They have all been sick-listed and have more frequently had psychiatric conditions of various sorts such as signs of psychic deficiency and lability. Thus they are basically a more fragile and disturbed group of people. These acts should not be disregarded or seen as isolated events. They are very serious on a deep level and often demand psychotherapeutic interventions well into late adolescence.

If there are few interesting studies, what about the clinical situation? I think it varies with the child psychiatric areas in the country, since the child psychiatric clinics in Sweden differ in their functions.

In my area, there is a population of 280,000 inhabitants. We have made an agreement with the four hospitals in the region that every youngster coming to the hospital because of a suicide attempt must be referred to our child psychiatric clinic. Since we have a clinic at one of the hospitals and policlinics at the other three, we can act rapidly. We go to the youngsters when they are in the intensive care department and usually let them go to one of our departments. They usually stay there about a week or two. During this time we have the possibility of coming into close contact with them and with other important persons, usually parents and girl- or boyfriends. We also make arrangements for their return to society, school, work, and friends. And, what is very important, since we know that the risk for a new suicidal act is particularly high during the first months, they must promise us never to do it again; if they feel unsure, they must promise to call us. We, on our part, promise to allow them to call us day or night, week or weekend, any time of year. This is why the child psychiatric clinic has its excellent opportunity to act. Very few organizations are open more than eight hours a day, and suicide thoughts do not peak between 8 a.m. and 5 p.m., but very often in the night. Every night there are three persons working in the clinic and a child psychiatrist on duty who is prepared to interfere.

Every young person who has attempted suicide ought to be sent to a child psychiatrist, who should be available at all hours of the day and night. Or, to express it the way a teenage girl who was admitted to our clinic did and who made renewed contact during the night when anxiety came sneaking up: "It is good to know that some of you are there, to feel that somebody is always awake at your place in the nights, someone I can always ring or come to if I want." Here in Sweden at least, medical care is superior because of its around-the-clock ability to look after this type of disturbance, which often demands acute efforts and individual and family therapeutic measures and support work for a lengthy period of time.

A group that ought to receive more of our interest consists of the parents of the children and adolescents who either have committed or attempted suicide. They are usually in a situation of intense crisis.

A Fairy Tale

Let us turn back to a poorer Sweden where many children were ill treated and foundered. Let us do it in company with the Swedish author Astrid Lindgren, famous for her books about Pippi Longstocking, among other things. She has written about children and death. Perhaps she does it most beautifully in the story "Sunnanäng," which means South Meadow, and which begins [2]

> A long time ago when poverty reigned, there lived a small brother and sister who were suddenly left all alone. But small children cannot live on their own in this world, they must live with somebody, and for this reason Matthias and Anna left Sunnanäng and went to stay with a farmer in Myra. He did not take them in because they possessed the brightest, nicest eyes and the most trusting little hands, or because they were beside themselves with sorrow for their dead mother. No, he took them for his own benefit. The hands of a child can work really well if one stops them from carving boats out of bark and making pipe whistles. ... And so the children were made to work and to slave. At school they felt ashamed of their clothes and their pauper's food box. Truly, nobody cared about them except each one for the other.

One day, when working in the forest, they came to a wall in which they found a gateway, and through it they entered into a wonderful summer with flowers, birds, and living streams, in other words, a paradise. In this land of dreams they met their mother. They wonder why the gate in the wall does not close. The answer they are given is that if the gate closes, it can never be opened again. (This land of dreams is naturally a symbol for the Kingdom of Death.) Out of a feeling of duty they go out again into the snow and the cold to the cottage where they live. And so they continue to live their miserable existence on the Myra farmer's farm.

One day they are once again out in the forest working. They are freezing, hungry, and tired. But they are guided by a bird once again to the gate in the wall. And at this point I would like to quote again to give you what I personally feel to be a very lovely description of the point where the longing for death takes preeminence over the will to live—when the children cannot stand it any more:

> The snow lay deep outside, but the cherry tree stretched its blossomy boughs over the wall, and the gate stood ajar.

"I have never longed for anything so much in all my life," said Anna.

"But now you are here," said Matthias, "you need long no more."

"No, now I need long no more," said Anna.

And Matthias took her hand and led her through the gate, into the eternal spring of Sunnanäng, where the fragile birch leaves quivered, where a thousand small birds sang and rejoiced in the trees, where children sailed their bark boats in the spring streams and where mother stood in a meadow and called "Come, all my children."

Behind them lay the cold, frosty forest and the approaching winter night. Anna looked back through the gate out into the dark and the coldness, and she shuddered.

"Why is the gate not closed?" she asked.

"Oh, dear little Anna," said Matthias, "if the gate closes, it can never again be opened, do you not remember that?"

"Yes, I remember it," said Anna, "never, never again."

And so they looked at one another. Matthias at Anna, she at him. They gazed long into each other's eyes and smiled gently. Then, silently and peacefully, they closed the gate.

References

1. Kreitman, N. Subculture aspects of attempted suicide. In *Psychiatric Epidemiology*, Hare, E. and Wing, J., Eds. London: Oxford University Press, 1970.
2. Lindgren, Astrid. *South Meadow*.
3. Otto, U. Suicide acts by children and adolescents. *Acta Psychiat. Scand. Suppl.*, 233, 1972.
4. Soubrier, N. Personal communication.
5. Stengel, E. *Suicide and Attempted Suicide*. Baltimore: Penguin Books, 1964.
6. World Health Organization. The Prevention of Suicide. Geneva: WHO Publication, 1968.

Adoption and Fostering as Preventive Measures

Michael Bohman, M.D.
Sören Sigvardsson, Ph.D. (Sweden)

In this paper I present some results of a prospective, longitudinal study of children who were registered for adoption at the time of their birth. For various reasons I restrict my presentation to the males in the population ($N = 329$). The purpose of my presentation is to analyze and discuss the possible preventive effect of adoption and fostering on the manifestation of social maladjustment among boys with a negative social heritage.

In other words, does the early placement of children from antisocial or otherwise socially insufficient families protect them from developing juvenile delinquency and/or social maladjustment? A large proportion of these boys were born to parents who exhibited social maladjustment, for instance, criminality and alcoholism. These boys have been followed and investigated from the time of their gestation through childhood and adolescence (11, 15, and 18 years). Our last investigation was undertaken when these boys were 22 to 23 years of age. The results of the investigations up to 18 years of age have been published elsewhere [1, 2, 5, 6, 7].

Subjects

The investigation presented here originated in a cohort of 624 children born in 1956–1957. They were born after unwanted pregnancies, and at the time of their births their mothers had reported to an adoption agency that they wanted them adopted. Subjects, family background, and so on, have been described at length elsewhere [1, 2] and only a short description is given here. Of the original cohort, 168 children (93 boys) were placed in adoptive homes before the age of one year (group I): 208 children (118 boys) were returned to their biological mothers (group II), most of them shortly after birth, and were brought up by them; and 203 children (118 boys) were placed in foster care (group III), most of them before one year of age. In these cases there was no clear decision about the legal status of the child from the beginning, but almost all of these children grew up with their foster parents and a majority were subsequently legally adopted by them. Accordingly, the three groups represent three alternative models of placement for unwanted children: group I, adoption; group II, care by biological mothers; and group III, care in foster homes.

From the very beginning of our study, it was clear that these three alternative placements provided an excellent opportunity to compare and evaluate the results and influences of child welfare decisions on the social and personal development of the subjects.

The adopted children in Group I were placed in homes that had been prepared thoroughly for this task through a series of interviews before placement. Many adoptive parents had a good social, educational, and economic standing. The children in the other two groups had less favorable placement conditions. The biological mothers who took care of their children despite their earlier decision to have them adopted (group II) were predominantly young, unmarried or alone, and mostly unskilled. In general, their financial and social opportunities were limited.

The foster parents in group III were on the average older than the adoptive parents. Their education and occupational status were similar to those of the general population. In contrast to the children in the other two groups, these children grew up in small communities or in rural areas. These parents were seldom prepared by the social authorities for their task as nonbiological parents in the way that the adoptive parents in group I were. Payments from the child welfare organization were also the rule, at least at the beginning of the placement and until legal adoption was consummated.

The Biological Background

A large proportion of the biological parents appear in the registers of criminality and alcohol abuse, indicating that this parent population was of a strongly negative social selection. Thus about one-third of the biological fathers were found in the criminal register, which is a substantial overrepresentation, the figures to be expected for a representative group of men of the same age being about 10 percent.

Registered criiminality differed somewhat, although not significantly, between the three groups, being lowest in group I (27 percent), somewhat higher (34 percent) in group II, and highest (40 percent) in group III. It should be noted that most cases concerned recurrent criminality, frequently combined with offenses under the Temperance Act (abuse of alcohol). Altogether, 37 percent of the fathers were traced in the Excise Board's register of offenses under the Temperance Act. This may be compared with a figure of 18 percent in a representative population of men of about the same age. There were substantial differences among the three investigation groups: 26 percent in group I, 39 percent in group II, and 48 percent in group III. ($p < .01$).

Among biological mothers, there was also a higher prevalence of registrations for crime or alcohol abuse than would be expected in a random group of women (group I, 3.0 percent, group II, 1.5 percent, group III, 9.7 percent). It is clear from these figures alone that the biological parents were a selected group with a high frequency of social deficiency.

Regarding the outcome in the three groups, it is obvious that the process of placement itself involved a certain amount of selection of the children. In all three groups there was a high incidence of negative social factors connected with the biological background, but this was most obvious in group III. Through the collection of social and medical background data, we tried to make it possible to control for such selective factors in our future analyses.

General Design of the Study

The study was planned as a longitudinal ex-post-facto experiment, starting at time of pregnancy. Studies have been performed for both boys and girls at 11 and 15 years of age (in their school situation by interviews with teachers or questionnaires). Boys were studied at 18 regarding information about medical and psychological investigation at the time of their enlistment for military service. Controls matched for sex and age have been selected from school or population registers. Finally, we have obtained information about the boys at 22 to 23 years of age from the Criminal Register and Excise Board Register for alcohol abuse. Table 1 illustrates the various steps in the investigation over the years.

Table 1. General Design of the Study

	Cohort of 329 Boys Born 1956–1957		
	Group I	Group II	Group III
	Adopted	Restored to Biological Mother	Foster Children
Birth	$N = 93$	$N = 118$	$N = 118$
11 years: Teachers-interviews, schoolmarks	$N = 93$	$N = 106$	$N = 69^a$
15 years: teachers-questionnaire, school marks	$N = 89$	$N = 109$	$N = 113$
18 years: Military enlistment procedure	$N = 79$	$N = 93$	$N = 91$
22-23 years: Registration of criminality and alcohol abuse	$N = 93$	$N = 118$	$N = 118$

^{a}One-year group only.

Results: Investigation at 11 Years

The results of the interviews with teachers at 11 years showed that the adopted boys (group I) manifested a high rate of nervous and behavioral disturbances compared to class controls. Thus 22 percent were classified as "problem children," compared to 12 percent among their class controls ($p < .01$). There were, however, very few among either subjects or controls who could be classified as severely maladjusted at this age.

The two other groups showed the same rate of disturbances as that among the adopted boys, with 20 percent for group II and 22 percent for group III (versus controls of 12 and 8 percent respectively). These results were somewhat unexpected and contradicted our original hypotheses, since we had expected fewer disturbances among the adoptees, who had been brought up in much better socioeconomic circumstances than the children in groups II and III. The disturbances were, however, more pronounced in groups II and III when we looked more closely at the cases.

Investigation at 15 Years

Four years later, when the boys were attending the eighth class of the nine-year Swedish comprehensive schooling, we sent a questionnaire to their class teachers. The instruments used in this study were rating scales in which adjustment and behavior of the pupils were scored on 7-point scales. This study showed that the difference between adopted children and their classmates were by now of little consequence. There was still, admittedly, a slight tendency for them to have lower scores of adjustment in different variables compared with their controls, but these differences were very small and only occasionally significant. On the other hand, a considerable proportion of the boys in the two other groups now displayed yet stronger tendencies of maladjustment than were found at the age of 11. Among the adopted boys, 4.5 percent were classified as socially maladjusted, compared to 5.8 percent among the controls (score of 1−2 on a 7-point scale). Among boys in groups II and III, social maladjustment was two to three times as frequent among probands as among controls. In group II, 13.9 percent of the boys, compared to 5.3 percent of controls, were classified as socially maladjusted, and in group III, 12.2 percent of proband boys compared with 4.1 percent of their class controls. The term social maladjustment here stands for cases displaying, for instance, repeated truancy, delinquency, criminality, or abuse of alcohol or drugs.

Boys in group I displayed somewhat lower mean grades than controls, but these differences were relatively small. On the other hand, there were often highly significant differences on these items between children in groups II and III and their controls. So far adoption seemed to have been successful in neutralizing the social heritage among the adopted boys.

Boys at 18: Investigation at the Military Enlistment Procedure

Results are given elsewhere in this series [5], but, in summary, the interviews, tests, and investigations during the military enlistment procedure confirmed our observations at 15 years of age in all three groups. The adopted boys in group I showed much the same achievements in different tests and assessments as their age-related controls did, and we have not found any clear tendencies toward a positive or negative deviation in this group. The dropout rate was of the same magnitude as in the control group, and the adopted boys were taken out and screened for military leadership in the same proportion as the controls.

In contrast, subjects in groups II and III had relatively high frequencies of exemption due to sociopsychiatric reasons compared to controls and did not reach the same level of achievement as their controls or as subjects in group I.

Investigation at 22–23 Years: Registrations for Criminality and Alcohol Abuse

For all subjects in the cohort of boys and their controls (from the 18-year investigation) a search was made for entries in the Excise Board register (registrations for alcohol abuse) and in the criminal register. The Excise Board register contains information about fines imposed for intemperance, records of supervision by temperance boards, and time spent in institutions for alcoholics. In this context, the incurrence of a criminal sentence of more than 60 "day-fines" constitutes criminality. The records cover the period from the subjects' sixteenth birthdays up to 1979 when they were 22 to 23 years of age.

RESULTS

Our findings are summarized in Figure 1, which gives the accumulated frequencies of registrations for criminality, alcohol abuse, and the combination of both in the three groups. The age-matched controls have been collapsed to one group, because there were no differences between controls in the three groups. It is obvious that there was fairly good agreement between controls (15.5 percent) and probands in groups I and II (18.0 and 16.5 percent, respectively, differences not significant), whereas probands in group III displayed a considerable increase of registrations (29.2 percent). Alcohol abuse—alone or in combination with criminal offenses—seems to be a characteristic of this group. Our results are somewhat contradictory, since we had expected boys reared in nonbiological foster homes to be less prone to social maladjustment than boys in group II, who to a large extent had grown up under insecure social circumstances, at least in their early childhood.

Discussion

The results so far indicate that the deviations and nervous disturbances, which we found at the age of 11 in all three groups, were to a large extent overcome among the *adopted boys* (group I) in the three subsequent studies. Their social prognosis has evidently been neither better nor worse than for boys in general, and their intellectual capacity, measured and classified during the enlistment procedure, showed about the same level as that of their age-matched controls. Registrations for criminality and alcohol abuse were also of the same magnitude as that of the general population. Regarding

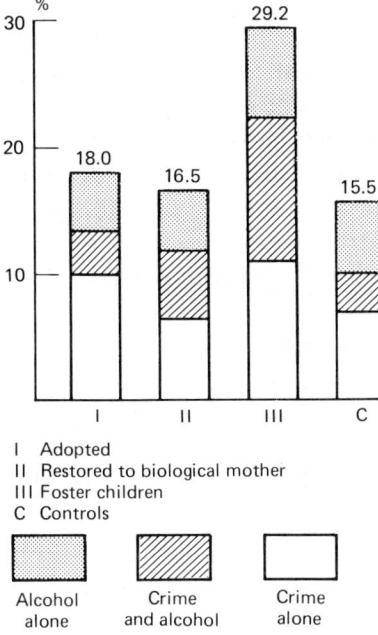

Figure 1. Criminality and alcohol abuse.

the high frequency of criminality and alcohol abuse among the biological parents of these boys, the conclusion is warranted that adoption largely reduced the risk of social incompetence among these adoptees. Accordingly, the "social heritage" seems to have been by and large neutralized by the secure placement that a well-prepared adoption offers.

The adoptive parents belonged to the higher professional and intermediate occupational groups. The controls, on the other hand, were randomly distributed, and thus it is conceivable that their parents' occupations corresponded to the distribution in the general population. For that reason the adopted boys could be expected to have higher intellectual capacity than did their controls (taking an environmental view). There may be various reasons for this failure to keep up with their social class level. Perhaps the adoptive situation in itself is fraught with complications that have had a negative impact on the general level of achievement. One explanation could be the influence of genetic factors. At present we do not have sufficient data to elucidate this question.

A somewhat unexpected finding in our study was the negative outcome among the foster children in group III. The socioeconomic status of the biological parents of these boys was significantly lower than that of the other two groups, which may explain the low school achievement to some extent, supposing a genetic influence. But, after all, these children were placed at an early age (mean age 9 months) in socially stable foster families, where they, with few exceptions, stayed permanently. The socioeconomic status of these families was fairly equal to that of the general population. A majority of these children were also subsequently legally adopted.

It is also true that other negative background factors such as perinatal complications, alcohol abuse, and/or criminality among biological parents were more common in this group of boys. However, our analyses at ages 11 and 15, taking such factors into account, did not give a sufficient explanation to the unfavorable outcome of this group.

The high frequency of registration for alcohol abuse and/or criminality possibly may reflect a genetically determined transmission. Recently published investigations of about 2000 adoptees [3, 4, 8] showed a high prevalence of alcohol abuse among the adopted-away sons of alcoholic parents, indicating genetic factors behind alcoholism. It is conceivable that the adopted boys in the present, younger sample of foster children have now reached an age when the exposition of the drinking habits in their environment also interacts with constitutionally genetic factors, increasing the risk of developing alcohol abuse and alcoholism. So far, however, our preliminary analyses do not support this conjecture.

Since alcohol abuse or criminality was common among the biological parents in all three groups, it is obvious that the boys in group III have reacted differently and much more negatively in regard to to their social heritage. One possible explanation of this strongly negative outcome among boys in foster homes may be connected with placement procedures. Foster parents in group III were seldom prepared before the placement of the child the way the adopting parents in group I were. There was also legal and psychological insecurity connected with the placement, since there was no guarantee that the child could not some day be moved back again to the biological mother. Many foster parents had to live with this feeling of insecurity for years, and this may have had a negative influence on the rearing situation. As a matter of fact, foster parents in interviews often expressed their concern about the insecure situation during the first years after the placement. It is conceivable that this situation may have affected the relationship between children and foster parents and impaired the healthy development of the former.

Our study also indicates a considerable risk for social maladjustment and school failure among children reared by their biological mothers, who were originally prepared to leave the child for adoption, but who later changed their minds and took care of their children themselves. Their social maladjustment did not, however, reach the same level as that of the children who were placed in foster homes, which may after all reflect a more stable personality development in this group of children compared to children reared in foster homes.

The implication of our study for the general policy of the care of children at risk is of course *not* that adoption is always the best solution for a child with social handicaps. Rather, the conclusion must be that early preventive work is important. Preparation and support should be given to everybody in charge of the child. But in the best interest of the child, decisions about the child's legal status should be made as early as possible, and prolonging the socially and psychologically insecure situation of foster care should be avoided [9].

When one looks at the very negative social heritage for the whole cohort of these unwanted children, it seems likely that the intervention and decisions made by parents, social welfare authorities, and the adoption agency at the time of the child's birth have had a very decisive influence on later life opportunities and careers, in both positive and negative directions.

References

1. Bohman, M. *Adopted Children and Their Families. A Follow-up Study of Adopted Children, Their Background, Environment and Adjustment.* Proprius, Stockhom, 1970.
2. Bohman, M. A comparative study of adopted children, foster children and children in their biological environment born after undesired pregnancies. *Acta Pediatr. Scand.*, Suppl. 221 (1971).
3. Bohman, M. Some Genetic Aspects of Alcoholism and Criminality. *Arch. Gen. Psychiatr.*, 35 (1978), 269–276.
4. Bohman, M., Cloninger, R., and Sigvardsson, S. Maternal inheritance of alcohol abuse: Cross-fostering analysis of adopted women. *Arch. Gen. Psychiatr.*, 38 (1981).
5. Bohman, M., and Sigvardsson, S. An 18-year, prospective, longitudinal study of adopted boys. In Anthony, E.J., Koupernick, C., and Chiland, C., Eds. *The Child in His Family*, vol. 4. Wiley, New York, 1978.
6. Bohman, M., and Sigvardsson, S. A Prospective, longitudinal study of children registered for adoptions: A 15-year follow-up. *Acta Psychiatr. Scand.*, 61 (1980a), 339–355.

7. Bohman, M., and Sigvardsson S.: Negative Social Heritage: Adoption and fostering as preventive measures: a prospective longitudinal study of boys of negative social heritage. *Adoption & Fostering*, 3 (1980b).
8. Cloninger, R., Bohman, M., and Sigvardsson, S. Inheritance of alcohol abuse. Cross-fostering analysis of adopted men. *Arch. Gen. Psychiatr.*, 38 (1981).
9. Goldstein, J., Freud, A., and Solnit, A. *Beyond the Best Interests of the Child.* The Free Press, London, 1973.
10. Jonsson, G.: Delinquent boys. *Acta Psychiatr. Scand.,* Suppl. 195 (1967).
11. Robins, L.N. *Deviant Children Grown Up: A Sociological and Psychiatric Study of Sociopathic Personality.* Williams & Wilkins, Co., Baltimore, Md., 1966.

A Site Visit to the Family Village at Skå-Edeby in Stockholm

Karen Madsen (Denmark)

The International Study Group members visited this treatment center for children and their families, which has been in existence for about 35 years. It was started by Dr. Gustav Jonsson, and he actively directed it until a few years ago when he retired, although still remaining a consultant. The directorship is now divided between Ted Winther, who has been the administrative leader for the last 30 years, and Bengt Borjeson, who is currently responsible for the treatment and research programs. Set in a wooded area and built on a cottage system, this unique Swedish institution has not only been a model for the residential treatment of children but has brought about many innovations in the approach to the multiple problems of neglected and deprived children and their families.

When Jonsson first started the village, he took in boys and girls between the ages of 7 and 15 years who had been unable to socialize in the conventional outside world.

In 1972, the institution changed its direction from a children's village to a family village that specialized in family treatment. It took in about 10 to 12 families a year. The shift from a child-centered to a family-centered orientation brought about concomitant changes not only in the treatment program but also in the areas of education and research.

The family units vary in size from a mother–child dyad to a family group comprising 11 members. Admission to the village is on a volunteer basis, at least in principle; parents who have been referred to the village by the Department of Social Welfare might well have their children removed from them and placed in foster homes should they refuse to participate. Fortunately, this is a rare problem, and the more common difficulty is to get families to return to Stockholm after the 10-month program offered by the village. Like many guests, they are reluctant to leave once they settle in.

In the past few years, there has been a change in the type of family referred to Skå: The children are younger, mostly below 7 years, and the parents are parents in spite of themselves and unable to cope with the problems of child rearing. The situation is further aggravated by the fact that most of them are drug abusers.

During their stay at Skå, the families receive money from the Department of Social Welfare, which is used to pay for their Stockholm apartment as well as their living expenses. The housing at the village is free. The parents generally are without jobs when they come but obtain employment at Skå as part of the rehabilitation process, and before they leave the village, attempts are made to find some employment for them. A social worker from the Department of Social Welfare visits every two weeks to attend case conferences, particularly with respect to families about to return to Stockholm. The children attend school at Skå and remain the school for a year following their families' departure.

One of the important goals of treatment is to render the families personally and socially acceptable to other families outside, so that the therapeutic task consisted not only of changing intrafamilial relationships but also of establishing a system of friendly "helpers." The village has obtained its best results with drug abusers who show some motivation to stop, families with drinking problems, and single mothers. They have been least successful with those in a primary phase of drug abuse or in physical and psychological marital conflict where the parental control systems are very weak, and marriages that are heading very rapidly toward divorce. The treatment at Skå tends to make it difficult for the mother to initiate change because of the good support system provided by the village, and at the same time the father seems more or less left out of the picture and worse off afterwards.

The professional group consists of psychologists, social workers, psychiatric consultants, and teachers, most of whom have their own homes as Skå, frequently close to the cottages housing the guest families. What is most refreshing about this center is the open-mindedness of the staff to new ideas, their readiness to discuss their methods and results, and their willingness to consider alternate approaches. This degree of flexibility seems to work very well in the treatment of multiple problem families. What is most surprising for an institution is that after 35 years, it is still advancing and thriving.

Discussion of Papers Presented at Gälöfsta

Chairman: Lionel Hersov, M.D. (U.K.)

E. J. Anthony (U.S.A.) addressed himself to the presentation by Jonsell on psychosocial risk factors in children. Although the investigation was focused on intergroup differences, he felt that there were a number of important prospective questions in the mind of the researcher of which the two basic ones could be formulated: Did physical complaints lacking a physical basis predict a serious psychosocial maladjustment at some future date, and could early screening and adequate interventions at the initial stage help prevent this? The third question concerns the "lost" child—the patients that are referred by pediatricians to the child psychiatrist but never get there. What happens to them on the way? The fourth and fifth questions are both highly pertinent to the liaison physician: Is reduced susceptibility to infection a function of psychosocial stress, and do the baseless somatic symptoms serve as a passport to the psychiatrist? The significant intergroup differences found by Jonsell have also been present in a number of other studies: broken homes, parent loss, teenage mothering, psychiatrically disordered parents, problem families, alcoholism, and families on welfare are all well recognized and well-documented antecedents to emotional disorders. However, why do some children from such settings somatize or "convert" their psychological stresses? The screening for psychological factors can be done very sensitively by trained clinicians or crudely by investigators with very little clinical knowledge of children. Symptom checklists have been a popular but somewhat simplistic method of exploring this psychophysical cluster of headaches, nausea, abdominal pain, palpitations, anorexia, and paraesthesias in combination with emotionalism, and the syndrome has been paraded under different names: Hysteria (Robins and O'Neal, 1954), conversion symptoms (Herman and Simonds, 1975), conversion reactions (Rock, 1971). The first study, based on children treated at a pediatric hospital, came up with a figure of 4 percent. The second study, based on children deferred from the pediatric to the child psychiatric clinic, gave a figure of 3.6 percent, and the third study, using the same criteria as the second study (baseless somatic symptoms, emotional triggering, psychiatric evaluation revealing psychological symptoms) produced a figure of 4.1 percent at a Hawaiian V.A. hospital. All these fit very well with Jonsell's findings. However, there was a consensus in the American studies that the incidence rates were determined by geographic and ethnic factors, criteria for diagnosis, the source of referral, and the nature of the egency delivering the services. There were other inconsistencies. In the Missouri study, incidence increased with age and was highest in the adolescent, whereas in the Hawaiian study, the reverse was true and the lowest incidence was at adolescence. Furthermore, in child guidance clinics, the incidence of hysteria is about 1.3 percent as compared with almost 22 percent of children seen in a pediatric in-patient service. Almost a third of the cases in the age range of 13 to 16 years on an in-patient pediatric ward were regarded as having a "hysterical" component. Jonsell mentions other aggravating factors interfering with psychosocial diagnosis: the pediatricians' notorious lack of time; the presence of an overriding somatic complaint that pushes the psychological factor to the periphery of awareness, and a lack of adequate contact among the physician, the parent, and the child. There will always be "psychologically blind" pediatricians, and there will always be parents who shudder at the very mention of the psychological and regard it as a stigma. The poor training in psychiatry given to students at some medical schools where lab technology is stressed is also a reason that some of these children remain undiagnosed and therefore often mistreated. Still other questions were raised by this thoughtful paper. Would adequate psychiatric coverage reduce unnecessary laboratory examinations and the concomitant expense? Would patients and their families feel less stigmatized if the pediatric and psychiatric clinics were coterminous and not segregated? Would a psychophysiological clinic run by pediatricians and child psychiatrists working synergistically and not competitively with one another make life smoother for the patient? Professional workers should keep two aspects constantly in mind: a physical illness is always complicated to some extent by secondary psychological reactions, and psychiatric illnesses in children invariably have some minor or major somatic expression. A third factor to bear in mind is that every illness in the child imposes stress on the rest of the family and can produce symptoms in other members. In one study, 14 percent of children between 6 and 19 years old suffered from recurrent abdominal pain and 20 percent from recurrent headaches. Over an eight-year period of study, the parents had similar somatic complaints. One might think of this as familial psychophysiological disorders, an "identification with an ill parent", or a somatically induced *folie à deux*. Different children develop different capacities for "body management" and different formations of a self-caring ego when reared by different parents. Some parents encourage the early development of physical autonomy, whereas others continue to cultivate somatic dependency. In the management of the psychosocial cases, children are often able to learn about their bodies and why they behave the way they do in response to certain stresses. One should also respect children's needs to understand their symptomatology and discuss with them their theories of illness. One should always complete a good physical examination and perform any necessary laboratory tests. One should always interpret the findings to the parents, carefully avoiding ambiguity and uncertainty. Unless there is definite evidence of physical disorder, one should present the parents and the child with a clean bill of health. One should endeavor to return the child to school if he or she is absent, correct any negative environmental conditions that are operating, and counsel the parents specifically with regard to management of the condition. At all times, one should maintain an ongoing communication among the child psychiatrist, pediatrician, parents, and school. One should never forget to inquire about the child's capacity to play and opportunities for playing, since this is an important barometer of both psychological and physical health in the child.

Dr. Lansdown complimented Dr. Otto on his multifactorial understanding of the nature of suicide in children and adolescents. He wondered if there were not some common factors in suicidal acts among the young and quoted Alverez (1971), himself a failed suicide: "I offer no solutions. I don't in fact believe that solutions exist since suicide means different things to different people at different times . . . The only conceiveable solution the suicide can hope for is help of one kind or another." The need for help around the clock is made clear in this paper, but perhaps we should not only look to the psychiatric clinics to provide this help. Nonprofessional workers have been able to work successfully with families that abuse their children, and the Samaritans set up their first emergency service in 1953 on a 24-hour basis. Psychiatrists and social workers are used as consultants, and perhaps a similar model might be applied to the problem of suicide. (In the United States, a call-in service operates in many cities and potential suicidal patients are encouraged to use the "hot line" that gets them a ready and sympathetic listener at the other end of the wire.) Lansdown also questioned the role of aggressiveness in suicides by young people, but here he did not differentiate between the suicidal attempt and the suicidal act. In 1910, Stekel said "no one kills himself who has never wanted to kill another, or at least wish the death of another." It would be surprising if there were any symptom unaffected by the process of development. It has been 83 years since Durkheim (1897) published his sociological study of suicide, but there still seems to be a dearth of good studies on children and early adolescents (except for David Shaffer's known work in Britain). Many clinicians feel that suicide at this age is passed off as an accident. However, bodies of suicides are no longer rejected for interment in Christian burial grounds, so the stigma has lessened. In the Middle Ages, a suicide was buried at a crossroads with a stake through the heart, presumably to stop the spirit from returning to damage others. Perhaps the denial of suicide in the young may represent a refusal to deal with the haunting effects aroused in such circumstances.

The I.S.G. was presented with an interesting but controversial account of the educational system in Sweden, and there was some question among our Swedish colleagues as to whether it accurately reflected what was actually taking place today in Swedish schools. There seemed to be two major themes in the presentation: the compelling necessity on the part of the educators to have the children learn, irrespective of their interest; and second, the need to provide help for those children who have personal problems leading to behavioral disturbances, the control of which lies beyond the skills of a classroom teacher.

The question of compulsion, with its deeper and wider implication of "social engineering" aimed at fostering social and intellectual equality, provoked a lively discussion. The "outsider's" view is summarized by Dr. Lansdown, and we have decided to print his remarks as being of more general interest.

References

1. Alvarez, A. *The Savage God: A Study of Suicide.* Random House, New York, 1972.
2. Durkheim, E. *Le Suicide; Etude de Sociologie.* Alcan, Paris, 1897.
3. Robins, E. and O'Neal, P. Clinical features of hysteria in children, with a note on prognosis; a two to 17-year follow-up study of 41 patients. *Nerv. Ch.*, 10,s (1953), 246-271.
4. Rock, N. L. Conversion reactions in childhood: a clinical study on childhood neuroses. *J. Am. Acad. Ch. Psychia.*, 10 (1971), 65-93.
5. Shaffer, D. Suicide in childhood and early adolescence. *J. Ch. Psychol & Psychia.*, 15,4 (1974), 275-291.
6. Stengel, E. *Suicide and Attempted Suicide.* MacGibbon & Kee, Bristol, 1964.

Richard Lansdown, Ph.D. (U.K.). First, on compulsion and social engineering: In Britain and, I suspect, in the United States and France, the school system can be seen to operate with a powerful hidden curriculum. The open curriculum has to do with math, English, history, cricket, and cookery lessons. The hidden curriculum has to do with the transmission of expectations (we can consider the meaning of the transmissions referred to by Dr. Cederblad) and operates by virtue of the extremity of the differences between schools. In Sweden the message is, we will compel you to be equal whatever your social origins. In Britain the message is, we will educate you in part according to your intelligence and in part according to your parent's purse. Approximately 10 percent of British children attend independent schools, and we perversely call the most expensive and elite of these public schools. Although some independent schools provide poor teaching in inadequate conditions, many of them are lavishly staffed, with ample libraries, laboratories, and playing fields. They are very expensive, costing about 12,000 crowns per year for a day school and three times that much for a boarding school, and they compare strikingly with the average state school, many of which are faced with financial cuts so severe that they can no longer afford to buy new books for their pupils. The public schools continue to provide a disproportionate number of undergraduates to Oxford and Cambridge, which remain in a socially different league from all other universities.

There is no doubt also that there are enormous differences between schools in the state system. We do not have the centralization that is evident in Sweden or in France. Every head teacher can, in consultation with the staff, decide what will be taught when, subject only to a compulsory religious education lesson. This can lead to anomalies of children in the same school being taught to read or to calculate by different methods according to the desires of their teachers. There are visits by school inspectors, and occasional glaringly bizarre activities are revealed (for instance, the lessons in a London primary school that consisted of children playing table-tennis for large parts of every day).

But do these differences really matter? Does the hidden curriculum exert any power, or is it simply an irritant to left-wing intellectuals? Teachers, in Britain at least, seem reluctant to agree to the idea that schools in themselves have any effect; instead they look to factors in the home and in society to explain variations in behavior and learning. Michael Power, a sociologist, offered evidence to suggest that in London school organization can affect delinquency rates. He was not allowed to set foot in a London school again. More recently, Michael Rutter and colleagues have offered similar evidence on attainment in secondary schools. The work has been widely attacked, especially by educators.

Perhaps both Rutter and Power asked the wrong questions. Perhaps schools do affect children, but it may be naive to say either that schools bring about social change or that society determines the educational system, because both statements are oversimplifications of a complex pattern of interrelated events. We should compare the findings on Northern Ireland: to look only to the events of the "troubles" to explain stress is to look only at part of the picture.

To move to the second theme, that of the provision for the disturbed or disturbing child, I would like first to throw out some random points. There was a note in the paper of increasing behavior problems but no mention of differences between town and country districts. I recently attended a conference in Somerset, a peaceful, beautiful county in the west of England. One speaker from an inner city school was introduced as "straight from the battlefield." Comparative work in Britain has suggested that rates of maladjustment in cities are at least twice as high as those in country areas. My own work in India has taught me that the urban–rural split there is even greater than in Europe. I was interested to hear that in Sweden you have 80 percent of your population in towns. In India it is a mirror image, with 80 percent in the rural areas.

Another random point is hyperactivity. In the United States more children are called hyperactive than in Britain, but is this because of a difference in diagnostic criteria or because American children are more active? Is the prevalence rising in Sweden? If so, can we begin to establish causes? Perhaps the concept of the aniara child is helpful here.

Finally, what effective help can be given to our schools? The Swedish system has ample money and many professionals. But are the professionals, the way they work at present, meeting the need? As Colette Chiland has said, increased provision seems to bring in its train increases in problems. The child guidance movement and the work of the child psychiatrist are both under fire in Britain at the moment, a key paper being one published several years ago in the London Educational Review by Jack Tizard. Child psychiatrists and the traditional model of the child guidance clinic are accused simply of not having delivered the goods. Educational psychologists now work far more independently of psychiatrists than they did even 10 years ago, but their therapeutic armory is often limited to what seems to me to be crudely applied behavioral techniques. If I am to believe the article in the current edition of the London magazine *Encounter,* the psychoanalytic contribution to mental health in America is declining fast, and the stage is set for a massive change in work on behavior problems in schools. If this change is to be effective, it must be monitored as carefully as any counterpart in physical medicine. Do we, though, have the tools to do this?

Reference

Rutter, M., et al. *Fifteen Thousand Hours,* Penguin Books, London, 1979.

Professor Rolf Zetterstrom presented a paper (which we are, unfortunately, unable to print) that raised the following interesting issues: Can feeding disturbances in children, ill enough to be hospitalized, act as a pediatric marker of probable psychosomatic illness and associated etiologic factors, particularly disorders in the mother and in her capacity to nurture her child? Can there be a possible link between the feeding disturbance and the etiologic factor through an inadequate bonding of the mother to her infant at the beginning of the feeding relationship? The discussion by Professor Gerald Caplan (Israel) had such a high order of pertinence to studies of this nature that we decided to publish it for its intrinsic worth.

Gerald Caplan, M.D. (Israel). It would be useful to explain the basis for this bonding disorder by collecting anamnestic data on early mother–infant interactive behavior to validate our current assumption that in many cases there has been an absence of frontal bodily contact and eye contact between infant and mother, or a current personality disorder of the mother that makes it difficult for her to build a healthy nurturing relationship with her baby. Contributing factors in the former case would be several weeks of bodily separation of infant and mother because of prematurity or early hospitalization of the infant, due to bodily illness.

The presentation indicates that in sick children with feeding disorders there is the empirical finding of an associated constellation of adverse psychosocial factors that Professor Zetterstrom believes to be of etiologic importance. I would prefer this constellation to be divided into three subgroups to allow for fruitful analysis.

1. *Long-term risk factors,* such as mental illness of a parent, alcoholism of a parent, one-parent family, chronic severe illness in a close family member, pregnancy or birth trauma, socioeconomic deformation, premature birth, and so forth.

Empirical studies have shown that children exposed to such risk factors have a higher incidence of mental disorder than a control group not exposed to such factors. *But* not all children exposed to even high levels of such risk factors become psychologically ill. To explain this we must take into account the next two factors.

2. *Current or recent life stress in the family.* Recent object loss or social deprivation or disruptive life change. Here too the outcome in terms of pathology is influenced but not determined by this factor alone.

3. *Current social supports.* Of importance are emotional support and cognitive guidance for the mother, such as from a loving husband, a nurturing family, and solicitous and helpful friends, neighbors, and community caregivers.

A number of recent, well-designed empirical studies have shown that a high level of risk factors and of recent life stress raise the incidence of physical or mental disorder *only* if there is a *low* level of such social support. This combination leads to a rise in nonspecific vulnerability to somatic or psychological disorders.

So, if indeed feeding disturbances in sick children constitute an effective marker for identification by pediatricians of children who are, or who will become, psychosomatically ill, the pediatrician should also collect anamnestic data on these three factors—preexisting risks, recent life stress, and current social supports—to illuminate a possible pattern of psychosocial burdens in children and their families that will help him or her understand the significance of what has been identified and plan preventive or remedial intervention.

It is important to alert pediatricians to the importance of these etiologic factors and to train young pediatricians to collect such anamnestic data. There is a difficulty in carrying out the latter because of the tendency of some parents to hide risk factors such as a history of psychiatric illness or social difficulties. Perhaps central computerized medical records can be tapped to reveal data that the denial or dissembling of parents may prevent their revealing during the initial anamnesis. Of course, either permission should be obtained from the parents for such a routine search of the computerized medical records of the family, or, if this permission is not given, the information must not be revealed to the parent. There is no intention of using it to confront the parent with noncompliance in the anamnestic investigation, since this would probably ruin the development of a trusting patient–doctor relationship.

Whatever the other psychotherapeutic or social welfare interventions that might be indicated by these anamnestic data, if direct observation by the pediatrician or nurses of mother–child interactive behavior on the ward (particularly in watching the mother feed her baby by breast or bottle or by an analogue with an older child) should reveal a disorder of bonding, this can often be remedied by appropriate retraining. The essence of the latter is to provide the nurturing parent—usually the mother, but sometimes the father—with repeated opportunities for frontal bodily contact and eye contact with the child; and also to provide a role model in the form of a nurse or child-care worker on the ward, or after discharge in the home, who demonstrates in action how to take care of the child in a warm and nurturant manner with a sensitive awareness of the behavioral cues that allow the child's needs to be identified and satisfied.

THE IBADAN CONFERENCE

The Mental Health of Children in Developing Countries

Phillip Graham, M.D.
Katherine Canavan, M.D. (U.K.)

Developing countries may vary in their characteristics, but, from the point of view of children, they share a number of unfavorable features. This makes it reasonable to consider them as a group, even though anyone planning services or practicing clinically in a developing country will be grossly handicapped without an intimate knowledge of the beliefs and attitudes of its people.

The adverse characteristics that damage the physical and mental health and indeed often prematurely end the lives of children must be summarized briefly. Widespread poverty results in inadequate stimulation of the developing child's mind. Malnutrition, present in from 400 to 1000 million of the world's population and most prevalnt among children, when it does not result in premature death, produces mild mental retardation and increased vulnerability to behavior disturbance. Acute and chronic infections, (not surprising when, for example, only about 20 percent of the population in Southeast Asia has access to a reasonably uncontaminated water supply) when they do no kill, frequently produce brain damage or dysfunction. Lack of available schooling contributes to low literacy rates, often around 20 percent in developing countries, in both parents and children. Inadequate employment opportunities in rural areas result in a population drift to towns and big cities where family support systems are lacking and children are readily neglected. If the goal of health for all by the year 2000 formulated at the joint WHO/UNICEF conference at Alma Ata is to be achieved, and if health for all includes the mental health of children, the ground to be covered in a short period of time is considerable. In addition, a public health approach to the problem rather than an approach geared to the provision of psychiatric services to individual patients is indicated. In so-called developed countries it may or may not be reasonable to spend time discussing the appropriate ratio of child psychiatrists to the child population. In developing countries, where poverty, malnutrition, infection, illiteracy, and family breakdown through forced migration are so widespread and so obviously militate against the enjoyment of mental health, such an approach surely seems wildly irrelevant.

Child Mental Health and Malnutrition

A useful distinction has been drawn between absolute and relative deprivation [18]. Absolute deprivation exists when the basic needs of an individual have not been met. Such needs include not only adequate food and protection from intolerable climatic conditions such as intense heat or cold, but also, in the case of a child, the provision of sufficient continuous and loving care to allow the development of the capacity to survive socially as well as physically. Such care is not a luxury but, as illustrated by the fate of those children in orphanages and in other circumstances who fail to receive it, a basic necessity for survival. In developed countries, where absolute deprivation is experienced by only a tiny minority of children, it is no longer considered by sociologists, who have concerned themselves with the description of poverty [24], to be a useful criterion for social or political action. The self-perception of the individual as deprived of necessary resources, or the suffering of multiple disadvantages on objectively defined criteria, are thought to be more relevant [20]. But in developing countries, individuals living in absolutely deprived circumstances are common, and, from a health point of view, the most striking indication of absolute deprivation is malnutrition.

In most developed countries, where there is an overabundance of food, even gross psychological disturbance in mothers does not, except very rarely, result in undernutrition in the child. This is not the case in developing countries where it is now generally recognized that psychological factors in the mother and in the child may be of major importance in determining malnutrition and its adverse effects. The scientific evidence for the behavior and cognitive sequelae of chronic undernutrition have been reviewed elsewhere

[9]. The association of poverty and material deprivation with malnutrition makes it difficult to identify the degree to which lack of food is, by itself, a cause of psychological deficit. Brothers and sisters of children who have been hospitalized for malnutrition perform almost as poorly as their hospitalized sibs on intelligence tests and show higher levels of behavior disturbance when compared to children reared in more favorable circumstances [17]. The importance of psychological factors in the development of malnutrition in areas where some parents manage to feed their children sufficient alimentation and others do not is now well established and can be regarded as of practical importance.

When the major causes of suffering in a child population are produced by poverty, malnutrition, and social disorganization, when so many children starve to death from lack of food and so many others are permanently impaired both physically and mentally as a result of early deprivation, is it reasonable to put any thought or resources at all into child mental health? It may be that psychological and social factors do determine to some degree who is malnourished, but, as the experience of developed countries demonstrates, where there is sufficient abundance of food, it is very unusual for even the psychologically most inadequate to suffer from malnutrition. Certainly it does not seem reasonable to suggest that concern for child mental health should take priority over concern for child bodily health, especially bodily survival. When a crop fails in a village and young children die as a result, one's thoughts must surely turn first to the relief of famine and to economic and social measures that might prevent a recurrence: improved agricultural techniques to increase food supply and the reduction of family size through family planning to ensure that there are fewer mouths to feed when the food supply again becomes tenuous. When, in a city, employment opportunities fail and men leave their homes to find work elsewhere and women and children are left to forage unsuccessfully for food after their departure, or when the breakdown of a traditional pattern of life in cities leads to family disruption and the wholesale abandonment of children in vast numbers, it is surely economic and social measures that should come to mind first in considering preventive remedies.

Unfortunately, however, effective economic and social solutions to these problems have not been found, and it would be optimistic indeed to consider that they *will* be found in the short-term future. This is partly because of the immensity of the problems that only recently have been thought of as a global responsibility. It is partly because the political institutions and social structures that exist contain strong built-in resistances to economic change, and because even when revolutionary transformations of political institutions do occur, the new governments merely reflect the interests of new elite groups, and there is little significant change in the lives of most people. Further, the social and psychological significance of traditional patterns of behavior such as dietary observances are so powerful that the injection of new knowledge threatening such belief systems is enormously difficult, even if such new knowledge (e.g., basic food and vitamin requirements) carries with it the key to physical survival.

In these circumstances it seems possible to justify a concern for child mental health in the following ways.

1. In areas where food is relatively scarce and the population is undernourished, greater awareness and understanding of the relationship between social incompetence and an inadequate food intake on the part of health workers and teachers is likely to improve the nutritional state of the population concerned. Starved children feed better when they are surrounded by those they love, and this is often not appreciated.

2. Measures to improve economic and social conditions in starvation areas will fail unless there is an understanding of the threat they pose to established patterns of behavior, including beliefs concerning child bearing and rearing. Someone has to be expert in identifying these patterns of behavior and beliefs.

3. Some measures to improve the physical well-being of the population will have coincidental beneficial effects on cognitive and emotional development. Others, such as those for improving the nutrition of children, which require disruption of bond formation and maintenance, will have a reverse effect. There is a need for a group of people who can advise government departments and other responsible bodies on the deployment of scarce resources with this in mind.

4. Children who are brain damaged or behaviorally disordered as a result of malnutrition and infection (e.g., those suffering from postencephalitic disturbances) have a right to assessment and treatment at least no less than adults similarly affected do.

5. People now look for improvements in their well-being at all social levels. It is futile to attempt to hold back progress among the relatively well-to-do until the less well-off have caught up. Experi-

ence from our own society suggests that amelioration of the living conditions in the poor is more likely to occur most rapidly when improvements for the rich have also been enjoyed. The revolutionary pursuit of total equality, which is an unrealistic aim, results in the creation of new power elites and little change in the distribution of goods. The reformist pursuit of greater equality is a realistic aim that, in the improvement in the standard of living of all social classes, often leads to the greater benefit of the poorer-off. Of course there comes a time when injustice and inequality are so widespread and reformist measures promise so little that revolutionary change may be justified. Discussion of the point at which this may be said to have occurred is, of course, beyond the scope of this paper. For our purposes it is only necessary to note that in sections of the population that are no longer preoccupied with physical survival, the psychological well-being of children is surely a legitimate concern. It also seems reasonable to expect those of us who have experience of the workings of the psychological and psychiatric services in developed countries to communicate our doubts regarding their structure and function so that the same mistakes are at least not automatically repeated.

Impact of Psychosocial Intervention on Nutritional State

It is now well recognized that protein−calorie malnutrition, the most important health problem facing children in the developing world, has a significant effect on cognitive development that interacts with social disadvantage but can also be seen to have its own independent effect [27]. Chronic malnutrition, according to Werner, appears to have "unique effects on attention, short-term memory, perceptual−motor development and motivation." Motivation is of particular importance because it is crucial in a vicious cycle: relative lack of food supply—malnutrition—impaired motivation—reduced chances of obtaining food in a situation of relative scarcity. This often ends in death but may be seen to change during a hospital admission when the first signs of a child's recovery from a malnourished state are an increase in energy and motivation, and a lift in affective state.

Psychological understanding of child development may contribute to the capacity to combat malnutrition in a number of ways.

Traditional Beliefs. It is common practice in many traditional societies for children to remain on the breast for two years or more until the birth of the next child. Malnutrition arises because readily available local foods are not introduced into the children's diets until weaning occurs. Therefore, weaning not only may be abrupt, but children may be transferred from the care of their mothers (with whom, because of the prolonged period of breast feeding, they have built up an unusually close relationship), to the care of relatives to whom they have only a slight attachment. The depression that may ensue for psychological reasons may then be compounded with the apathy arising from a less than adequate diet to initiate the vicious cycle outlined. A knowledge and understanding of these processes may assist the primary health worker to identify children at special risk for malnutrition (because separated from their mothers) and to suggest measures that might prevent or ameliorate the situation. Such an approach is not currently emphasized in primary health worker training.

Prevention. Measures to teach uneducated mothers living in rural or slum areas the importance of an adequate diet for the health and well-being of their children have not, in the past, met with conspicuous success. The introduction of new beliefs and practices has met strong resistance and suspicion. However, various efforts have been reported that, although perhaps not based directly on psychological understanding, have nevertheless involved a greater acknowledgment of psychological mechanisms than has hitherto been the case. The Road to Health card devised by Morley [14] is an example. This card, which is ideally given to and kept by the mother with the assistance of the primary health worker, enables the mother herself to chart the physical growth of her child and to detect a dropoff in physical progress at an early stage. This is an example of how individuals can be stimulated to take more informed responsibility for their own family care.

Hospital Admission. The treatment of malnutrition has improved considerably over the past two decades, and this improvement has not been limited to physical or biochemical considerations. In many crowded, understaffed hospitals, uneducated mothers, after instruction, have been given considerable responsibility in the maintenance of fluid intake for their malnourished infants, and it has been realized that infants thrive better if their mothers continue to be involved in looking after them. Further, it has been demonstrated [6] that improving the quality of environmental stimulation from nurses actually reduces the length of admission in malnourished babies.

Outpatient Care of Established Cases of Malnutrition. Ramsey, [16] has described a procedure for dealing with children admitted to the hospital for malnutrition which, he claims, not only reduces the likelihood of recurrence, but also has an impact on the total level of nutritional problems in the population. After the child's admission to the hospital unit, the guardian is interviewed by a nurse on details not only of diet but also of home circumstances. After the child is discharged, the nurse visits the home and appraises the situation, giving advice on homemaking where necessary. Particular efforts are made to help families with socioeconomic problems, the aim being to prevent a recurrence either in the identified hospitalized child or in the sibs. Community surveys carried out before the program was instituted in 1969 and after it was terminated in 1975 revealed a decline in the number of infants falling below the third percentile for height and weight from 16.5 to 10.2 percent. Over the same period, the infant mortality rate declined from 54.1 to 29.1 per 1000 live births. Before the study began, readmission for malnutrition had been necessary for one in four of the children admitted. After the program had been under way for some time, the need for readmission disappeared completely. Doubtless factors other than the program played some part in this considerable improvement, but it seems probable that the program was at least partly responsible.

Group Self-Help. The Road to Health card is one example of how greater individual self-help in infant nutrition can be achieved. In a recent publication [10], a number of initiatives are described from centers as far afield as Colombia, the Cameroons, and Senegal, in which mothers have themselves dealt with the unsatisfactory child arrangements normally made while women work in the fields. In these circumstances it is common for young children only 5 to 6 years old to be left to supervise even younger children and babies. Dissatisfied with this situation and stimulated by educators and primary health workers, mothers have grouped together in villages in each of these countries, although doubtless not on a very wide scale, to improve the situation. In Senegal, for example, mothers now operate day centers set up to help during the two months that they work in the rice paddies on a year-round basis. They take turns looking after the children and share knowledge with the local teacher and primary care workers on improvement in hygiene, diet, and the stimulation of learning processes.

It must be emphasized that in the improvement of child nutrition in the developing world, psychological intervention of the type just described must never be regarded as any sort of substitute for the most urgent masures required to deal with the situation. These have been listed [25] as involving supplementary feeding in pregnancy and during lactation, encouragement of breast-feeding, prevention of nutritional deficiency diseases, dealing with moderate forms of malnutrition, and treatment of severe protein–calorie malnutrition. Nevertheless, in the achievement of these goals, in the engagement of parents in measures to help themselves on both an individual and a group basis, in improvements in out-patient and hospital care, and in overcoming traditional beliefs and practices that disrupt bonding and promote unsatisfactory feeding habits, it is clear that psychological understanding could well have some part to play.

The mental health professional in a developing country probably has rather little input into health policies concerning measures to combat malnutrition at the present time and is similarly not likely to be involved in measures such as family planning, vaccination, and immunization programs that have a vital role in sustaining the health of the child population. Nevertheless, psychiatrists dealing with children are by no means as cut off from the diagnosis and management of organic disorders as are their counterparts in Western Europe and North America. In particular, they are likely to spend a great deal of time dealing with children suffering from epilepsy and mental retardation who, in the Western medical structure, tend to be dealt with by pediatricians or family doctors.

It is probable that rates of epilepsy are higher in developing than in developed countries [9], and a small number of comparative epidemiological studies confirm this view [5]. This well may be because certain infections such as malaria, not occurring in the West, are a frequent cause of febrile convulsions sometimes leading to epilepsy, and other conditions like measles occur in a much more dangerous form in developing countries—again with febrile convulsions and subsequent brain dysfunction as a common outcome. In Western countries, sufferers from epilepsy are stigmatized, for example, sometimes unnecessarily placed in special schools when they could be educated in ordinary schools. This situation is slowly improving. It is not surprising that in many traditional societies the strange and sudden nature of the epileptic fit has given rise to beliefs that result in the sufferers being virtually outcast from ordinary life. Billingshurst et al. [2] have described how in some African village societies epilepsy is thought to arise as a result of witchcraft. Children are kept away from sufferers of epilepsy, including child sufferers, because the condition is thought to be infectious. Children with epilepsy are automatically thought to be of low intelligence even though there may be very little evidence for this view. Their fits are taken to indicate that they are especially likely to show violent behavior. It is probable that these beliefs sometimes produce their own confirmation. It would not be surprising if children neglected and outcast as a result of stigmatization sometimes reacted with seriously aggressive behavior. If, as Billingshurst et al. [2] report, even in areas where education is universal, only 25 percent of children with epilepsy are allowed to attend school, it is surely only to be expected that a myth will become perpetuated that these children are of low intellectual ability.

Severe mental retardation is the other organic condition seen as within the province of the psychiatrist and other mental health professionals in a developing country. The prevalence of mental retardation has not been the subject of study to any great degree, but it seems probable that the low standards of perinatal care, especially in some rural areas, and the high rates of infection often involving the brain occurring in early childhood, produce many children with this problem. Axton and Levy [1], on the basis of their experience with African children in Rhodesia (now Zimbabwe), suggest that many children with severe retardation in developing countries succumb at an early age. This is particularly likely to occur if the children suffer from associated psychiatric disorders, and Lotter [12] has suggested that autistic syndromes are less common in African mentally handicapped children than in handicapped children living in developed countries.

It is likely that, as material standards of living and the quality of health care improve in developing countries, the incidence (number of new cases) of severe mental retardation will rise, but the prevalence (frequently of occurrence in the general population) will remain about the same because more handicapped children will survive. Doubtless there will then be a demand for better community facilities for educating such children. It seems important, however, for those living in developing and developed countries to achieve better ways of sharing the enormous burden that such children present to their families. Institutionalization, which it is now agreed, is an inappropriate way to deal with the problem, did at least achieve a sharing of the burden. If this approach is to be discarded, how can greater sharing of the load be achieved in the community? This remains an unsolved problem.

Mild and moderate degrees of mental retardation are probably very common in developing countries, but experience in developed countries might make one wonder in which way this should be regarded as a matter for concern. In Western countries it has become clear that the large number of children with intelligence quotients from approximately 60 to 75 are suffering from temporary disabilities imposed on them by the schooling system. If universal schooling did not exist, or if children at the lower end of the achievement scale were not regarded as "problems," it is doubtful whether the mass of these children would ever come to professional attention. Certainly most children of this level of ability grow up able to obtain gainful employment and to marry and have children. The cause of their school problems lies usually, although not always, in the social conditions in which they are reared. Poverty and lack of cognitive stimulation result in a poor capacity for learning and especially for abstract thought. The demands made on them by school teachers are very different from the more practical requirements they meet in their everyday, out-of-school life. They are expected to use a linguistic code for communication at school that has little similarity with the language they use at home. In developing countries, where linguistic diversity is even greater and where, for example, a child living in an African city may be exposed to a number of different tribal languages at home and yet another language at school, one might imagine that frequent labeling could occur of even very bright children as intellectually slow because of a failure of communication between teacher and child. Improvement of this state of affairs is not likely to occur on a large scale as a result of better identification of slow-learning pupils, but more from gradual amelioration of the living conditions of the poor together with greater understanding by teachers of the social and cultural background of such children.

Not all slow-learning children are suffering from sociocultural deprivation. It is common for psychiatrists working in cities of developing countries to be faced with disappointed middle-class parents of a child who, for some genetic reason or because of some form of brain damage, is functioning at a below-average level. An I.Q. of 85 in a child with ambitious, upwardly mobile, middle-class parents is a greater tragedy to the parents than a child of the slums with an I.Q. of 70 is. Parental rejection of children whose below-average ability fails to meet parental expectations can be a difficult phenomenon to manage helpfully. Often there is little a professional can do to help except to point to the child's positive capacities and to encourage the parents to value the child despite their disappointments.

Emotional and Behavioral Disorders

For the Western-trained psychiatrist, whose own professional work is likely to provide no experience with malnourished children and little experience with children suffering from brain damage or severe mental retardation, the main area of interest in developing countries lies in the nature of childhood psychiatric disorders. Until recently, these problems have been little considered by health professionals working in developing countries, but it is now clear, as evidenced by the very positive reception of the report of the WHO Expert Committee [28], that those concerned with planning health services in developing countries now wish to give more attention to matters relating to emotional disturbance in childhood. The most likely explanation for this change in attitude is that problems of older children living in big cities, especially drug problems and delinquency, have now become so obtrusive that those involved in planning policy can no longer avoid them, especially when they are bound to have concerns that their own children will become affected. Further, there are other good reasons for taking emotional and behavioral problems seriously and, once the major causes of mortality have been eradicated, according them high priority. Surveys in developed countries have revealed that the presence of such problems markedly impairs the quality of family life in at least as powerful a manner as do many of the main causes of physical morbidity.

The natural response by health planners when faced with problems such as these is to set up treatment services on as wide a scale as possible to deal with affected children. This approach characterized attempts to deal with child psychiatric problems in the Western world and resulted in the development of very large numbers of child guidance clinics and child psychiatric departments. It has been realized for many years that such an approach may not be the most appropriate. Only a highly selected minority of affected children and their families will attend. Little impact is made on the mass of those who suffer, and little effort goes into preventive measures. In the absence of validated treatment methods, expensive personnel spend their time in therapeutic endeavors of doubtful efficacy. In these circumstances it would be wise to advise those considering action not to rush into services imitative of those in Europe and North America. *Some* level of service does of course have to come into being to provide a nucleus of a professional staff whose main preoccupation and area of interest lies in this field. But what should the main tasks for such a core group of people be?

The WHO Technical Report [27] makes a number of recommendations for action and places a good deal of emphasis on the need for the acquisition of knowledge. Knowledge already exists [9] to suggest that the rates of psychiatric disturbance in children living in developed countries are not greatly different from those in the developing world. Indeed, in some instances such as suicide in children, rates in developing countries actually appear to be higher [22, 23], although in most countries such information is not available. It would be inappropriate to generalize from the few studies carried out and to use such data as a basis for planning services. One of the first requirements in the field of child mental health must be the conduct of surveys to establish the rates and types of disorders and the factors associated with them. Concepts of deviance developed in Western Europe and North America may or may not be applicable here. It has now been reasonably well established that the WHO multiaxial classification scheme [19] with its five main elements (clinical psychiatric syndrome, intellectual level, specific delays in development, underlying or associated medical conditions, and psychosocial environment) is appropriate to the needs of developed countries. It is probably also relevant to the classification of disorders in children living in big cities in developing countries, but it is by no means established that this is an appropriate framework for children living in traditional societies.

There are daunting problems facing those who wish to carry out surveys in developing countries. The identification of the population at risk presents particular problems where only a proportion of children attend school. The acquisition of information also presents difficulties. Unfamiliar interviewers may be treated with suspicion or given misleading information. Linguistic diversity may present problems, not just because it may be difficult for interviewers to understand informants and vice versa, but also because data obtained using different languages may not be comparable. Nevertheless, as already indicated, a number of surveys have been carried out in developing countries. Further, it does seem particularly urgent that such studies are carried out to establish the effects of change on the rates and kinds of mental disorder [27]. It is widely thought that compulsory education, the drift of population from rural areas to big cities, and the breakdown of traditional beliefs and attitudes all result in increased rates of disorder, but some studies have suggested that rates of problems are just as high in traditional societies. There would be important policy implications whatever the findings from comparative studies.

All of those working in the field of child health in developing countries seem agreed that urbanization is a main factor associated with high rates of child psychiatric disorder. Comparative studies from Western Europe confirm high rates of disorder in city children [19], but the phenomenon is not universal [11]. It might be possible to identify certain features of urban life such as social isolation, or, conversely, degrees of overcrowding that make family life intolerable. Gatere [7] has already shown how the pressures of city life in Nairobi reduce interaction between mothers and children. Sixty percent of mothers contacted in that city were spending less than two hours a day with their children. He has suggested that parents reexamine their motives for going out to work when their children are under 3 years old, leaving them in the hands of housemaids who are uneducated and may not even speak the same language. He also suggested encouragement of mothers of young children to work part-time. In addition, there seems to be a need for more intervention programs promoting mutual self-help, similar to the programs fighting malnutrition.

One of the reasons so much emphasis is placed by professionals on problems in big cities is that most of them work in such places and have very limited experience of the stresses and strains on children of traditional village societies. The comfortable assumption that extended family networks protect children in these situations is not borne out by the limited evidence available [13, 15]. This is also an area for further investigation. Most studies of child-rearing patterns and child behavior in traditional societies have been carried out so far by social anthropologists much more interested in establishing the usual patterns than in identifying deviance.

Schooling

The continuing failure to provide universal education for the school-age population in developing countries has produced psychiatric problems in children in developing countries very different from those seen in the Western world. Serpell [4] has described the highly competitive ethos in Zambian schools in a situation in which only 50 percent of those completing three years of secondary schooling can find places to complete the last two years. Students failing to complete these last two years apparently are stigmatized as dropouts and "emerge into the world of work with a sense of frustration and unpreparedness." A similar position has been described to me in other parts of the developing world such as

Singapore. Further, as Chintu and Haworth [4] have pointed out, the emergence of a school system in developing countries has produced a new population of failures: children with learning difficulties who previously would not have been perceived as in any way deficient yet now have no special provision made for them. Experience in the Western world suggests that special provision by no means overcomes the sense of failure and stigmatization experienced by children with learning problems and that the creation of a sense of failure in children is an inevitable experience in schools with an atmosphere of individual competitiveness. Bronfenbrenner's contention [3] that an emphasis on cooperative activity in learning can overcome this dilemma needs to be taken seriously.

Patterns of Professional Services for Children with Mental Health Problems

The WHO Expert Committee [28] proposed that certain principles should be considered by assessing the value of different possible types of preventive action. It suggested that the main emphasis should be placed on the most prevalent mental health problems (not, for example, on psychoses), but that preventive action should be based on empirical findings and that long-term actions were more likely to be effective than brief interventions in situations of chronic deprivation. If at all possible, early intervention should be undertaken before fixed maladaptive patterns of behavior have been established. The Committee suggested that a number of measures could be introduced immediately on the basis of existing knowledge. General health measures included improvements in maternal and obstetric care, better nutrition, effective immunization programs, reduction of accidents, improved physical and social conditions, and better care of the chronically handicapped. Social welfare measures included the avoidance of unstable and discontinuous patterns of parenting, improved conditions in daycare facilities as well as hospitals and other residential institutions, a reduction in the number of unwanted births, and enhanced public awareness of children's needs.

Treatment measures recommended by the Committee included behavioral methods applicable to a variety of common problems, focused short-term counseling, and, for a highly selected group of children, medication. Other measures thought to be probably effective but recommended with less enthusiasm because more costly include hospital treatment, special educational services, and specialized psychotherapy.

Who is to perform these manifold tasks? It seems likely that all those involved in child care—parents and other family members, friends, and professionals at all levels and of all disciplines—must be involved. It would not be appropriate to describe possible patterns of service in any detail, but it is those professionals who are in daily, or at least very frequent, contact with children and families who are often in the best position to help. School teachers fall into this category for school-age children, and health-care workers for younger children.

The primary health-care worker, defined in a recent WHO publication [28] as "a man or woman who can read and write, and is selected by the local community or with their agreement to deal with the health problems of individuals and the community," seems to have a massive task. On the basis of a recommended six- to eight-week official health service training with minimal subsequent supervision, he or she is expected to cope with all health problems, including mental illness and the learning difficulties of childhood. The proposed curriculum for these workers contains a suggested approach to learning problems in children but makes no mention of equally common problems such as headaches, stomach aches, soiling, wetting, weakness, and tiredness for which no physical cause is found.

A WHO-supported study based on primary care centers in four different countries—Sudan, Phillipines, India, and Columbia—has demonstrated that children with mental health problems are commonly present in such centers and that the adults who bring them report such difficulties when simple systematic enquiry is made [8]. However, primary care workers only recognize between 10 and 22 percent of the cases thought to show significant problems by experienced psychiatrists. The results of this study have been used to design training courses in child mental health for primary care workers participating in the study.

The role of child psychiatric specialists in countries where one or two people represent the entire resource in the subject is clearly very difficult to delineate. Heavy service demands compete with requests for teaching more and more disparate groups of professionals concerned with children, and it is amazing that any research is conducted at all. Yet among all the various demands made on child mental health professionals, surely one of the most worthwhile must be the instruction of those concerned in teacher and primary health worker training in the emotional needs of children in the developing world.

References

1. Axton, J.H. and Levy, L.F. Mental handicap in Rhodesian African children. *Dev. Med. Child Neur.,* 16 (1974), 350–355.
2. Billingshurst, J.R., German, G.A., and Orley, J.H. The pattern of epilepsy in Uganda. *Trop. Geogr. Med.,* 25 (1973), 226–232.
3. Bronfenbrenner, U. *Two Worlds of Childhood.* Russel Sage Foundation, New York, 1970.
4. Chintu C., and Haworth, A. *Mental Health Services for Children in Zambia.* Unpublished paper, 1979.
5. Chioialo, N., Kirschbaum, A., Fuentes, A., Cordero, M.L., and Madsen, J. Prevalence of epilepsy in children of Melpilla, Chile. *Epilepsia,* 20 (1979), 261–6.
6. Cravioto, J. and Arrieta, R. Stimulation of mental development of malnourished infants. *Lancet,* ii (1979), 899.
7. Gatere, S. Child-rearing patterns in Kenya (City of Nairobi). In Kiev, A., Muya, W.J., Sartorius, N., Eds. *The Future of Mental Health Services.* Excerpta Medica, Amsterdam, 1980.
8. Giel R., Arango, M.V. de, Climent, C.E., Harding, T. W., Ibrahim, H.H.A., Ladrido-Ignacio, L., Murthy, R.S., Salazar, M.C., Wig, N.N., and Younis, Y.O.A. Childhood mental disorders in primary health care. *Pediatrics.* In Press.
9. Graham, P. Epidemiological approaches to child mental health in developing countries. In Press.
10. International Children's Centre. *Children in the Tropics.* International Children's Centre, Paris, 1979.
11. Kastrup, M. Urban–rural differences in 6-year-olds. In Graham, P., Ed. *Epidemiological Approaches in Child Psychiatry.* Academic Press, London, 1977.
12. Lotter, V. Childhood Autism in Africa. *J. Child Psychol. Psychiat.* 19 (1978), 231–244.
13. Minde, K. Psychological problems in Ugandan school-children—a controlled evaluation. *J. Child Psychol. Psychiat.* 16 (1975), 49–59.
14. Morley, D. *Paediatric Priorities in Developing Countries.* Butterworths, London 1973.
15. Ramanujam, B.K. Psychiatric problems of children seen in an urban center of western India. *Amer. J. Orthopsychiat.* 45 (1975), 490–496.
16. Ramsey, F.C. Nutrition indicators and the Barbados school-child: Nutrition Intervention Program. In US Department of Health, Education and Welfare, *Evaluation of Child Health Services* DHEW Publication No. (NIH) 78-1066 (1978), 169–92.

17. Richardson, S.A., Birch, H.G., Grabie, E., and Yoder, K. The behavior of children in school who were severely malnourished in the first two years of life. *J. Health Soc. Behav.* 13 (1972), 276–284.
18. Runciman, W.G. *Relative Deprivation and Social Justice.* Penguin Press, Harmondsworth, 1972.
19. Rutter, M., Cox, A., Tupling, C., Berger, M., and Yule, W. Attainment and adjustment in two geographical areas—The prevalence of psychiatric disorder. *Brit. J. Psychiat.* 126 (1975), 493–509.
20. Rutter, M., and Madge, N. *Cycles of Disadvantage.* Heinemann, London, 1976.
21. Rutter, M., Shaffer, D., and Shepherd, M. *A Multi-axial Classification of Child Psychiatric Disorders.* WHO, Geneva, 1975.
22. Sathyavathi, K. Suicide among children in Bangalore. *Ind. J. Pediat.* 42, (1975), 149–157.
23. Shaffer, D. Suicide in childhood and early adolescence. *J. Child Psychol. Psychiat.* 15 (1974), 275–92.
24. Townsend, P. *Poverty in the United Kingdom.* Penguin Press, Harmondsworth, 1979.
25. United Nations Economic and Social Council. *Priorities in Child Nutrition in Developing Countries.* New York, UNICEF Executive Board, 1975.
26. Werner, E.E. *Cross-Cultural Child Development.* Brooks/Cole, Monterey, California, 1979.
27. World Health Organization. *Child Mental Health and Psychosocial Development.* WHO, Geneva, 1977.
28. World Health Organization. *The Primary Health Worker.* WHO, Geneva, 1980.

Some Aspects of Disruption of the Attachment System in Young Children: A Transcultural Perspective

Klaus K. Minde, M.D.
Regina Minde (Canada)
Seggane Musisi (Nigeria)

Since the 1950s, increasing effort has been devoted to understanding the nature of early parent–child interaction and its role in later development. Although initially the mother's contribution to this interaction was emphasized [4, 36], more recent work has stressed that even the very young infant has cognitive and perceptual abilities, previously unrecognized, which make him or her an active partner in any interaction context [3, 24, 29]. Researchers and clinicians also have become interested in the effects that specific stressful environmental events have on both the current parent–child relationship and on the child's future coping skills [14, 22, 34]. Although a number of epidemiological studies have stressed the complexities of external factors that can affect the normal emotional development of the young child [19, 34], some authors such as Ainsworth and Bowlby continue to see the presence of a reliable adult with whom the child can form a stable attachment as one of the most formative influences on later life [1, 5–7].

Since transcultural observations can provide one method of clarifying the importance of basic psychological principles governing development, this paper integrates both positions. We first consider some of Bowlby's basic concepts about the loss of the primary attachment figure and enlarge on these by employing a more ecological point of view. The resulting multilevel framework is then used to discuss the effects that various forms and degrees of disruption of this attachment system may have in children of different cultural backgrounds.

Bowlby's Theory of Attachment

Central to Bowlby's work is the notion that children universally suffer both short- and long-term consequences from the temporary or permanent inaccessibility (i.e., separation or loss) of their attachment figures [6, pp. 72–73; 7, p. 22]. Following separation or loss, children are said to develop specific anxieties, symptoms compatible with mourning, and particular defensive reactions (e.g., rejection of the mother after the reunion). Bowlby is especially concerned about such defensive reactions, because these, if they persist, represent one mechanism by which loss may hinder future adaptation. Although loss may be traumatic at any age, he believes that children between the ages of six months and three years are particularly vulnerable to its effects. He writes that "in infants and children, it appears, defensive processes once set in motion, are apt to stabilize and persist" [7, p. 21].

The evidence that pathological mourning and defense decrease as children grow older is not clear in Bowlby's exposition. Indeed, during this early period of susceptibility the young child has only a limited appreciation of temporary as opposed to permanent conditions, and it may be of little practical value to distinguish between separation and loss.

Although the use of terms such as loss and mourning suggests the relatively circumscribed situation of parental death or desertion, Bowlby believes that small doses of everyday separation are simply at the other end of a continuum of maternal inaccessibility. He also stresses that the mother may be physically present but emotionally absent if she is "unresponsive" to her child's need for mothering. A regular experience of such parental unresponsiveness or inaccessibility due to a brief separation may then be as pathogenic as parental death.

Referring to Ainsworth's observational studies [1], Bowlby notes that the responsive mother provides her infant with a secure basis from which the young child can explore and adapt to a wider world. As a result, the young child gradually develops positive cognitive expectations about the availability of the mother and feelings of security, both of which contribute to confident adaptation. In contrast, an unresponsive mother does not support her child's adaptive exploration and thus inhibits the internalization of positive cognitive expectations and felt security—essentials for secure adaptation later in life. This will leave her child overly dependent and fearful (i.e., "anxiously attached"). As other studies suggest, the child may, in extreme cases, even learn to avoid such a mother to defend against her rebuffs [25].

Cognitive processes play a central role in Bowlby's analysis of attachment and loss. They are believed to mediate attachment and responses to separation or loss in two main ways. First, the development of general cognitive skills provides some of the necessary conditions for phases of attachment in infancy and early childhood to take place. An example of such cognitive skill is the infant's developing belief in the permanence of objects or persons. In other words, the infant must have at least a primitive understanding that the absent mother still exists to enter the phases of attachment marked by a search for mother or separation distress upon her absence.

A secondary role of cognition is the increasing control of the attachment system by mental models or expectations specifically relating to the attachment relationship. These models are built up through experience with the attachment figure, and their contents may affect the child's subsequent perception, feelings, thoughts, and actions. For example, the insecurely attached child may adopt expectations about the mother's unresponsiveness that carry into later relationships and will also exacerbate the effects of disruptive loss. However, regardless of the initial quality of attachment, certain events such as parental death will always require reorganization of a child's mental models of attachment relationships and, through them, of the world in general.

In summary, it appears that Bowlby emphasizes mechanisms within the child to explain the effects of loss. Even though in his most recent volume [7] he seems more sympathetic to the role ecological variables such as family support may play in the child's adaptation to loss, the individual child's attachment system remains the focus of his thinking. Bowlby also suggests that the external interruptions of the attachment of a child to primary caretakers will invariably lead to specific symptoms, which in turn influence future adaptation. However, this may not necessarily be the case, since there is evidence that the impact of at least short separations can be softened by making certain changes in the setting where they occur. For instance, when children are left with interesting new toys, they will miss their mothers much less than when only routine play materials are available [12, 32]. In addition, modifications in the effects of separation have been demonstrated when children were prepared sensitively and well nurtured during their mothers' absence [33]. These observations suggest that other secondary variables may play a role in modifying the effects of disruption or deficiencies in childrens' relationships with their parents.

Bronfenbrenner [8] refers to such secondary variables when he describes an "upper" and "lower" layer that make up the child's ecology. The upper layer (i.e., the immediate setting) consists of the space in which things may happen to the child, in which significant others act and interact in ways meaningful for the child. The lower, or supporting, layer relates to the surrounding structure in which the immediate setting is embedded (the physical setting or social system). The relations both between and within these two systems may, according to Bronfenbrenner, influence the relationship between the child and the caretakers in various ways and therefore affect the child more or less directly.

Bowlby does not address himself directly to such issues, but the kinds of experiences he discusses suggest that "loss" may be analyzed at very different levels.

The Attachment Level. At this level, loss refers to activation of attachment behavior without termination such as following parental death, producing mourning and persisting defensive reaction. Loss can also, however, refer to activation of attachment behavior in response to insensitive or unresponsive mothering, producing insecure attachment.

The Level of Children's Social Cognitions—Their Belief Systems. In addition to denying termination of attachment behavior, events such as the caretaker's death, desertion, or emotional unavailability will also violate expectations about the social world that are part of the mental models organizing the attachment system in the older infant and young child.

The Parents' Social Cognitions as Related to the Child. Although this level of analysis has received little attention in the literature on attachment, it appears logical that the expectations and interpretations of those around the child will modify their interactions and therefore the child's experience of the loss. For example, in the case of parental desertion, the remaining parent's interpretation of the child's response to this traumatic event obviously would affect subsequent interactions.

Ecological Factors. The ecological factors are the environmental variables outside of the attachment relationship. When there is a disruption within the child's family, there are often associated changes in the child's immediate social and material environment and possibly the wider surrounding system. For example, relationships with siblings or peers may help compensate for the loss. On the other hand, adverse environmental events may preoccupy the parents to such an extent that the parent–child interaction may suffer.

The Garden of Eden Principle. Although the levels of analysis listed above deal with loss in terms of disruption and deficiency, one can argue that certain generally accepted yet nevertheless less-than-optimal child-rearing conditions may also be defined as loss. The Garden of Eden principle focuses on the degree of discrepancy between accepted practices and theoretical or clinical judgment regarding what is optimal. These judgments may be more or less informed by research. An example would be Bowlby's notion of the biologically given norm of close contact between the infant and a responsive mother, on which he bases his interpretation of what "man's environment of illusionary adaptiveness" must have been like.

Cross Cultural Implications of Bowlby's Work

In the second part of this paper we use the multilevel framework developed above to examine some specific situations involving loss or separation.

1. At what level or levels can loss be defined most clearly?
2. Can specific interventions be related to the levels at which the loss is most significant?

The situations of loss we examine were chosen because they occur frequently and have been traditionally of concern to the practicing clinician, although few of the effects have been studied with scientific rigor.

UPROOTING OF THE CHILD

Violent Disruptions. Examples of violent disruptions of the attachment systems are not difficult to find in our age. Although there are few reports documenting the long-term effects of such disruptions in a scientific manner, we have a good number of careful, clinical observations that help us understand the response and attempted coping mechanisms of individual children. For example, A. Freud and D. Burlingham reported on their wartime nursery experience with almost 200 infants and young children (aged one week to five years when first admitted) who were separated from their parents to protect them from the dangers of living in wartime London. The authors noted that invariably the children found it easier to live in bomb shelters with their parents with little material comfort than to cope with the separation from their parents. In fact, all the children suffered intensely and clearly showed the various stages of mourning described by Bowlby. These stages could last days, weeks, or months, and seemed to depend on the children's ages and on the form the separation had taken (i.e., the more abrupt the separation, the more problems the children had [17]).

A more dramatic example of disruption of the attachment system and continuing loss involves the experiences of six three-year-old concentration camp survivors described by A. Freud and S. Dann [16]. These unrelated children had been separated from their parents when only a few months old and had been passed from hand to hand during much of their first year until they were admitted to the Tereczin concentration camp ward for motherless children. There they were looked after by other inmates under appalling conditions. After their liberation almost three years later they were again uprooted three times until they arrived at Bulldogs Bank, a country home given to them for a year. Here they were cared for and prepared for a new life by S. Dann and her coworkers. Freud and Dann described these youngsters as hypersensitive, restless, very aggressive toward adults, and very difficult to handle. Yet possibly because of their strong attachment to each other they were not mentally deficient, delinquent, or psychotic. In the authors' words, "they had found an alternative placement for their libido and, on the strength of this, had mastered some of their anxieties and developed social attitudes" [16, p. 165].

If we were to relate the losses experienced by these children to the various levels of loss outlined in this paper, we would have to say that, although all five levels were affected, the attachment level was the most severely disturbed.

Thus in the case of the separated children as well as the concentration camp survivors, treatment was directed at the lack of attachment behaviors. For example, the children were allowed to express their grief, rage, and frustration, and their caretakers' responsive and sensitive "mothering" encouraged them to form new attachment relationships. Unfortunately, not much is known about the later development of these youngsters beyond one single case reported by one of the substitute mothers. This case involved a girl, aged two years eight months at the time of separation, who had been so depressed that her substitute caretakers had been much concerned about the long-term effect of the experience. However, she grew up to be a well-adjusted young adult [20]. Of the six Bulldogs Bank children, the three girls are all married and allegedly happy and good mothers to their own children 35 years later. One of the boys has a family and appears to be well settled, another is divorced and reportedly very unreliable, and the third never married [13]. It well may be that the seemingly good outcome of these children following such an obviously violent early separation experience is related to the sensitive treatment supplied by S. Dann and her staff.

Children who witnessed the maltreatment and arrest of one or both of their parents are others whose attachment systems had been disrupted by outside interference. In a recent report, Allodi [2] describes a total of 232 children of South American families who experienced such events. The children were under the age of 12, with one group of 28 Argentinian children between six months and four years old at the time of their parents' torture and imprisonment. Examination three years later revealed about 75 percent of the younger children showed signs of fearfulness and withdrawal, and the older children (above age seven) displayed a great deal of aggressiveness, especially toward adults outside the immediate family. It was felt that the emotional withdrawal of the younger children was related to the remaining parent's preoccupation with his or her own loss, fear, change in status, and the fate of the detained family member, which in turn led to a "psychological unavailability of the other parent to the young child." In contrast, the older children appeared able to "hate" and in this way externalize and project feelings of rage and abandonment.

Very similar clinical examples have been experienced by the authors in their contact with children in Uganda who witnessed the abusive treatment or murder of one of their parents. In virtually all cases, the older children "hated the enemy" and appeared to be reminded continuously to do so by the remaining members of their extended families. Yet as long as the killings or murders could be seen as part of a particular policy directed against "their tribe" or "their profession," the children remained kind and considerate to their peers and other adult tribal members.

It should be stressed that in the literature on children who have experienced violent separation from a parent, little mention is made of the many other pathological factors that habitually accompany such an event. For example, the remaining family members often have no legal status on which to appeal, and, because the fate of the detained or disappeared person is uncertain, no mourning can take place. In addition, in many of the documented cases of parental torture, the families later emigrate to other countries and face yet another range of stresses associated with migration. For example, follow-up data from Amnesty International [9] of 75 Chilean children now living in Denmark with their reunited families show that even two to six years after the trauma, 36 percent of these children still show clear signs of anxiety, 35 percent experience insomnia, 16 percent are depressed, and 17 percent show consistently aggressive behavior. Both Cohen et al. [9] and Allodi [2] suggest that the most effective treatment in these cases seems to be regular group meetings with similarly affected individuals, that is, interventions designed to deal with the effects of the traumatic events at a cognitive level. Such meetings allow both the children and their parents to share their experiences within a wider forum and hence help them overcome their sense of social isolation and withdrawal. This in turn may facilitate the giving up of severe defensive reactions and consequently permit the children to experience the world anew and finally adjust to their new country.

Disruption of the Attachment System Due to Changes in the Immediate Family Situation. Changes in the immediate family situation leading to the uprooting of a child may or may not be part of a culturally acceptable custom and tradition. For example, in some societies in Africa and the Caribbean, even very young children may be sent to spend long periods with members of their extended family far away from their biological parents. Such arrangements, although obviously disrupting to the basic attachments of the child concerned, will not be seen as a loss in terms of the parents' and maybe even the child's social cognitions, (i.e., loss on the levels of the parents' and children's social cognitions), as long as they are based on the mutual agreement of all family members. However, moving to the same grandmother's house because of the desertion or death of a parent and the consequent disintegration of the family violates the expectations of both adults and child.

Are such "culturally specific" differences reflected themselves in the behavior of the children both following their initial separation and during later childhood? Although only a few specific data are available, clinical evidence provides us with some possible answers.

In a number of studies, the first author examined the incidence and types of psychiatric disorders in various school and clinic populations in Uganda [26, 28]. The results are shown in Table 1.

Among primary school children who scored within the abnormal range on Rutter's Teacher Symptom Screening Test [34] translated into the local language, as many children had lost one parent through death as did a matched low-scoring control population (8.3 versus 10.4 percent). An almost equal number of children (58 versus 54 percent) had also been sent away for more than two weeks to a relative before the age of six for culturally sanctioned reasons (a grandmother wanted them, a sibling was born, or the school was too far away from the biological parents' home). Since the rate of definite psychopathology of children identified as deviant by this screening test was largely confirmed by a standardized psychiatric interview (about 80 percent), one can conclude that a separation from the biological family, if it occurs within a culturally acceptable frame of reference (at least in southern Uganda), does not lead to an increase in later psychopathology. This does not mean, of course, that a more thorough examination of the children would not have discovered certain psychological difficulties. Also, the exclusion of children who stayed for less than two weeks with other people may have unwittingly not taken into account those who were the most seriously affected by their separation. For example, clinical and personal experience clearly indicates that Ugandan adults generally *know* that children who are asked to live with relatives will not be happy there. Nevertheless, the children are expected not to complain. As a consequence, a child who is seriously upset by the move

Table 1. Background Variables in Various Ugandan Populations

	School		Psychiatric Clinic
	Problem	Control	
Broken homes	39.5	14.5	44.4
1 parent dead	8.3	10.4	18.5
"Bad" moves	41.6	12.5	22.2
"Good" moves	58.2	53.9	51.8
	$N = 48$	$N = 48$	$N = 27$

will often express the conflict not by complaining but through rapidly developing physical symptoms such as paralysis of the legs, aphonia, and so forth. In Buganda such symptoms are then interpreted as a sign that the spirit of a dead person does not want the child to be with the nonbiological family. The standard treatment of this condition is the return of the child to the biological family within a week, and the symptoms usually disappear almost immediately. What is important in this example is that the affected child will not be blamed for the "illness" and that the treatment is part of a culturally accepted pattern.

Table 1 also indicates that sending a child away for other than culturally sanctioned reasons (the "bad moves") was clearly associated with later psychopathology. Bad moves included moves following the structural breakdown of the family due to parental separation or desertion, at times leading to a total abandonment of some children.

To help these totally uprooted children in Uganda, we used a two-stage treatment process in our clinical practice that was designed primarily to provide the children with a more growth-enhancing environment. In practice this meant that these youngsters, who were frequently collected from local jails by the first investigator, were placed in a home run by a middle-aged couple. The children were kept there for two to four weeks to (a) assess them for malnutrition, medical illnesses, or other obvious symptoms of neglect; (b) reexpose them to a traditional Buganda family structure and permit them to relearn ways to interact appropriately with elders and peers; and (c) provide them with the basic reassurance that they were welcome members of a clearly defined society. Since the family usually would have not more than four or five children at their home at the same time, each youngster received a good deal of personal attention. Following this group rehabilitation the children were placed into the homes of individual rural families, and their foster parents received the equivalent of $5 per month for one year. We hoped that following this period the parents and children would like each other sufficiently well to make it possible to maintain the child within the family. Follow-up visits indicated that after two years, some 75 percent of the 120 children who remained with these families helped them with agricultural chores, and 25 percent had received some additional schooling. Although this program obviously depended on the relative intactness of the society in the rural areas, it led to few new disruptions (about 10 percent) and restored a number of normal expectations to these children.

UPROOTING OF THE FAMILY UNIT

Distinctions between culturally sanctioned and nonsanctioned losses also may help us understand the problems of young children whose families never had definite homes (e.g., migrant workers who follow the crops) versus those who for whatever reasons were forced to emigrate and in the process experienced significant changes in their social and economic support structures.

Although data in this area are again sketchy, a number of specific predictive factors seem to emerge. For example, R. Coles, a child psychiatrist who lived among North American migrant workers, describes the stresses these children are exposed to, for instance, not being allowed to establish roots since they never remain in one place long enough or being looked at with suspicion by the foremen in the fields and the local population [10]. Moreover, all the children and parents Coles interviewed were resigned that these children would follow in their parents' footsteps and be migrant workers later on, implying that the restrictions of their present-day lives appeared to preclude even the thought of any alternative course of action in the future.

In this particular condition, loss may best be defined through the Garden of Eden principle, since the instability of the wider ecological field contributes not only to parental preoccupation but also deprives these migrant children of a world and social system to grow into.

It is interesting to note that these migrant children who were frequently born by the roadside and, according to Coles, received very little physical and virtually no medical care were nevertheless breast fed for an average of 18 months, that is, had intimate physical contact with their mothers for a prolonged period. In fact, their mothers repeatedly stressed that this period was the best time they ever had with their children [10, p. 10] and established a true closeness between them. From the time of weaning, however, when the parents became unavailable, these migrant children quickly learned to switch over to their older siblings for comfort and guidance. Unencumbered by the protective restrictions normally applied by parents, these children initially seemed to thrive, ready to take on almost everything that might come their way [10, p. 15]. After age eight, however, they were seen to be apathetic, to be weighed down by a feeling of powerlessness, and to have the feeling that "their fate is of no real concern to others" [10, p. 74]. Since Coles never reports any signs of "active" psychopathology in any of the children he examined, one may argue that we deal here with yet another type of "culturally acceptable" loss that may lead to a negative attitude toward life but not necessarily to active psychopathology.

However, Coles' study also may point to yet another phenomenon associated with loss in childhood. He reports that the migrant children interviewed became increasingly apathetic when they reached school age, and suggests that the failure of society at large to validate them at that age may have been responsible for that. It is of interest here that sociologists who have studied the adjustment of children of foreign workers or immigrants in Germany, France, and Israel [31, 35] have also found that children's educational and cultural adaptation to their new country was best when the migration occurred before the age of six, or after the age of 11. Inbar and Adler, for example, studied 103 Moroccan children who had settled in Israel, and 106 who had gone to France, as well as 29 young Rumanian immigrants in Israel. These authors found that 40 percent of children up to five years old at the time of immigration, versus none who had migrated during the ages of six and 11, entered college later. On the other hand, 22 percent of children aged 12 to 15 and 36 percent of those older than 16 at the time of immigration enrolled in college. In discussing these results, Inbar and Adler talk about a "vulnerable age" between six and 11 for immigration because, under normal circumstances, children of that age are expected to cope with novel situations or events only within the familiar cultural setting—they have not yet acquired sufficient skills to adapt easily to a drastically different culture.

Whereas these studies define adaptation exclusively in terms of later educational achievement, others have focused on the emotional and social adjustment of immigrant children. In our own study [27], which examined 51 Ugandan Asian children of primary school age whose families had been expelled from Uganda and settled in Toronto, we found that 53 percent of these children showed psychological adjustment problems one year after leaving Uganda. In one-third of these children, the difficulties were of a serious nature and by parents' reports had not been present prior to expulsion. Although temporary separations of parents and children in the wake of the expulsion had been brief (none longer than eight weeks) and did not seem to have a negative effect on these children's later mental health, Table 2 shows that the presence of general family discord was highly correlated with the clinical diagnosis of a psychiatric problem.

Table 2. Family Adjustment and Psychopathology in Children in Percent ($N = 51$) [27]

	Family Adjustment		
	Good	Medium	Poor
Psychopathology present	46	14	12
Psychopathology absent	4	10	14

$\chi^2 = 9.65$; df = 2; $p < .01$

These findings are confirmed by data from Switzerland and Sweden suggesting that migration per se is not detrimental to children [15], particularly if they remain with their families. On the other hand, longer separations associated with migration seem to result in deviance later on. For example, reports on physical disorders in the children of West Indian immigrants in Great Britain show that a high percentage of those first left behind with the maternal grandmother following their parents' immigration were later more often referred to child guidance clinics because of antisocial disorders [19, 30]. In these cases, however, the children had suffered an accumulation of losses, beginning with the separation from their biological parents, followed by the separation five to six years later from their substitute caretakers and familiar social and cultural tropical environment, only to join their half-forgotten parents and foreign-born siblings in a cold and strange city thousands of miles away. In addition, these children were supposed to compete in a society that demanded very different behaviors and coping strategies than they had been exposed to before. This, of course, is similar to the behavioral changes that are demanded of children within Africa who migrate from the village to the slums of the burgeoning cities.

In general, it seems that among uprooted children, those of preschool age can enter into a new peer group system fairly easily. Such children consequently may experience less of a loss on both the adult's and child's level of cognition. Adolescents in turn may be cognitively better equipped to search for alternatives of resocialization within their new world and in this way be less vulnerable to losses brought about by migration.

Migration is, of course, a risk factor not only for children. Parents, especially mothers, may be no less vulnerable. For example, if migration is associated with a complete change in the family structure (e.g., from extended to nuclear), the parents' coping ability in job requirements or other social demands may be overtaxed and, as a result, their parenting abilities may be seriously affected. For example, Goshen-Gottstein [18], in a study of 60 Yemenite families with infants aged two to 19 months, found that a significant number of mothers of these children had become very aggressive and abusive toward their infants, frequently cursing and threatening them and actively discouraging exploration and play. The author suggests that these abnormal behaviors were related to these mothers' loss of their previously assured support networks and their ignorance regarding monomatric child-rearing demands, leaving them easily frustrated and angry.

What do these studies suggest to us in terms of remediation? Although research provides few clear guidelines, it seems important to examine how many of the parameters of loss described are affected by the trauma at hand, and at which stage in cognitive development the child experiences disruption or deficiency. For example, it may be most beneficial therapeutically to deal with the uprooted school-age children's expectations about their social world, because at this developmental stage children's expectations may be more crucial for their further development than are shifts in caregiving routines or a disruption in parental social recognitions. On the other hand, disturbances or disruptions in the attachment process between children and their primary caretakers and the parents' expectations and interpretations of traumatizing events may be most crucial for the emotional welfare of the one- or two-year-olds.

MULTINUCLEAR FAMILIES, POLYMATRICAL CHILD REARING, AND "LOSS"

One of the questions initially raised by Bowlby and later emphasized by Klaus and Kennell [23] following their experience with families and infants is the ability of a parent to attach him- or herself to two children simultaneously. Bowlby felt that the commitment a parent makes to an infant could not be divided between two children. He called this the principle of monotrophy.

By the same token, the question arises whether the polygamous type of family found in many African countries will impede the development of a child, since it violates the Garden of Eden principle of one mother and one child. In contrast to this potential "loss" are some statements in the literature suggesting that the plurality of personal exchanges within a multinuclear family gives the child a particular security not available to children raised in nuclear families [11]. Although there are too few hard data to settle this issue definitely, the first author, in his work in three Ugandan primary schools, showed that children who came from extended (one mother and other female adult relatives) or multinuclear (one husband and one or more wives) families were clearly overrepresented among the problem children (see Table 3).

Although we have stated previously that the association of potentially adverse background factors with later psychopathology does not mean that the behavioral abnormalities are specifically caused by a disturbance in the attachment system of the infant, clinical vignettes and common folklore seem to suggest at least the possibility of such an explanation. Thus there is a clear awareness, at least among Ugandans, that among polygamous families there are more jealous arguments (e.g., mujja, the word for co-wife in Luganda, is the same for jealousy). As a consequence, a married woman will generally avoid disciplining or involving herself in the care of the children of her co-wives. The practice is at times used by youngsters to escape reprisals for socially unacceptable behaviors (e.g., a truanting child may hide in the co-wife's house with the knowledge that she will not force him to go to school). Children in such families usually develop a clear hierarchy of loyalty toward their various caregivers; they feel much more attached to their biological mother than to any other woman within the household. Thus again we have a situation where a culture provides a potentially hazardous situation that can, in some circumstances, cause maladaptive behavior.

Some confirmation of these clinical impressions comes from the work of Reed and Leiderman [31] with Gusii children in Kenya. Leiderman and his colleagues tested 28 Gusii infants, ranging in age from six to 27 months, in a modified Ainsworth paradigm on their attachment to their mother, a regularly available child caregiver, and an unfamiliar adult. The authors repeated the same procedure 3 months later when the infants ranged in age from nine to 30

Table 3. Family Constellation in Psychiatric Clinic and Control Children in Uganda

	Nuclear	Extended	Multinuclear	One Parent Only
Controls $N = 35$	16	5	11	3
Problems $N = 47$	13	12	17	5

months. They found that (a) the Gusii infants showed specific attachment behaviors toward both their biological mothers and familiar caretakers from about 9 months onward; (b) the infants showed indiscriminate attachment behaviors toward the stranger up to the age of nine months but none thereafter; and (c) the infants invariably were more attached to their biological mothers than they were to the other familiar caretakers.

This means that the development of differential attachment behavior for polymatric infants is similar to that observed in monomatric societies. This similarity in the pattern of infant attachment behaviors across cultures and between caregiving figures suggests that the behavior is less culturally or socially influenced and more developmentally determined.

In terms of practical management of the disturbed behavior of children from multinuclear families, it appears that the strengthening of the child's ties toward the biological mother is both the culturally most acceptable and therapeutically most effective method of treatment.

Conclusions

In the present paper, by using a particular framework for the analysis of loss we have attempted to examine the possible short- and long-term impact that a number of negative features of the child–environment interaction have on children's behavior and development. However, in doing so we have unwittingly emphasized the stressful components of live events and their associated negative outcome in children and their families. Yet in reality all the changes associated with disruptive events are not necessarily negative. The death of a parent may draw the surviving parent and child closer together. In a similar way, deficient conditions may also produce compensatory processes. As an example, we have seen the culturally sanctioned ways of reuniting severely distressed children with their families as practiced in Buganda, or the enormous resourcefulness encountered in so many African children who are transplanted into "detraditionalized" cities. We hope that the ecological approach to loss that we have outlined in this paper will sensitize us to both positive and negative aspects of loss.

Another clear gap in what we have presented is that we have discussed loss in terms of the child–environment interaction but have not dealt in depth with what the child brings to this interaction. Again, these characteristics could have positive or negative consequences. To take just one example, the child who has an easy temperament or who has satisfactory previous interpersonal experiences may be better able to withstand disruptions or any of the other upheavals we have described.

A final shortcoming of this paper is obviously the dearth of good research data that can substantiate some of our clinical impressions. Again, one may suggest that both the levels of analysis we have proposed and the severity of the disruption pertaining to each level may be used in future research studies to examine the impact of disturbances in the attachment system on children and their families. It is obviously easy to say that we need prospective studies with multiple levels of analysis to arrive at an understanding of the various losses we have touched upon in this paper. It is harder, of course, to do such research. Nevertheless, we propose that the kind of framework outlined here may aid in this endeavor.

References

1. Ainsworth, M.D.S., Blehar, M.C., Waters, E., and Wall, S. *Patterns of Attachment. A Psychological Study of the Strange Situation.* John Wiley, New York, 1978.
2. Allodi, F. The psychiatric effects of political persecution and torture on children and families of victims. *Can. Ment. Health,* 28:3 (September 1980), 8–10.
3. Bell, R.Q. A reinterpretation of the direction of effects on studies of socialization. *Psychol. Rev,* 75 (1968), 81–95.
4. Bowlby, J. *Child Care and Growth of Love.* Penguin Books, Harmondsworth, 1953.
5. Bowlby, J. *Attachment and Loss, Vol. 1: Attachment.* Hogarth Press, London, 1969.
6. Bowlby, J. *Attachment and Loss, Vol. 2: Separation, Anxiety and Anger.* Penguin, Harmondsworth, 1975.
7. Bowlby, J. *Attachment and Loss, Vol. 3: Loss.* Basic Books, New York, 1980.
8. Bronfenbrenner, U. Developmental research, public policy, and the ecology of childhood. *Child Dev.,* 45 (1975), 1–5.
9. Cohen, J., Holzer, K.I.M., Koch, L., and Severin, B. *An Investigation of Chilean Immigrant Children in Denmark.* Amnesty International, Danish Medical Group. Unpublished Manuscript, 1979.
10. Coles, R. Uprooted Children—The Early Life of Migrant Farm Workers. University of Pittsburgh Press, Pittsburgh, 1970.
11. Collomb, H., and Valentin, G. The black African family. In Anthony, E.J., and Kopernik, C., Eds. *The Child in His Family, Vol. 1.* John Wiley, New York, 1970.
12. Corter, C.M., Rheingold, H.L., and Eckerman, C.O. Toys delay the infant's following of his mother in an unfamiliar environment. *Dev. Psychol.,* 6 (1972), 138–145.

13. Dann, S. Personal communication, 1981.
14. Douglas, J.W.B. Early hospital admissions and later disturbances of behavior and learning. *Dev. Med. Child Neur.*, 17 (1975), 456–480.
15. Ekstrand, L.H. Migrant adaptation: Cross-cultural problem. A review of research on migration, minority groups and cultural differences with special regard to children. *Educ. Psychol. Interactions*, 59 (1977), 104.
16. Freud, A., and Dann, S. An experiment in group upbringing. *Psychoanal. Study Child*, 6 (1961) 127–168.
17. Freud, A., and Burlingham, D. *Infants Without Families. Reports on the Hampstead Nurseries 1939–1945*. International Universities Press, New York, 1973.
18. Goshen-Gottstein, E.R. Treatment of young children among non-western Jewish mothers in Israel: Socio-cultural variables. *Am. J. Orthopsychiat.*, 50 (1980), 323–340.
19. Graham, P.J., and Meadows, C.E. Psychiatric disorders in the children of West Indian immigrants. *J. Child Psychol. Psychiat.*, 8 (1967), 105–116.
20. Hellman, I. Hampstead Nursery follow-up studies. 1. Sudden separation and its effect followed over twenty years. *Psychoanal. Study Child*, 17 (1962), 159–174.
21. Inbar, M., and Adler, C. The vulnerable age: A serendipitous finding. *Socio. Educ.*, 49 (1976), 193–200.
22. Kendrick, C., and Dunn, J. Caring for a second baby: Effects on interaction between mother and firstborn. *Dev. Psychol.*, 16 (1980), 303–311.
23. Klaus, M., and Kennell, J. *Maternal Infant Bonding*. C. V. Mosby and Co, Saint Louis, 1976.
24. Lewis, M., and Rosenblum, L.A. *The Effect of the Infant on its Caregiver*. John Wiley, New York, 1974.
25. Main, M., and Stadtman, J. Infant response to rejection of physical contact by the mother: aggression avoidance and conflict. *J. Acad. Child Psychiat.*, 20 (1981), 292–307.
26. Minde, K. Child psychiatry in East Africa. Some lessons learned. *East Afr. J. Med. Res.*, 3 (1976), 149–159.
27. Minde, K., and Minde, R. Children of immigrants: The adjustment of Ugandan Asian primary school children in Canada. *Can. Psychiat. Assoc. J.*, 21 (1976), 371–381.
28. Minde, K. Children in Uganda: rates of behavioral deviations and psychiatric disorders in various school and clinic populations. *J. Child Psychol. Psychiatr.*, 18 (1977), 23–37.
29. Moss, H.A. Sex, age and state as determinants of mother–infant interaction. *Merrill-Palmer Q.*, 13 (1967), 19–26.
30. Nicol, A.R. Psychiatric disorder in the children of Caribbean immigrants. *J. Child Psychol. Psychiatr.*, 12 (1971), 273–287.
31. Reed, G., and Leiderman, P.H. Age related changes in attachment behavior in polymatrically reared infants: The Kenyan Gusii. In Field, T., Leiderman, P.H. et al., Eds. *Culture and Infant Interaction*. Lawrence Erlbaum, New York, in press.

32. Rheingold, H.L. The effect of strange environment on the behavior of infants. In Foss B.M., Ed. *Determinants of Infant Behavior. Vol. 4.* Methuen, London, 1969.
33. Rutter, M., Tizard, J. and Whitmore, K. Education, Health and Behavior. Longmans, London, 1970.
34. Rutter, M. Protective factors in children's responses to stress and disadvantage. In Kent, M. Whalen, and Rolf, J.E., Eds. Primary *Prevention of Psychopathology*, Vol. 3., *Social Competence in Children.* University Press of New England, Hanover, N.H., 49–74.
35. Schrader, A. The "vulnerable" age: Findings on foreign children in Germany: A comment in Inbar and Adler, Sociology of Education. *Sociol. Educ.* 51 (1978), 227–230.
36. Winnicott, D.W. *The Ordinary Devoted Mother and Her Baby.* Tavistock Publications, London, 1949.

The Nigerian Family in Transition

A. O. Sanda, M.D. (Nigeria)

Contemporary Nigerian society has become a complex society. The roots of its complexity involve a number of social, economic, and political forces that have combined to modify the traditional socioeconomic and political organization of Nigeria since the era of colonialism. Nigeria's complexity is particularly observable in the emergent class structure, the multiethnic composition, and the internal political restructuring that has taken place since 1960.

Within the context of Nigeria's social system, it is necessary to recognize the Nigerian family with the understanding of the possible variations occasioned by increasing class differentiations [11] and persistent ethnic pluralism [22] in Nigerian society. The formation, structure, and function of the Nigerian family have been affected over the years by social class restratification and ethnic heterogeneity.

In this paper, we emphasize the Yoruba family and its transition since the 1960s. Similar contributions with respect to other ethnic groups can be consulted in Nzimiro's work on the Ibo [14] or Daryll Ford on the Yako [7].

Whether the subject of emphasis is the family within a particular ethnic group or Nigerian families in general, certain forces or factors of change have affected the whole society in the last 100 years, and such changes also have had modifying effects on Nigerian families. For example, factors of industrialization and urbanization, population change and migration, the dynamics of political and sociolegal changes, the elements of culture contact and formal or institutional education, as well as economic growth, all have had their visible impact on the formation, structure, and functions of families, however conceived or defined, in contemporary Nigerian society [4].

In this paper an attempt is made to provide a brief description of the traditional precolonial Yoruba family including its structure and functions, and subsequently the changes in the traditional structure and functions of the family will be highlighted, along with the dominant factors responsible for the transformations. Finally, the social consequences of the process of change in the Nigerian family are discussed.

The Yoruba Family Before Colonialism

The Yoruba family before the early twentieth century was a collection of several individuals who claimed descent from a common ancestor or progenitor; such a family usually consisted of three or more generations of related nuclear families, in which the great-grandfather, the grandfather, the father, and the children, together with various spouses were often in common residence. An author like Schwab would refer to such a family as the segmentary lineage system [24]. Other authors like Aldous or Olusanya refer to this type as the extended family [2]. According to Aldous [2]

> The concept of the extended family itself developed from studies of African peoples. Life in the tribal village follows a traditional pattern. *The person is important only as he contributes to the extended family unit.* In return, he is given the security of not one, but many fathers, mothers, brothers, sisters, uncles and grandparents. Such a social organization results in strong group solidarity with an attendant communal spirit. (emphasis added)

Writing specifically of the Yoruba extended family, Aldous further notes:

> Though living long before colonial times in cities of up to 100,000 residents, the Yoruba have maintained their traditional extended family patterns. Individuals continue to feel strong obligations to give economic assistance to relatives, while maintaining social ties and the customary residential unit remains the lineage.

Aldous itemized four crucial empirical referents of Yoruba extended family: the *common residence* of two or more related nuclear families; the pervasive nature of *joint activities* among the members in economic, legal, welfare, and leisure matters; the mutual or *reciprocal rendering of assistance* dictated by the traditional normative expectations of the Yoruba (for example, in the education of the young or the support of the aged); and the existence of *friendship networks* that derive from membership in such an extended family.

The description of the traditional Yoruba family by Imoagene [10] is also instructive. The emphasis on location in a common residence for different generations of relations and the predominance of group orientation and general interdependence are also clearly portrayed.

> Essentially, Yoruba families were organised in compounds and were three or four, sometimes more generations deep. They were extended units which included a man, his wife (or wives), his brothers, sons and sometimes grandsons with their wives. There was a feeling of belonging in the family group, and individual activities were (or supposed to be) oriented towards the achievement of the group objectives. *Common interests and goals took precedence over individualism and self-interests.* An important point to note about this system is that the obligation to support kin members was directed not only to parents but also to brothers, uncles, aunts, and cousins of all descriptions.

It is the same group orientation of the traditional Yoruba family that ensured that marriages consisted of unions between families rather than between individuals. Indeed, the long process of involvement and reciprocal investigations of the families of prospective partners ensured an almost total and permanent union. When a marriage proposal was received by a family, the head of that family authorized a fact-finding study of the history and reputation of the family members of the prospective partner. In particular, efforts were made to find out if any member of the family had been afflicted with any type of incurable disease like leprosy or advanced psychosis, or whether any of the family members had been found guilty of any criminal offense. Once the family was cleared, the arrangements could continue. The practice of widow inheritance additionally guaranteed the continuance of the marriage even after the death of the original husband.

The family unit, being a semiautonomous political unit, took charge of its internal administration. The head of the family adjudicated in disputes over resources like land and between husband and wives or between siblings. Succession to political office, even outside the family, was largely dependent on the position of the aspirant within his family.

As a link between the living and the dead, the head of the traditional Yoruba family was also the religious head of his family, performing funeral rites and ancestral rites as the occasion demanded, and he was believed also to possess the spiritual support of the ancestors, which he could invoke against erring family members. He was the keeper of family land and in control of the total family resources. Such economic resources like land could also be granted to new members of the family. In essence, therefore, there was considerable interdependence between the Yoruba family and the traditional political, religious, and economic systems.

With regard to the traditional extended family as an economic unit, Olusanya [19], in his study of Lagos Yoruba, made a minor modification:

> Traditionally, although the large extended family comprising a couple, their married sons, and the wives and children, as well as the unmarried ones (that is, the three generation type of household) as a single economic unit is very rare among the Yoruba (the main group in the city of Lagos), the same building or compound can and often does accommodate more than one nuclear family. Usually on the marriage of a son, he is given a portion of land for use, and he automatically becomes the head of a separate economic unit, though mutual help among the children and between them and their parents continues. He may continue to live in the same house with his parents if there is sufficient space, but usually moves to his own separate building as soon as, and provided he can afford to build.

Olusanya's position represents a variation of the same theme. As observed by Morris [13], the manifestation of mutual obligation by members of the family represents an outstanding characteristic of Lagos social life.

It must be noted that in spite of the dominant position of the patrilineal head of the Yoruba family, the women also contributed to the traditional family. Such contributions included custodial and developmental care of the children and informal, functional work. Most Yoruba women were either traders in the domestic environment, where they could combine child care with remunerative work, or they took part in farm harvests and the sale of their husband's farm products. There were, however, clear divisions of labor between the sexes within the traditional Yoruba family.

Parental power and authority over the children were almost total; this characteristic of the traditional Yoruba family was reflected in the dominant role that parents usually played in the selection of spouses and work for their children. The nature of parental power and authority were also evident in the moral upbringing and general socialization of the children in the values and behaviors of their immediate community. The female children were consciously prepared for their marital roles in later life, and the male children were trained or socialized to develop into family leaders and breadwinners. For both sexes, the norm of chastity before marriage was enforced by the parents on behalf of the community, and the children were expected to avoid causing embarrassment to the parents on their marriage day through strict adherence to the "no sex before marriage" ethics.

Finally, the traditional Yoruba family believed in and encouraged the production of as many children as "the lord gives them." This orientation may have resulted partly from the economic production requirement of the times when the father depended essentially on his wives and children for much of the farm labor and partly from the high mortality rate occasioned by hazards of war and inadequate medical facilities.

In the traditional Yoruba family, therefore, the group was at the center of both the individual's efforts and the family's collective efforts. The structure of authority, the network of mutual help and friendship, the claim to property, and the call on spiritual power of the ancestors were all interwoven in and deriving from the peculiar form and functions of the Yoruba extended family. This was the prevalent situation before certain factors brought about transformations in the form and content of Yoruba family life.

Major Factors of Change

Significant changes have occurred in the composition, functions, characteristics, and attitudinal orientation of Nigerian families since the 1880s. Of all the salient factors of change, perhaps the first and most influential is the factor of cultural contact and the diffusion of nonindigenous values and attitudes within Nigerian society. Authors like Schwab [24] suggest that such cultural contact of the Yoruba dates back to 1900. However, colonial history indicates that as far back as 1861 the Yoruba in Lagos were already in contact with the West. This contact of Nigerian indigenes in general and Yoruba people in particular with foreign traders, colonial administrators, and missionaries of both Christian and Islamic religions led to the gradual modification of the people's attitudes on the family.

For example, the orientation of the Christian converts toward the monogamous family unit of the missionaries conflicted with the basically polygamous households that antedated the coming of the missionaries and colonial administrators. White-collar jobs requiring the literacy of indigenes and introduced by the colonial administrators conflicted with the traditional location of the individual within the domestic environment while simultaneously engaged in works that may be rewarding. The introduction of new legal, political, and economic structures or institutions gradually subverted not only the basis of the authority of the family head but also many of the bonds uniting the members of the traditional family.

Even the belief in ancestral cults became weakened as a result of people's contact with the Christian and Islamic religious beliefs and rituals.

A second major factor of change that brought about gradual modification of the Nigerian family in general and the Yoruba family in particular was the introduction of Western education and the exposure of both sexes and the very young to it. The comparatively significant position that education occupies as an agent of change can be seen from this statement by one of the veterans of Nigeria's educational system [6].

> Education is still the largest industry and the most labour intensive in this country today. It has twenty Ministers and Commissioners of Education, twenty Permanent Secretaries, twenty Professional Heads, at least 2,000 Administrative and Professional Officers, Principals, Headmasters, Head Mistresses, Librarians, House Masters and Mistresses, Sectional Head Registrars, Engineers, Bursars and Catering Officers, 400,000 Teachers, more than 50,000 schools and institutions, some 12.5 million pupils ... and some 100,000 students in Universities, Polytechnics, Colleges of Education, etc. ... Indeed, education in Nigeria, as in many countries of the world, is not only the biggest industry, it is also everybody's business. *It is the only enterprise that touches the life of every citizen.* You are either a pupil, a student, or a parent, a guardian, or an education official, or at the most, you have a brother, sister, or aunt whose child or children go to school. (emphasis added)

From 1842 to 1882, education in Nigeria was in the hands of the missionaries. But from 1882 onward the colonial government became involved. In 1905, the first colonial Department of Education was established. As early as 1914, there were 49 government and six native administration schools with a total enrollment of 9649 boys and 1000 girls; in addition, there were 269 mission or private schools with about 36,780 boys and 10,080 girls and 2440 unassisted mission and private agency schools with 72,250 boys and 8874 girls. This implies that already by 1914 there were about 138,633 pupils in formal, primarily educational institutions in Nigeria.

By the same year, there were only two government schools—Queens College and Kings College in Lagos with 142 boys and 39 girls, and 17 mission-assisted secondary schools with 442 boys and 11 girls. Also, only four government teacher training colleges existed by this time with an all-male student population of about 90. The mission teachers training colleges already had about 375 boys and 41 girls enrolled [6].

As early as 1914, therefore, education had assumed its pervasive impact as a potent agent of social change. The content of this education led to tremendous diffusion of Western culture and the modification of Nigerian social structure and values as well as the gradual disruption of family ties and orientation. The growth in education has continued throughout the era of educational expansion in the 1950s (with the western and eastern regions' free universal primary education) to the era of free universal primary education along with the student explosion and inadequate university places for qualified students. It is only since 1970 that serious efforts have been made to address the issue of relevance of the educational content for Nigeria's social and economic development purposes.

A third major factor that has affected the family in its process of transition in Nigeria concerns the twin process of urbanization and industrialization [12]. In 1931 only Lagos and Ibadan had grown to a population of 100,000; by 1952–1953 census, only seven towns (including Kano in the north and six towns among the Yoruba) had attained a population of 100,000. By 1963, about 24 towns had populations of 100,000. Indeed, the last 50 years have witnessed accelerated rural–urban migrations, especially in the Yoruba area, and by 1963, about 51 percent of Yoruba people lived in towns with a population of 20,000 or more, about 40 percent lived in communities with 50,000 people, and about 25 percent lived in towns with 100,000 or more. The rate of urbanization has continued unabated. According to Imoagene [9], just as there are forced migrants who have been compelled to migrate to the industrial and capital cities for economic reasons, there are also psychosocial migrants who have left their rural origins because of their dissatisfaction with the rural social life and the attraction of the cities.

The development of the industrial sector was given an impetus by the 1955–1962 Development Plan, and a further drive toward industrialization was contained in the 1962–1968 plan. As small as the industrial sector may have been in the past, it has grown to become a major employment-generating sector in all major Nigerian towns. The earliest industrial enterprises were canning factories, fruit and vegetable processing, sugar factories and refineries, soft drinks, tobacco, and, recently, breweries and vehicle assembly plants. In spite of its stage of infancy, the industrial sector has contributed in no small way to the diversification of the economy.

The creation of new states in Nigeria, the rapid industrialization of the major cities, the introduction of new employment opportunities, and the growth of the population have all combined to produce rapid urbanization with attendant problems of family instability and dislocation. The spatial mobility of family members

Table 1. Growth Rate of Selected Industrial Towns in Nigeria 1931–1963[a]

1963	1952 (taking 1931 as base)	Annual Growth Rate Between 1931 and 1952	1963 (taking 1952 as base)	Annual Growth Rate Between 1952 and 1963
Sapele 100 (4,143)	812 (33,658)	33.9	181.2 (61007)	7.4
Enugu 100 (12,959)	488 (63,212)	18.5	219 (138,457)	10.8
Aba 100 (12,958)	452 (58,251)	16.7	225 (131,003)	11.4
Lagos 100 (126,108)	325 (409,959)	10.7	204 (834,625)	9.4
Port Harcourt 100 (15,201)	387 (59,548)	13.7	302 (179,563)	18.4

[a]From O. Imoagene. The Impact of Industrialisation and Urbanization on the People of Nigeria. Paper presented at the Symposium on Nigeria and Black Civilization, 1974.

has weakened both the form and content of traditional family in Nigeria in general and among the Yoruba in particular.

A fourth major factor that can be linked directly to the emerging distortion of the traditional family type in Nigeria concerns the process of political and legal transformation in the society at large. Elsewhere we have treated the problems attendant on ethnic politics in the society [23]. It is, however, relevant to mention here that both ethnic politics and party politics and the three-year civil wars in Nigeria (1967–1970) have left their indelible marks upon the family, particularly in the war-affected areas.

Additionally, the legal provisions on contractual marriage, the place of marriage by ordinance or through native law, and the legal revisions of the matrimonial laws (under the military) have had their varying impacts on membership within the family unit and the roles and responsibilities of principal members.

The study by Adewoye [1] has shown rather vividly the fact that the English law and courts introduced during the colonial times were instrumental in the growth of individualism and the alteration of the status of women. In addition, the courts were most instrumental in imposing the norm of one man, one wife and the general subversion of the traditional family system in Nigeria, particularly in southern Nigeria.

> The administration of justice by native rulers on the advice of British officers who are resident in the native states is gradually resulting in the absorption of the family by the state through the supercession of the paternal power. The court may

uphold the child who will not marry at the choice of his parents, it may enquire if a punishment of the child by the father has been excessive, and the father may be punished therefore; the neglect of a child may be punished with the death of the parents ... The basis of the imported English law is individual responsibility in contrast with the traditional jurisprudence which placed high premium on family or even communal responsibility in place of the "collective responsibility of the extended family and to some degree of the kindred for the conduct of its members"; the British-established courts and the imported English common law were concerned only with the individual in so far as his acts or omissions were called in question in particular cases. It is for this reason that the breakdown of family ties among the Yoruba has been attributed with some justification to "the enforcement of English social laws" and to "the individuality of English life" as reflected in the imported legal system [1].

The promulgation of the marriage ordinance of 1863 was the most obvious evidence of the deliberate attempt of the colonial administrators to impose English marital ethics on Nigerian society. The Nigerian marriage ordinance of 1863 was a replication of the English Matrimonial Causes Act of 1857, and marriage under the act is supposed to be monogamous. It is also the more recognized of the two forms coexisting (i.e., as opposed to customary forms of marriage). The provisions on inheritance under the ordinance also differed from the customary provisions: "The concept of the extended family has no place in the English law" [1].

Social Consequences for the Yoruba Family

The combined effects of the processes indicated above were, over the years, to transform the Nigerian family from its traditional structure and to attenuate and distort some of its traditional functions. As noted by Aldous with regard to the Yoruba, "The city's effect on the family consequently is to strip it to its bare essentials. The nuclear family of father, mother, and children replaces the extended family" [2]. This view, however, contradicts the one by Schwab, who suggests that in spite of all the forces of change, the lineage system and the concept of the lineage persist [24]. As far as Colson is concerned, the residential extended family has had to accept some adaptations that have been imposed on the family [4]. In the view of Imoagene, however, the salience of the extended family, both in terms of control of members and reciprocal involvement in common activities, varies from the politicians to the businessmen and the bureaucrats in that order [10].

It is possible to identify specific spheres of family form and process in which changes have taken place. First of all, studies tend to suggest that women have been increasingly attracted to white-collar jobs that take them away from their family environment for long hours during the day [3, 16, 19]. The high cost of living, the induced needs for many modern amenities, and the attempt of family members to cope with socioeconomic demands imposed by change compel many women to leave their family and to take up permanent employment. This process leads to the erosion of functions that were performed previously by the extended family. Fadayomi et al., [5], in their study of seven states in Nigeria, suggest that "what is being observed is an emerging conflict between mothers' increasing participation in gainful employment and motherhood, especially in the case of pre-school children." The procurement of employment outside the home and very often also outside the town of birth not only means disruption of the residential pattern of the extended family but also the weakening of its socialization functions. Women's role in children's early socialization has become delegated to house helpers and daycare centers.

The introduction of numerous and different avenues of making money has eroded the authority of the family head in some ways while enhancing the status of women. The fact that a young man or a wife does not have to depend on the financial support of either the father or husband has conferred great measures of autonomy on both the youths and the women. This point was emphasized by Ottenberg [20] for the Afikpo Ibo women whose economic independence came with the introduction of cassava into their ethnic community. The situation clearly contrasted with what existed in Afikpo before 1902 when women were physically and economically dependent on their husbands. In spite of the reduced authority of men, Ottenberg further noted:

> Men's position of religious, moral and legal authority is in no way threatened. In other words, *though change in the relative economic positions of men and women in Afikpo has contributed to conditions of instability in relations between husbands and wives*, it has not altered the traditional division of economic responsibility for the maintenance of the household upon which the survival of the family and the society depends. (emphasis added)

Among the Yoruba, the acquisition of Western education and the procurement of stable occupation by the emergent women of the middle class have occasioned several challenges to the traditional conceptions of women's roles within the family. The same process has created strains between husbands and wives, especially in regard to the expressions of freedom and claims of equality by the women. The legal provisions have helped enforce these. For instance, in the event of a man's death intestate, the properties now go to the wife and children, whereas in the traditional setup the properties went to the male heirs.

In the Yoruba as well as in other Nigerian families, the group-centeredness of the traditional family is gradually being replaced by individual-centered families in the contemporary context. This is not to say that members of the family do not now cooperate as of old in the performance of funeral ceremonies, naming, and elaborate marriage ceremonies. However, the implication is that in the final analysis, whether the family survives as a unit or breaks up as a result of divorce, separation, or desertion now depends to a greater extent on the individual parties to the union. The dispersal of members of the family, which has been helped by urbanization and industrialization, the spread of market values, the increasing acceptance of individual values, and continuous contact of family members with total strangers continue to make the traditional group-centered family an anachronism.

The family, as a result of these changes, has changed from being one economic unit. In many cases, the increasingly monetized economy has produced families in which husbands and wives keep separate bank accounts. Joint business ventures between husbands and wives still occur, either with the husband being the owner of the business and the wives working for him as of old (but paid salaries), or with the wives having shares of a joint venture.

In terms of family members' attitudes toward issues like premarital sex, birth control, and the like, Olusanya [19] noted, "Urbanization, rural-urban migration and the dispersal of members of the extended family have brought about not only structural changes within the family but also changes in the functions, responsibilities and attitudes of members." His comparative study of different socioeconomic classes in Lagos revealed that families were not only becoming increasingly nuclear in composition but also that the traditional attitude of "unlimited procreation" is losing favor among the Surulere high-status respondents to whom the small family idea was already becoming attractive. On the other hand, low socioeconomic educational status groups still adhere to large family ideals. Women in the study were not in favor of postponing employment during the period of child bearing. Even though the high status groups "overwhelmingly approve family planning, a large majority of the control group disapprove" [19].

The norm of chastity is fast giving way to the recognition of premarital relations and trial marriages as inevitable steps before marriage. In some situations, many of the prospective husbands insist on the spouse becoming pregnant before marriage. The pattern has recently compelled a church leader to threaten not to conduct church marriages for couples whose spouses were already pregnant before coming to the altar.

The traditional custom of reciprocal investigation of the families of prospective spouses has become less important, and in some cases this has been given up entirely. Prospective partners are frequently brought together by accidental location, either in educational institutions or in employment offices, both of which constitute the great levelers in society. However, recent research reveals the strains and stresses occasioned by the loss of people's dependence on traditional families, and the emergent hybrid families (neither Nigerian nor Western) in the contemporary context are still struggling to cope.

Conclusion

The discussion of the transformations taking place in many spheres of Nigerian family life has endeavored to demonstrate certain tendencies. First, there is the dual experience of persistence and change by the Nigerian family, which, as a consequence, is fast becoming a family type with hybrid characteristic structure and functions, and in which the members consistently manifest a marginality of role relations, attitudes, beliefs, and socio-psychological orientations. This development cannot be ignored in any attempt to provide necessary support for family members.

For example, it is most probable that the increasing adult patronage of the Aladura, Christ Apostolic, and Celestial churches in southwestern Nigeria is not unrelated to the emerging instability and marginality of the family and may be a direct manifestation of family members' desire to seek alternative sources of socio-psychological anchorage. Nor is the proliferation of such syncretic churches in Nigerian urban centers unrelated to the degree of family disruption in those locations.

Second, society, in particular the government and professionals in sociology, social work, and psychiatry, cannot afford to ignore the dysfunctional consequences of the family's change for children and youths. Many young mothers have spent all their premarital life mostly in formal educational institutions ranging from daycare centers to nurseries, primary and secondary schools, and finally the university. In urban centers like Lagos, children are "bundled" into vehicles as early as 6:00 a.m. on their way to school, and, because of the exigencies of traffic and transport, the children and the parents often do not cross paths again until night falls. The contribution of the family to the preparation of such young people for life may be so inadequate that it constitutes sources of marital maladjustment in later life. At a recent marriage ceremony, a father-in-law was quoted as requesting his new son-in-law to be understanding and never to complain about the fact that the bride-to-be did not have any home training. This, according to the father, was due to the fact that the daughter had spent all her time in school, and immediately after graduation from the university she decided to get married. As far as the father was concerned, he, as a parent, did not have enough time to prepare his daughter for her new status and related roles. In a traditional family context, other members of the family would provide the missing links.

However, if the trend toward nuclear families is as irreversible as Olusanya and others would make us believe, and if the structure and functions of the extended family continue to be weakened and distorted, what substitute social institutions are to be provided so social change in the family may not continue to create unresolved social problems for Nigeria?

One possible option is for the compound *(Agboile)* concept of family living to be revisited with a view to adapting the concept in the residential designs and living conditions of Nigerians. It must be noted that apart from the protective cover that the structure provides against various kinds of robberies and burglaries, the compound concept of living will provide many of the extended family's informal means of psychological or emotional and moral support to the adherents.

In addition, the family laws and public service "general orders" guiding antenatal and postnatal relations of women to their employers require a new look. It was possible in the past for educated women in Nigeria to terminate employment voluntarily to get married and take proper care of children. The soaring cost of living and the new race for materialism have made this practice an anachronism. Perhaps the government may want to consider granting leave without pay for two or more years to nursing mothers (on demand).

In the long run, however, the formal educational institutions will have to be used to transmit indigenous values and attitudes compatible with the type of family desired for Nigerian society at large.

In the sphere of political authority of the family head, the institutional differentiation in society has made the change in this direction irreversible. Even the town chiefs and village heads are already dwarfed in stature and authority through constitutional politics and the modern political process.

In the realms of religion and the economy, the contemporary position and roles of the family cannot compare with the positions, structures, and functions of organized Christian churches or Islamic sects on the one hand, and the usurpation of the function of economic planning and development by the state on the other.

The Nigerian family has undergone considerable transformation of structure and functions as a result of numerous social, cultural, economic, and political changes. The changes have resulted in the development of new attitudes and functions by the family and new problems for the family and society. The response of society to these developments will determine the extent of negative or positive functional consequences that may emerge from the Nigerian's family transition.

References

1. Adewoye, O. Courts of law and socio-cultural change in southern Nigeria: 1854–1954. *Nigerian J. Sociol. Anthropol.*, 1, 1 (1974), 62.
2. Aldous, Joan. Urbanization, the extended family and kinship ties in West Africa. In Van den Berghe, P.L., Ed. *Africa; Social Problems of Change and Conflict.* Chandler, San Francisco, 1965.
3. Arowolo, O. *Female Labour Force Participation and Fertility. The Case of Ibadan City, Western State of Nigeria.* Changing African family Monograph No. 4 Dept of Demography, Research School of Social Studies, The Australian National University, Camberra, 1976.
4. Colson, Elizabeth. Family change in contemporary Africa. In Middleton, John, Ed. *Black Africa; Its Peoples and Their Cultures Today* Macmillan, New York, 1970.
5. Fadayomi, T.O. et al. *The Role of Working Mothers in Early Childhood Education: A Nigerian Case Study.* UNESCO/NISER Report, 1977.
6. Fafunwa, B. The administration of some key services: Education paper presented at the National Conference on 20 years of Nigerian Public Administration. University of Ife, Ile-Ife, 1980.
7. Ford, Daryll. Double descent among the Yako. In Radcliffe Brown, A.R., and Ford, D., Eds. *African Systems of Kinship and Marriage.* Oxford University Press, New York, 1964.
8. Green, L. Migration, urbanization and national development in Nigeria. Paper presented at 11th International Seminar on Modern Migration in West Africa, Dakar, March 27, 1972.
9. Imoagene, O. Psycho-social factors in rural–urban migration. *Nigerian J. of Soc. Econ. Stud.*, 9, 3 (1967).

10. Imoagene, O. Extended family detachment among the new elites in emergent society. A strategy of social closure in class armation *West Afr. J. Sociol. Pol. Sci.*, 2, 1 and 2 (1976/77), 65.
11. Lloyd, B. Education and Family life in the development of class identification Among the Yoruba. In Lloyd, P.C. Ed. *The New Elites of Tropical Africa,* Oxford University Press, London, 1966.
12. Mabogunje, Akin. L. *Urbanization in Nigeria.* University Press, London, 1968.
13. Morris, P. Slum clearance and family life in Lagos. *Hum. Organ.,* 19 (1960).
14. Nzimiro, I. Family and Kinship in Ibo land Cologne.
15. Ohadike, P.O. Urbanization; growth transition and problems of a premier West African city (Lagos, Nigeria) *Urban Aff. Q.,* 3,4 (1968), 74–75.
16. Okediji F.O. Some social psychological aspects of fertility among married women in an African city. *Nigerian J. of Econ. Soc. Stud.* 9, 11 (1967).
17. Olusanya, P.O. Status differentials in fertility attitudes of married women in two communities of western Nigeria. *Econom. Dev. Cultural Change* 19, 4 (1971).
18. Olusanya, P.O. Reflections on the relationship between extended family obligations and the standard of living of members. *Int. J. Contemp. Sociol.* 12, 3 and 4 (1975).
19. Olusanya, P.O. Nursemaids and the pill: A study of household structure female employment and the small family ideal in a Nigerian metropolis. Population Dynamic Programme, University of Ghana and University of Northern Carolina, Chapel Hill. (forthcoming).
20. Ottenberg, Phoebe. The changing position of women among the Afikpo Ibo. In Bascom, W.R., and Herskovits, Melville J., Eds. *Continuity and Change in African Cultures.* Phoenix Books, The University of Chicago Press, Chicago, 1962.
21. Sanda, A.O. "Education and Social Change in Africa: Some Problems of Class Formation" *UFAHAMU*
22. Sanda, A.O. Ed. *Ethnic Relations In Nigeria.* Caxton Press, Ibadan, 1976.
23. Sanda, A.O. Ethnic interest and political fragmentation in Nigeria. *Nigerian Behav. Sci. J.,* 2, 1 (1979), 53–68.
24. Schwab, W.B. Continuity and change in the Yoruba lineage system. In Middleton, J., Ed. *Black Africa; Its Peoples and Their Cultures Today.* Macmillan, New York, 1970.

Effects of Rapid Socioeconomic Change on the Nigerian Family

R. Olukayode Jegede, M.D. (Nigeria)

Nigeria, the most populous country in Africa, is located on the west coast of the African continent. Its population is estimated to be somewhere between 80 and 100 million people. There is a high proportion of children and adolescents, and the dependency ratio (the number of persons who are too young or too old to work divided by the number of those in the working-age group) is high. General living standards are on the average low, but extensive socioeconomic changes are occurring at a rate that probably never has been matched by any other country. Most Nigerians are either Christians or Moslems, but a small but significant proportion practices traditional religions. Owing to widespread illiteracy, most people are engaged in subsistence-level agriculture and other occupations requiring little skill and have meager incomes.

In Nigeria, four kinds of marriage are available, all of which have legal status. Marriage according to traditional custom and Moslem law permit polygyny. Church marriage and registry marriage impose monogamy on the married couple in theory but in practice many men who subscribe to these types of marriage acquire additional wives without any legal repercussions. (It should be noted that having more than one husband is not allowed in the male-dominated Nigerian society.) In the traditional and Moslem forms of marriage, especially in the past, the female partner need not give her consent. Her parents or their representatives (if the parents are unavailable) are the ones whose consent matters.

Until one or two decades ago, most men were farmers and they had several wives, many of whom provided manual labor on the farms in addition to rearing children. The men lived in compounds with their wives, their children, their own parents, and other older relations such as uncles and aunts. Thus a compound often had three or more generations living under the same roof. A woman did not just marry her husband but was seen as being married to his extended family as well, the entire membership of which owed her, and to whom she also owed, important obligations. She and her husband were therefore not regarded as solely responsible for the upbringing of their children. In fact, a young couple had little say about how their children were raised, since the husband's parents and other elders in the compound constituted the final authority when matters such as discipline and provision of treatment during sickness arose. A mother usually had older and more experienced women around to assist her in taking care of her children. This was of immense value, especially to the young, inexperienced mother who might doubt her ability to take good care of her offspring. Even for the older and more mature mothers, the assistance of other women in the compound came in very handy.

Until about 10 to 20 years ago, the birth rate was generally high, although about half the children died before the age of 10, due to largely preventable conditions such as malaria, infections, and malnutrition. Children were expected to assist their parents as much as possible. Thus a male child usually continued working on his father's farm until, when the father was too old, control of the farm passed to him. Children were obliged to provide financial and other support for their aged parents and other relatives in need. Even persons who lived far away from their place of birth continued to fulfill their obligations by sending money and other materials and by appearing personally when necessary.

In summary, the Nigerian society until recently was characterized by a broad conception of family membership emphasizing the extended family. A strong sense of loyalty existed, which made help readily available at all times. Child rearing (including discipline) was the duty of parents, other adults, and older children in the household. Although the society as a whole was patriarchal, women had an important say in many matters. In general, apart from child rearing and other functions performed by the family elsewhere, the Nigerian family executed those functions that social security and similar agencies carry out in the present-day, technologically developed countries of the West.

Recent Socioeconomic Changes

During the past 20 years, since Nigeria's independence in 1960, numerous socioeconomic changes have been occurring. These changes vary not only in the rate at which they occur but also in their effects. Perhaps the most important single change is in the field of education. Educational facilities at all levels have expanded by leaps and bounds. In the last few years alone the number of universities increased from 6 to 13. The introduction in 1978 of the Universal Primary Education program, the ultimate aim of which is to make school enrollment cover all school-age children, is perhaps the greatest single index of the increasing importance attached to education. The program has resulted in the expansion of existing schools and the building of new ones in urban and rural areas. The ever-rising demand of young people for education and government recognition of the role of education in manpower development serve as the impetus to provision of more educational facilities. The availability of petroleum-generated funds has made the ambitious educational programs possible.

Another major socioeconomic factor is industrialization. Nigeria is eager to become an industrialized country, as evidenced by the fast rate at which industries, ranging from giant cement manufacturing factories to textile mills, are springing up, mostly in the urban centers. Highly skilled technical manpower needed to operate the new industries is provided by training in Nigerian institutions and abroad. In 1980 alone thousands of young Nigerians went to Europe and America for such training.

Occupying a prominent place in Nigeria's development program is the provision of transportation facilities. Thousands of kilometers of highways have recently been constructed, and many more are being built throughout the country. Several airports are under construction, and seaports are also being developed. As a result of this, journeys that lasted days in the past now take only hours.

Urbanization has been increasing steadily since the 1970s. Many previously large urban centers such as Lagos and Ibadan have increased enormously both in size and in population. This expansion also affects towns and villages, many of which, owing to the establishment of industries or administrative headquarters, attract large numbers of people. In addition, new cities are being built or are in the planning stage.

Effects of Socioeconomic Changes on the Family

IMPROVEMENT OF LIVING STANDARDS

One major consequence of the socioeconomic changes described is the improvement in living standards of a substantial proportion of the population. Thanks largely to better educational opportunities, social mobility has been facilitated greatly. Thus the majority of young people, at the completion of their professional training or university education, find themselves earning incomes undreamed of by their parents. Along with the incomes go relatively high living standards, characterized by, among other things, access to better food, housing, and medical care. These are important considerations in a society where malnutrition and infectious disease, along with their neuropsychiatric sequelae, are common. In spite of the advantages accrueing from socioeconomic changes, there are potentially deleterious effects on the family. Such changes do not operate in isolation, but they interact in a complex manner.

WORKING MOTHERS AND CHILD REARING

Social and geographic mobility leads to many young married couples living far away from their parents and relations. As a result, the influence of the extended family is diminishing, whereas that of the nuclear family appears to be increasing. The psychological support traditionally provided by the extended family in times of stress or crisis is not available to these young people. Worse still, no equally effective alternative is provided by the society at large.

A related issue pertains to child rearing. As women receive better education they become qualified for better jobs. Many of these women have fulltime jobs, a role that they combine with the domestic duties of looking after husbands and children. In many cases this multiple role is performed admirably well, but in many others problems arise. Adolescent domestic servants and/or badly run, overcrowded nurseries act as mother substitutes while the natural mothers are at work. The growing children are thus deprived of the traditionally warm environment provided by their own mothers and other women of the extended family. The consequences of poor mothering and inadequate supervision of children are too many to be discussed here. Suffice it to mention that juvenile delinquency and other behavior disorders are among the psychiatric disorders in which poor parenting is believed to play an etiological role. The effects of maternal employment on Nigerian children, the mothers themselves, and the families as a whole is an area in which research is badly needed. However, there is evidence from research done elsewhere [2] that:

1. The working mother provides a different role model than the nonworking mother.
2. Employment affects the mother's emotional state, which in turn influences mother–child interactions and child-rearing practices.
3. Working mothers provide less adequate supervision than nonworking mothers.

Nigerian children, and African children in general, traditionally are breast-fed until rather late, sometimes until the age of three or four years. With increasing modernization, Nigerian women of all social classes began to see breast-feeding as out-of-date and bottle feeding as fashionable. In the case of educated women, this did not cause any major problem, but the children of illiterates or those with little formal education (who constitute the majority of the population) suffered immeasurably. Owing to ignorance and poor hygiene, feeding bottles were not properly cleaned, resulting in gastroenteritis, which killed off many infants. Mothers fortunately are now being persuaded to return to breast-feeding.

Discipline of children and adolescents recently has been given much attention in Nigeria. Government leaders and others have identified the widely prevalent behavior problems, including delinquency, as symptomatic of indiscipline. Although there is unanimity in diagnosing the problem, there is much debate over how to solve it. The cause of behavior problems, however, have not received the attention they deserve. It appears there are multiple causes, including rural–urban migration and marriage practices that militate against proper upbringing of the young.

MARITAL RELATIONSHIPS

In registry and church marriages, monogamy is obligatory, but in practice many men have other wives. Almost invariably these other wives are expected to have children. These women and their children often live together in one house while the men with their legitimate wives and the children borne by the latter live elsewhere. In many cases the affected men have to divide their time between their two homes, and one of them, usually the legitimate one, is neglected. Consequently, many children are deprived of adequate paternal attention. Cases of severe reactive depression precipitated by their husbands' relationship with other women are by no means rare among educated married women. It should be pointed out that there are many cases in which a man, his original wife, and subsequent wives with all their children live together in such a manner that all parties are more or less contented and proper child rearing is possible. The fundamental problem in the case of men who formally opt for monogamy but subsequently practice polygyny appears to be symptomatic of a society in transition. Monogamy was introduced into Nigeria by Europeans who came to evangelize or colonize Nigeria. However, monogamy stands in sharp contrast to traditional African polygyny. The majority of educated Nigerians today are either the first or the second generation of educated (Westernized) persons in their families. Hence the typical educated person is more or less strongly attached to African traditions, including polygyny. The tragedy of the problem facing the monogamist-turned-polygynist African male is that he does not enjoy the advantages of monogamy long enough before he rushes into polygyny. He is denied the advantages of polygyny for various reasons such as the need to appear a monogamist and the fact that he is unable to live under the same roof with all his wives and children.

RURAL-URBAN MIGRATION

Modern amenities such as electricity and pipe-borne water are introduced to the urban areas where jobs are also concentrated, and the cities attract young men and women who are eager to leave their villages for better standards of living. These young people usually have at least some primary school education, as a result of which they come to regard working on the farm with their fathers (as well as living in villages) inferior and undignified. That villages lack such city attractions as electricity, plumbing, and cinemas is an important factor in motivating rural-urban migration among youth. The primitive methods of agriculture, in which the hoe and the cutlass constitute the major tools, is another factor that makes farming, and by implication village living, unacceptable.

Rural-urban migration affects the family in several ways. In the cities many young people attain a better standard of living. But for others, and they are probably in the majority, the cities are not the get-rich-quick places the youth think they are; jobs are too few, and, even when they are available, the new migrant lacks the necessary skills. In addition, accommodations are limited. These factors are largely responsible for the rapid growth of slums in big cities such as Lagos. Slums are known everywhere for their deleterious effects on child rearing and family stability. The frustration experienced by those young people, whose dreams of life in the big cities are shattered because of joblessness and related factors, may be important in the genesis of mental disorder [3].

One of the effects of rural–urban migration is that the migrants are now on their own. The emotional support from members of the extended family is no longer readily available, due to the physical separation that migration has created. Another effect of rural–urban migration is that married men leave their wives and children in the villages while they search for jobs in the cities. In other cases, even men who live in urban areas may have to leave their families behind in the cities when they work on construction sites where only temporary accommodation is possible. Part of the problem of absent fathers is contributed by employment practices, characterized by husbands being transferred frequently from city to city. Many such men decide to keep their wives and children in one town to save them the trouble of having to move too often. These men commute to visit their families on weekends. The responsibilities of child rearing thus devolve largely on the wives. The importance of having fathers available to join mothers in the upbringing of children has been emphasized repeatedly with little empirical support. Recently, there is increasing evidence to show that fathers influence (1) the moral development of their children, (2) their tendency to express or inhibit aggression, (3) whether they become delinquent, and (4) their overall adjustment [5].

SUPPLY OF ESSENTIAL SERVICES OUTSTRIPPED BY DEMAND

Due to the fast rate of expansion and to the shortage of managerial skill and inadequate resources, the supply and delivery of essential services are outstripped by their demand. Traffic jams, in fact traffic chaos, is the order of the day in the largest cities. For the same reason, irregular supply of water and electricity and frequent disruption of telephone service are regular features of urban living. It is not difficult to imagine some of the psychological effects on parents of spending several hours daily in the sun as they go to and from work in the interminable traffic jams. Getting home late, tired, and irritable is to be expected from such parents. Not only is the time available for family interaction thereby reduced, but the quality of the interaction itself is adversely affected.

THE CURRENT STATUS OF WOMEN IN NIGERIA

In traditional Nigerian society, women felt relatively secure in the extended family. Even when her husband died, a woman was sure that her children and she would be looked after by members of the extended family, despite the fact that she had no basic rights to the house or landed properties she and her husband had used. A similar situation occured in Tanzania and in many other African countries. One of the consequences of modernization for the Nigerian woman is that she can no longer depend on the extended family of her husband for support should he die prematurely. Some of the more educated women are able to resist the hostility of their deceased husbands' relations. In general, the uneducated women and perhaps a proportion of the educated easily yield to pressure to give up their husbands' possessions.

It appears that Nigerian women have attitudes different from men's toward modern changes. For example, women (whether or not educated) readily accept monogamy, whereas many educated men practice polygyny. Lloyd [4], who studied the educated elite of Ibadan, one of the largest Nigerian cities, reported that husbands and wives have little in common, since they spend their leisure time apart, each with his or her own friends. The differences in outlook vis-à-vis modernization may impose severe stress on marital relationships [1].

The march, or rather the rush, to modernization in Nigeria has brought mixed blessings in its wake. On the one hand, considerable improvement in the living standards of many people has occurred. But on the other hand, several untoward effects have resulted. Although reliable figures are hard to come by, the divorce rate and the incidence of juvenile delinquency and drug abuse are widely believed to be on the increase.

The Future of the Nigerian Family

Nigeria is a country undergoing very rapid change. Many traditional African customs are being replaced by Western values or modifications of them. The extended family system that worked so well under an agrarian economy is being threatened seriously as a result of a complex interaction of urbanization, industrialization, and formal education. Parents and their children are participants in and are affected by the process of socioeconomic and sociocultural change. The major problem facing the family at present and in the near future at least is how to maximize the gains of modernization and minimize the undesirable effects.

An overview of the state of the Nigerian family suggests that it is probably the greatest loser, in terms of stability and other variables, in the rush to modernize. Should the present trend continue, the Nigerian family is likely to fare worse in the future. It is possible, although it is not going to be an easy task, to salvage the Nigerian family. This would require concerted action by mental health professionals, the government and its various agencies, politicians, and others. Mental health personnel have the responsibility to advise government on preventive measures to minimize the negative effects of socioeconomic development on the family. Assistance by the federal or state governments in providing well-run nurseries can relieve working mothers of the burden of looking after their young children. This will also save the children from being physically and emotionally battered by domestic servants and other poor mother substitutes. Government assistance should include training of nursery teachers, funding, licensing, and regular inspection of nurseries. The status of women should be enhanced through appropriate legislation and through unified action by women themselves to make society more responsive to their needs. Many husbands need to be helped to see that it is their duty to provide for their wives and children. These and other measures will make women feel more secure, thereby facilitating performance of their roles as mothers, wives, and members of the society at large.

As part of the process of ensuring a better future for the Nigerian family, efforts should be made to decongest existing towns, especially Lagos (the federal capital), where there is a large concentration of industries, which are among the major causes of rural–urban migration. Through tax relief and similar measures, relocation of industries to less populated areas can be encouraged. Certain defects of the existing towns such as poor sanitation, shortage of parks and other recreational facilities, and overcrowded schools should be avoided in the new towns being planned in Nigeria.

Apart from advising government and various agencies on preventive actions of this type, mental health professionals are faced with the challenge of providing treatment for the casualties of the modernization process. These are the adults and children who may need treatment either as individuals or as families. A systematic approach to helping disturbed families is yet to be formulated by mental health professionals.

Conclusion

Nigeria is a country in transition. Although events there may appear dramatic because of the rapid rate of change, other African countries also have been undergoing considerable socioeconomic and sociocultural change, especially during the last two decades. Thus what has been said for Nigeria is applicable with some modification to other African countries [6]. It is hoped that Nigeria can become industrialized without permanent loss of those aspects of traditional African life such as the responsibility of women for their children that have served Africans so well in the past.

References

1. Gugler, J. The second sex in town. *Can. J. Afr. Stud.* 6(1972), 289–301.
2. Hoffman, L.W. The effects of maternal employment on the child: A review of the research. *Dev. Psychol.*, 10, No. 2 (1974), 204–228.
3. Kleiner, R.J., and Dalgard, O.S. Social mobility and psychiatric disorder; A re-evaluation and interpretation. *Am. J. Psychother.*, 29, No. 2 (1975), 150–165.
4. Lloyd, P.C. The elite. In Lloyd, P.C., Mabogunje, A.L., and Awe, B., Eds. *The City of Ibadan.* Cambridge University Press, Cambridge, England, 1971.
5. Lynn, D.B. *The Father: His Role in Child Development.* Brooks/Cole, Monterey, Calif. 1974.
6. Whiting, B.B. Changing life styles in Kenya. *Daedalus,* 106, No. 2, (1977), 211–225.

Clinical Aspects of Adolescent Problems in Nigeria

Ayo Binitie, M.D. (Nigeria)

It is important in a discussion on the problems of adolescents in Nigeria to discuss the cultural milieu and the African view of the cosmos both in the traditional form and in its modern Afro-European context. It is only then that an understanding of the problems of the adolescent can be placed in context, and a meaningful analysis, which takes into account the various factors impinging on young persons, can be made.

The African World

Imokhai (1979), writing about Uzairue society, described the universe seen by the people of Uzairue. He showed a hierarchical structure of the society in terms of age groups from birth to old age and death. At the top of the hierarchy were the elders. These elders were the intermediaries between the present generation and the departed ancestors. The ancestors in turn held communion with God. The citizens of the Uzairue saw a continuity between all these forces of nature, namely, there is God Almighty, then spirits, then the ancestors.

The immediate departed ancestors keep a watchful eye over the affairs of the present generation. They watch, protect, and guide the present generation; they are the avenging angels for misdemeanors of breaking taboos and violating customs. Extensive studies of the belief system of Africans have found this common theme.

Radcliffe-Brown and Daryll Forde [8], Daryll Forde [2], and Fortes and Dieterlen (1965) have published reports from various parts of Africa on the Yorubas, Binis, and Hausas from Nigeria; the Ashanti of the Gold Coast (now Ghana); the Fon of Dahomey; the Dogen of French Sudan; the Lovedu of the Transvaal; the Abeluyia of Kenya; and the Lele of Kasai. Fortes [3], writing on ancestor worship, said:

> One might perhaps generalize and say that they are deemed to be primarily benevolent when social life is running its normal course, but when individual misfortune or threat to social order supervenes, then they are believed to be punitive in the interest of restoring well-being and order. In this connection, one of the more interesting ethnographic facts was the animosity usually attributed to the ghost left out in the wild. Ancestor spirits have to be brought home in the appropriate way for them to be accessible to prayer and persuasion.

Ancestors play an important and even crucial role in the life of Africans. Since they represent the continuity between one generation and the next. The ancestral representatives on earth are the traditional priests, elders, and seers, who interpret their wishes and, through appropriate sacrifices, minister to the needs of the spirit world and hence to God.

Ancestral spirits are not remote, impersonal gods. They are a living force, omnipresent and constantly watching over the present generation. There is thus a holistic reality to the presence of ancestors within the social fabric. This living presence—although invisible—is the main agent for social cohesion and maintenance of law and order.

Piddington [6], in a review after observing traditional societies, stated, "instead of anarchy and chaos, a well ordered social system in which tradition, taboo and the cake of custom laid down certain rules which members of the community invariably obeyed. Hence arose the artificial misconception of the savage automatically obeying the traditional rules of his society either from his own goodness of heart or because of some almost mystical quality of primitive social behavior such as group consciousness or communistic organization. This perception of the universe is maintained by the realistic misfortune that visits malfeasants. The visitation of punishment by ancestors is swift and effective. There is evidence that some of it is contrived by the elders through agents such as masquerades, rituals, placing of curses, recitation of incantations, and so on. Whatever the case, psychological anxiety is created, which reinforces the prevailing social system."

This account of family life in Edo land was obtained by speaking to elders who are 60 years and above. At the turn of the century, families were much more homogeneous, and frequently three or more generations lived together, that is, the head of the family and his wives and children (who are married themselves). In addition, grandchildren and great-grandchildren may be found in the household. Benin City itself was known as Oredo and was of moderate size. The majority of the inhabitants within the city walls were chiefs and their descendants and were skilled craftsmen, traders, hunters, and native doctors. Not much agricultural activity took place within the city, which depended on the surrounding villages for sustenance.

The focus of social life was the Oba's palace. Craftsmen and hunters worked for the glorification of the Oba and his court. A close relationship existed between children and their parents. Children had not only their own biological mothers to look after them but frequently had grandmothers, grand aunts, co-wives, uncles, and older cousins to guide them in the culture of the land. What the society demanded—uprightness, strong character, and physical strength—was simple, and it was relatively easy for young persons to conform, because of the presence of so many adults to look after them and also because of taboos, the violation of which gave rise to dire consequences.

Traditional religion provided an effective system of social control in the society. It was common to leave yams at the side of the road and have nothing happen to them, because there was a traditional belief that the curse placed on someone who stole the yams would result in the death of all who partook in the eating. The effect was that both the culprit and even innocent participants might pay penalties for the sin of their relative or friend. This strong religious overtone was reinforced by ritual ceremonies and constant worship. Powerful social control was the consequence. Parents were restrained in their behaviors as a result of strong religious beliefs, and they in turn, as carriers of the culture, ensured that their children conformed.

The training of children was by active participation in the trade or occupation of the father. If the father was a bronze worker, who would be found even in this day at Igun Street in Benin City, the children simply accompanied their father as assistants, doing minor chores, learning the trade by direct participation, observation, and practical work until sufficient mastery has been achieved. Even then, the child continued to serve the father, although he might undertake minor contracts of his own. Children of chiefs who were

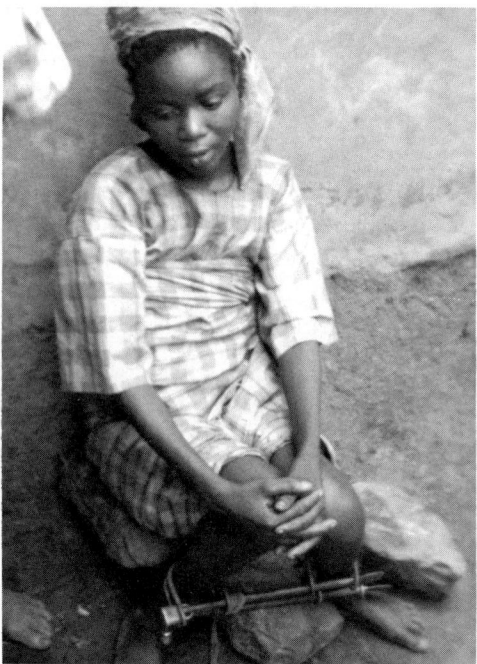

Figure 1

courtiers in the Oba's palace accompanied their fathers as pages to the palace daily. While the fathers were busy with the affairs of state, the children included wrestling and running for the proper development of future warriors. When these children were sufficiently grown, they were introduced into the palace and entered any of the palace societies. They continued their training there and, depending on what skills they showed might be sent by the Oba on various expeditions. Outside the city, where people were mainly farmers, children accompanied their parents to the farm and there learned directly practical aspects of their future occupation.

This pattern was generally similar for most areas in Nigeria. The important thing to note in this form of training is that there was direct contact between parent and child, and the objective and purpose of training was immediately obvious.

The social changes that took place at the turn of the century have had far-reaching effects on the upbringing of children. The main factors that brought about this social change are the introduction of schools and the effect of Christian religion. The impact of religion was the more pronounced and more dominant, since it challenged the very foundation of many traditional beliefs. We have seen earlier in this paper that one of the systems of social control was taboos and fear of visitation and punishment by unseen forces such as ancestors, witches, wizards, and various household gods. The Christian religion (and to some extent the Moslem religion), backed by modern Western technology, was able to challenge successfully the traditional systems. Indeed, many of the shrines, gods, and goddesses were destroyed and some of the gods burnt. People could see that nothing happened and that the Western religion was the more powerful. The basic problem was, that, although these manifestations of Western religion were absorbed, the far-reaching moral ethic that went with them was not. The Western religion, therefore, was taken at face value, and behind this facade of Christianity, many of the traditional beliefs and values were practiced. One example is that polygamy was presumably abandoned by converted Christians. Secretly, however, polygamy continues to be embraced. The effect on the Nigerian population—parents as well as children—is the presence of conflicting values. This shows itself in the form of paying lip service to Christian morality but at a more profound level behaving socially in the traditional manner. Indeed, because belief in the Christian religion lacked roots, gaps in learning that have occurred have been filled in by the Edo social system. Thus in the 1980s, a modern Edo youth is in conflict, trying very hard to resolve the conflict within two separate and different cultures.

The parental generation absorbed some of the Western ideas and manner of behavior, but on the whole are more steeped in traditional practice. This point of culture conflict has had tremendous impact on the overall body politic of Nigeria. Thus in the traditional system a strong feeling toward the community and for the welfare of all the members in it has broken down. This has not been replaced by a fully Western mode of thinking with a strong Protestant ethic of work. Another important aspect of the Western way is individualism. Edos, therefore, like other Nigerians, fall between two stools and have not yet integrated completely the Western and the traditional.

Lest this argument become too theoretical, a practical example will illustrate the difficulty. In the past, when you wanted to build a house, you summoned your friends and neighbors who assisted you. In return, when they wanted to build their houses, you and your friends went along and assisted them. There is no doubt that in more remote areas, this is the practice to this day. In larger urban centers, however, it has been abandoned, and building houses is done by individual contractors for fixed fees.

The other social change at the turn of the century was the introduction of schools. Children now must go to school for long periods in pursuit of an occupation which they may have no knowledge of whatsoever. And indeed, their parents may have no such knowledge to guide them. Many youths must rely on what they hear from their friends and members of their peer group to come to a decision about their future careers. What is more, they must be away from home for long periods, out of touch with their parents and out of contact with any adults who are thus not in a position to give them guidance. The children have to rely on themselves. The problem is further compounded in that many of the parents do not know what goes on in the institutions where their children are trained. Far from giving the children guidance, therefore, the parents must be instructed by their children.

Spiritual Upbringing

Side by side with this formal education, further processes of acculturation at a spiritual and more profound level are going on. The children would have witnessed ritual at various family shrines. The solemnity, songs, and dances and the mystical invocation of ancestors would have been performed often enough that these spiritual forces become embedded firmly and permanently in the psyche. The harmony with nature, the continuity between the present and past, and the ever-watchful presence of the ancestors now become second nature. The existence of supernatural forces, witches, and wizards receives regular reinforcement in the multifarious festivals involving masks and impressive dance rituals. To be in harmony with nature, to avoid giving offense, and to be at peace with one's neighbors represent the greatest good. The majority of African youths go through this spiritual experience. Even those whose parents are completely Westernized come to acquire this African ethos by association and contact with others.

Clinical Problems

Over the years, adolescents with a number of problems for clinical analysis and proper management have come to our attention. Their complaints fall into the following broad categories.

PSYCHOTIC SYMPTOMS

These patients are usually brought in by parents, who complain of aggression, dirty habits, negative behavior, talking to self, running into the bush, restlessness, and aimless wandering. The illness may be of insidious onset or may start suddenly. These are clearly psychotic symptoms. Management is along traditional lines—the phenothiazine group of drugs followed by rehabilitation. Our clinical experience suggests that in the majority of young persons, the illness runs a benign course—the patient recovering fully and returning to a useful life.

SOMATIC SYMPTOMS

These are the most common presenting complaints. The symptoms are myriad, diffuse, and affect all parts of the body. There is heat in the head, heat in the body, heat along the spine, worms crawling all over the body, worms in the throat, peppering sensation in the body, pain in the eyes, pain in the forehead, chest pain, dizziness, dry mouth, dry throat, abdominal pain, nausea, vomiting, diarrhea, noises in the abdomen, dysmenorrhoea, poor vision, poor concentration, and a legion of other symptoms. Our experience shows that clusters of similar symptoms tend to come from a particular institution. Thus one school will have a preponderance of heat in the head and chest pain, another headache and peppering sensation, and so on. Other symptoms are present if asked for. Many writers have commented on these bodily symptoms (Field (1960), Lambo (1956 & 1960), Collomb et al. [1], Leighton et al. [4] Binitie (1971)). Prince [7] coined the term "brain fag" to describe the association of these symptoms with scholastic difficulties. It is to be noted, however, that the symptoms are distress signals, and all forms of psychiatric diagnoses may be encompassed within them. Over time, and with the realization that the symptoms are more specific, Nigerian psychiatrists now use the appropriate diagnostic terminology to describe each clinical case.

BEHAVIOR DISTURBANCES

These present special problems to parents. The child is unreliable and unpredictable. In any given social situation parents are unable to decide what is actually going on because of previous deceit. The complaints of parents include lying, truancy, pilfering, fighting, uncontrollable temper, promiscuity, poor school work, and running

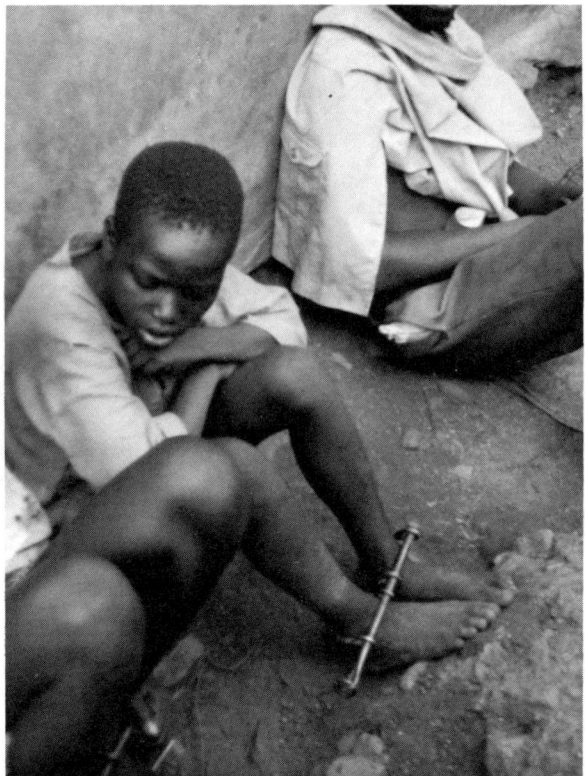

Figure 2

away from home. To these may be added drug taking and smoking of marijuana.

These, in our experience, are the ones that are very difficult to manage. There is an understanding of the social norm and expected behavior, which the child may even accept as standards. The youth is, however, unable to keep these standards. Our theory is that the impulse for libidinal gratification is so powerful and demanding that discharge is obtained at all costs with resulting delinquent behavior.

There are those adolescents who behave in a socially acceptable way but are poorly motivated in terms of searching for a career or pursuing educational goals. These are children of middle- to upper-class families. The parents seek advice from educational authorities on how to motivate these children and give them direction. In the majority of cases there is no abnormality as such; only the desire for comfort. These children just drift and are not impelled toward achievement or a career. These are young men and women in search of a cause. The danger is that they may fall into the hands of unscrupulous persons and be led to antisocial behaviors. In some instances, this strange inertia is accompanied by drug taking.

Children in this group frequently are the children of professional middle class groups or the moneyed classes.

Clinical Examples

CASE 1

Patient A, a female, was 19 years old when first seen. She had just completed secondary school and taken a job six months prior to the index date. She was single and had been brought by both parents, who complained of sudden wild and uncontrollable behavior accompanied by aggressive acts. She did not sleep, talked wildly and at random, and had to be forcibly restrained with shackles.

The illness started about one month prior to the date of consultation. She lost appetite, did not sleep, and lacked energy. No history of fever was obtained. Nevertheless, the parents suspected the illness to be malaria and arranged for two shots of chloroquin to be given intramuscularly on successive days. The dose given was not known, but the father reported that the content of one ampule (probably 40 mg base) was given on each occasion. A few days after the injections the patient burst out into the wild uncontrollable behavior described.

The parents were alarmed at the turn of events. They rushed the patient to a prayer house, convinced that she had been possessed by evil spirits. They were convinced this must be so since no member of the family had ever suffered from psychiatric problems. The patient, in accordance with the custom in these churches, was enrobed in white with a suitable white hat, and prayers invoking the holy spirits were offered. Both parents were invited to participate in the religious ceremonies, which involved, in addition to the prayers, the burning of incense to ward off evil spirits and the lighting of candles on the principle that when there is light, darkness disappears. In addition, there was drinking and bathing with holy water, singing and dancing to hymns in a rhythmic fashion, clapping, and regularly saying halleluya. The mother bore the brunt of these activities, staying with the patient and nurturing her. The father went to his work but came regularly after work to visit.

During this two-week period, the violent acts of the patient disappeared. This was replaced by weeping, slowing speech, staring vacantly, and posturing. More prayers were said and more fasting initiated. The parents were informed that indeed it was the evildoers and the devil that had taken possession of the soul of the patient. In particular, it was the people at her place of work who were jealous of her who were at the bottom of it all. In spite of all efforts at prayers, the patient made no further progress. The parents then consulted relatives, who suggested the patient be taken to see a psychiatrist. This the parents did one month and four days after the illness started.

The psychiatrist obtained the following additional information. The father is a lawyer of many years' standing and was in his late forties. The mother was a trader in her early forties. She was an only wife. There are six children from the marriage, four girls and two boys. The patient is the eldest of the children. She was brought up at home by the parents. She was well looked after by the parents and as a family they were close to each other. She was above average at the primary school level but was an average student in her secondary school. She was a pleasant girl of easy disposition, got on well with her teachers and school mates, and was well liked by her colleagues. She obtained a Grade Three school certificate, not good enough to go straight on to the university. She therefore obtained employment as an officer in the Department of Customs, with the responsibility of catching smugglers and preventing smuggling. It must be stated that in Nigeria this is no mean undertaking. These duties involve occasional night patrols, mounting of roadblocks, and other operations. She appeared to be coping with these tasks before her breakdown and to lead a moderate social life. This job took her away from home, so she had to live in the company of a few friends in a house within the city. However, on weekends when the demands of her job permitted, she went home to her parents. She was generally in good health, having the occasional attack of malaria for which she usually received chloroquin, until the events described occurred.

When seen by the psychiatrist, she had a zombielike gait, stared vacantly, and wept and postured. The psychiatrist, on the basis of the typical features, made a diagnosis of catatonic schizophrenia and started her on chlorpromazine, 100 miligrams, three times a day as well as fluphenazine decanoate (Modecate), 25 miligrams. Tablets of 2-miligram benzhexol were given three times a day two days after the commencement of therapy when Parkinsonian side effects were observed. A few days after the commencement of treatment the patient was able to narrate her experiences further. "I hear a woman and a little girl telling me to dance and then I begin to dance. I see a crowd of people, some whom I know and some of whom I do not know." The mother who accompanied her complained that the girl was dancing in the absence of music and in addition kept gesticulating to people she could not see. She complained that the behavior was embarrassing.

The patient improved following treatment and returned to her work three months after she was first seen by the psychiatrist. The father decided that she had had enough of that work and shipped her off to England 10 months after she was first seen for advanced studies. She embarked on her undergraduate education at a polytechnic insititution in the United Kingdom. She was joined there by her two younger sisters. She completed the first part of her diploma but broke down again with a similar illness three months before her final examination and was repatriated to Nigeria.

The clinical picture was similar to that for which she was hospitalized four years earlier and again she made a rapid recovery. She is presently in Nigeria. Her psychiatrist has advised the postponement of examinations until the next academic session.

CASE 2

Patient B is a 14-year-old male adolescent. He attends a grammar school in the city and is in the fourth year of the five-year school certificate course. The patient was accompanied for the visit by both parents, who gave the account of what had happened.

The patient previously attended a boarding school about one hour from the city of Benin. This is a prestigious institution, most parents struggling hard to get their children into the school. The parents were delighted when their son was admitted to this school. All went well for awhile then the patient felt vaguely ill, had no appetite, did not sleep well, could not concentrate, and was fearful. He went directly to the head of the school and asked permission to go home to his parents. Since the school takes pride in the welfare of its students, the principal advised him to see his house master, who put machinery into action for treating and hospitalizing any students who fell ill.

The student left the school compound and wandered off. Apparently, his behavior gave room for suspicion about the state of his mind. Someone found him and took him to the police station. The police kept him until the next day. By this time the patient had become fully aware of where he was, correctly identified himself, and asked to be allowed to go. No crime had been committed, and the patient was now in complete control of his faculties and spoke intelligently. The police allowed him to go.

While the events with the police were going on, the school authorities observed the absence of the patient and telephoned the parents in Benin to find out if he was at home. He was not. The father went quickly to the school to assist the school authorities in searching for the patient. When the search in the school compound and in the town was to no avail they informed the police. After a search in their records, the police informed the father that such a young person had been found wandering and exhausted but was allowed to go back to school after 20 hours or so at the police station. They felt that the boy must be in school by that time. The father went back to the school but could not find the boy. After some further search in the town, he returned to Benin to bring in some relations to assist. The police were asked to be on the lookout for the boy. He was found again 48 hours after he was first reported to be missing. He was found close to a stream, looking ill. He had lost some weight, was unkempt, and kept holding his throat. He could not talk and could not tell the parents what had happened. The parents took him home to nurse him, thinking that he looked so ill because of the ordeal he had been through. His physical health improved, but he had now become dependent and childlike. He followed the mother everywhere she went and begged for forgiveness. He was quoted as saying regularly, "I beg you now, forgive me. A devil is worrying me. I wish to be born again. I should not have done it. I should not have done it." The parents, after family consultation, came to the conclusion that this was no ordinary sickness. They were convinced that the illness was due to "African science" and therefore called for treatment in the traditional manner. Western-trained doctors were no use for this kind of illness. The parents took the child home to the village and obtained the services of a traditional healer. In accordance with custom, the traditional healer consulted the oracle, who found that the boy indeed had been poisoned at school by jealous school mates. The traditional healer administered an emetic which caused the patient to vomit copiously. He also administered a purgative. This treatment improved the health of the patient. He was able to return home, after staying approximately one week at the traditional treatment center.

The father decided that the patient should leave the school where he had enemies ready to do him in. He contacted the principal of the school and asked for a transfer to Benin. After a period of convalescence at home, the youth started at a school in Benin City as a day student.

As soon as he was told he had been admitted to a new school the illness started again. He again lost weight, was restless and fidgety, and could not sleep. He returned to following his mother everywhere she went, was afraid, and held on to her. He would not eat; he gazed at his mother. He could not explain what the trouble was and again pleaded with her, "Mummy please, mummy please." Out of the blue he announced he wished to be a priest. This time, the parents decided to see a Western-trained doctor, who administered diazepam. The patient improved and was able to resume school. He was again not eating one month later and complained of headaches and weakness. The father immediately took him back to the general physician who referred him to the psychiatrist.

The psychiatrist obtained the following additional information. The father is a professional surveyor in private practice. He previously worked for the government but left to set up his own business. His wife described him as an intensely private person, with a strong will and determination. He is not given to much talking. The patient's mother worked for a time as a civil servant but left when the children became too many to manage without additional help. She has stayed home ever since to look after the children. The patient is the eldest of seven children—two boys and five girls. The last born is the other boy. He is aged two years; the patient is aged 14. The patient was born in the hospital and was precocious in that he started talking at 14 months. He has always been a quiet, serious boy, in many ways like his father. He did well academically. He does not like domestic work. After completing his primary education, he went to a good boarding school where he continued to do well academically.

Of his childhood, the young man remembered that his mother frequently sided with his sisters in any quarrel and would beat him for things he did not do. The mother, on the other hand, said that the patient spoke very little and occasionally got angry and beat his sisters. She beat him to control these eruptions. She mentioned that in school, food and other things sent him by his parents would be stolen or taken from him. The patient never reported this to his parents but rather kept his own counsel. The mother only discovered these things much later.

The young man said that it was his view that many students in the school did not like him. He told of his experiences. "One night I was almost sleeping; one of the boys stood by my window, called my name and then began to laugh." Three boys really upset him in school. These students were close to him. They began to spread "news" about the patient. These three students were the kind of people that like to put themselves on top. They talked about the patient, implying that he was bush, meaning that he was not civilized but a native from the jungle. "I was sure what the boys were saying was not true but I just kept quiet. I don't know why I take the views of these people seriously. Nevertheless, I did and responded by refusing to speak to them. The boys came round to speak to me but I would not talk to them."

These were the events that immediately preceded the first episode of his illness. The psychiatrist observed that the events reported by the patient were the kinds of things that happen in a grammar school. It is possible, and indeed likely, that the boys called him bush, but these are everyday occurrences in a school of this type. The offended party normally makes a report to the school authorities or replies with another joke at the expense of the students concerned.

The reaction was inappropriate and the psychiatrist made a diagnosis of a paranoid illness. There were dynamic factors at work that favored this kind of response. At an earlier time, the mother "took sides with the sisters" when the patient had done nothing wrong. The activities of the three boys must have awakened this repressed rage originally directed against the mother and sisters and now against the three boys.

The patient was given redeptin and the paranoid symptoms cleared. Counseling was undertaken. The patient has remained well and in school.

CASE 3

Patient C is a 15-year-old female. She is in the final year of a secondary grammar school in Benin. She is a Christian. She was brought to see the psychiatrist by both parents on the advice of the school principal. She had been at home for the four weeks prior to the index date. She had been sent home for lovemaking on the college premises. A precondition for readmission was that the parents should sign an agreement that there would be no recurrence of such behavior in the future. The parents were unwilling to give such assurance since they had problems with the girl dating back 10 years. There was a long list of complaints about her behavior, including lying, pilfering, disappearing from home for days, running away from home, and promiscuity. In addition, she was untidy and lazy and always preferred other people's things to hers.

The patient's father is an accountant in private practice, in his early forties. The mother is the only wife, although the father had a daughter by another woman before marrying the patient's mother. This half-sister is now aged 18, three years older than the patient. The mother is in her middle thirties and goes out to work. The patient described her as strict. There are two other children from the marriage, boys aged 11 and nine. The full siblings got on well together, but the patient did not get on with the half-sister, who only came to live with the family about two years back.

The patient was born in England and lived with both parents who were then students in England. To allow the mother to go to school, it was decided by both parents to send the child back home to Nigeria to the care of an uncle and his wife. This uncle had children of his own and two other children of relatives. His wife was uneducated but looked after the children to the best of her ability. As is the habit in many poorer families, the children were given money to buy food in the neighborhood. The patient was given this facility in the same way as other children. The children had great freedom and a happy time. There was much dancing. The patient herself felt she was well looked after there and agreed she had unrestrained freedom, going and coming without hindrance. Said the patient, "We were free to do anything there." She stayed three years with the couple until she was five, when the parents returned from the United Kingdom.

The mother expressed shock at the physical appearance and behavior of the child. When the parents and their child were reunited, the mother set out with a will to improve the physical appearance of the child and, more important, to introduce discipline. The freewheeling days of the patient were to be terminated and replaced by order, cleanliness, and discipline. "I began to have problems with her immediately. It was very hard. She wouldn't take correction. It was all very strange to her. I had to be very careful so I wouldn't scare her away." The pilfering started almost as soon as they took her home in 1970. In spite of the emotional problems that the mother was doing her best to correct, the patient continued to do well in school and was able to pass on merit to one of the best girls' boarding schools in Nigeria. She began to have trouble almost as soon as she got there. In addition, she began to go with boys. Apart from having problems with discipline, she also frequently fell ill. The parents decided to withdraw her from the school to a local one in Benin City so they could exercise greater control over her. These changes did not much alter the patient's pattern of behavior. She would disappear from school for three days and stay with boys. The mother said she would have even accepted this behavior if there were only one boy. But she went about with many boys with no steady boyfriend. Pilfering has continued, although the frequency has diminished. She has continued to get through school examinations in spite of truancy. Her performance has deteriorated. The behavior of the patient gives her parents much anxiety.

On the advice of relatives, she was taken to their home town for two days and sacrifices offered to the gods and ancestors so that the ancestors would be appeased and the "hot spirit" of the girl cooled. This did not achieve the desired effect.

The patient is the victim of conflicting values: one traditional, the other Western. The child was raised at the crucial period of her life in the traditional manner of easy discipline, plenty of freedom, and much spontaneity. The parents, on the other hand, as a result of their sojourn in Europe, acquired the ethics of the West and also the European style of child rearing. This they tried to apply to the child, who failed to respond and became maladjusted. It is of interest to note that in seeking a solution to the problem of maladjustment in this child, both the traditional and Western approach to treatment have been adopted. Neither has produced a satisfactory result so far.

Discussion

A spectrum of the problems seen in adolescents in Nigeria has been presented. The management of psychotic problems follow closely the usual therapeutic regimen seen in Western Europe. An analysis of the contents of delusions and hallucinations show that even in the most Westernized adolescent there are cultural influences operating in the background that impart a peculiarly traditional African belief system into the presentation of disorder. The African belief in the cosmos, the forces of good and evil immediately present, make their appearance in the presentation of psychopathology. The voices patient A heard were commanding. The explanation offered is within the context of the African belief system. It is the envious neighbors through magical means that produced the patient's problem, not the rigors of a tough occupation. In times of crisis Nigerian patients return to their roots.

The role of cultural factors in the genesis of neurotic behavior disorders is even more notable. In Case 3, traditional child-rearing practices came into conflict with Western European patterns. Resolution was impossible, the child taking flight into delinquent behavior. Another important observation concerns body language as a system for presenting emotional disorder. Lopez Ibor [5] has noted similar presentations of symptoms in his description of masked depression among Spanish peasants. It is noteworthy that in many of the Nigerian languages, emotional distress is expressed by reference to the body. "He made me very angry" could be translated literally as "he made me so angry my head is boiling."

It is important to be aware that such points of cultural conflict may precipitate disorder in vulnerable persons and that signals of distress may be expressed in body language.

References

1. Collomb, Henri. *Conditions psychosomatiques en Afriqu.* Transcultural Psychiatric Research, 1964, 130–134.
2. Forde, C. D. *African Worlds: Studies in the Cosmological Ideas and Social Values of African Peoples.* Oxford University Press, New York, 1954.
3. Fortes, M. The character of kinship. In , Goody, J. (Ed.) Cambridge University Press, 1973.
4. Leighton, D., Harding, J.S., Macklin, D.S., Macmillan, A.M., and Leighton, A.H. *The Character of Danger: Psychiatric Symptoms in Selected Communities.* Basic Books, New York, 1963.
5. Lopez Ibor, J.J. *Schizophrenia as a Life Style.* Springer Publishing Co., 1974.
6. Piddington, R. *Kinship and Geographical Mobility.* E.J. Brill, Leiden, 1965.
7. Prince, R. *France and Psychological States.* R.M. Bucke Memorial Society, Montreal, 1968.
8. Radcliffe-Brown, A.R. and Forde, C.D. *African Systems of Kinship and Marriage.* Published for the International Institute by the Oxford University Press, New York, 1950.

Discussion of Dr. Graham's Presentation

Chairman: Norman V. Lourie (U.S.A.)

Dr. Graham's presentation and the discussion that followed emphasized that poverty and inequality, with all their consequences, were among the most violent exposures endured by children. They also bred violence in children and engendered future disturbances that were especially characterized by hostility and aggression. The social, personal, and familial implications were among the most important confronting the International Study Group at this meeting. There was unanimous agreement on the major thrust of the paper. The discussion that it stirred, however, concerned not the prime etiological elements but the use of mental health manpower.

The group was concerned lest the scarce sources might be lost to treatment if the mental health workers assumed major roles in the prevention of poverty and other social ills. No one questioned the fact that these professionals had a significant contribution to make in this area in which psychosocial indicators were among the earliest to predict malnourishment; in which an increase in the understanding of negative influences at work in child rearing, such as the separation of children from their families, could be conducive to more positive mental health; and where the education of policymakers on mental health issues could actually bring about improvements in mental health practice. In countries where many families are displaced, many children are separated from their parents, and many children do not receive adequate nourishment, it is vitally important to convey the basic message that to become resilient and competent, children need to be physically well and remain attached to their families.

The group agreed that clinical services and clinical research should not be depleted through the absorption of clinicians into preventive work, but they were unanimous in advising that mental health clinicians, like biomedical professionals, should be encouraged to participate in some type of public health activity such as training, consultation, and techniques of intervention. It had to be borne in mind that not all mental health workers were clinicians. Some were engaged in community mental health, others in community development, and others in public policy careers. However, both clinicians and nonclinicians could influence policymakers, program planners, service providers, and administrators.

Graham had been involved in a multicontinental WHO effort to assess the total picture of mental health problems in the world's children, and he discussed with the group the strategy of using "primary health workers" in case finding, "primary helping," and preventive programs. ISG supported the idea as a means to offset the lack of mental health personnel, but once again expressed caution about expecting too much from such strategies. It is important that primary care workers do not go beyond their capacities and that their training and supervision should be continuous, not limited to one short term as had been suggested.

It was pointed out that changing familial and child-rearing practices as well as changing the mental health policies of developing nations should not be the exclusive task of one professional group, since "change agents" were to be found in other professions. What mattered was the ability of the different professional and interest groups, in both public and private sectors and across cultural and ethnic lines, to formulate common goals and work purposefully together. Territorial issues often deterred the cooperation and coordination of efforts. The problems were so large that they required all one's diagnostic skills to bring about changes not only within our own professional groups but also among the powers that were responsible for policy.

In setting up the training of mental health professionals, it is necessary to teach them how to translate their clinical findings into social policy and social change strategies. Schools of public health and social work and departments of community psychiatry in medical schools have paid heed to the necessity of mental health workers to learn about community development, planning, and organization.

Apart from warning against expecting too much from primary workers and of overloading clinicians when massive case findings are undertaken, the I.S.G. also emphasized the need for long-range planning to provide adequate numbers of clinicians and researchers. There was also a reservoir of ancillaries such as teachers, pediatricians, obstetricians, nurses, midwives, and even native healers who could be mobilized to assist in the work of prevention.

The I.S.G. bemoaned the fact that the transfer of knowledge was so slow and that we know much more in theory than we can make operational. Some developed countries have had much experience with preventive programs, and it is important to learn from their mistakes as well as their know-how before transposing their programs to developing countries. Too often, the latter are urged to mirror the Western methodology without giving sufficient attention to historical, cultural, and ethnic modifying factors.

One last important area is stressed: The need for reaching parents early and of teaching parenting skills in conjunction with useful native habits. One could also make more use of parents in early childhood education by providing them with some understanding of basic child-rearing procedures (again in concert with successful clinical patterns), as well as some knowledge of infant psychiatry and its findings, especially in relation to the identification of parents and children at high risk.

Discussion of Dr. Minde's Presentation

Chairman: Peter B. Neubauer, M.D. (U.S.A.)

The stimulating discussion that followed this paper was wide ranging and opened many theoretical and service-oriented considerations. The paper addresses itself to a basic developmental sequence which anchors clinical, sociocultural, and biological areas and thus allows the organization of data in a meaningful spectrum. External events can be seen as they relate to the internal experience of the child and its impact on developmental organization.

It may be necessary to add to the paper's propositions the role of individual differences among children and to differentiate those children who had never had the opportunity to make an attachment from those whose attachment was interrupted. It was suggested that one may consider a respective timetable such as the period from birth to three months, from three to six months, from six months to three years, and from three to six years.

Furthermore, it was suggested that the concept of the Garden of Eden principle needs clarification. If it implies that full gratification is expected, then development itself implies that the child experiences a loss in moving to the restraints imposed by reality. If, on the other hand, the concept refers to the optimal or at least average expectable environment, then we need an outline that follows the interaction between stages of developmental organization and the environmental conditions. Thus the question was raised whether the concept of loss as presented was too wide and whether it was equated with stress, since it did not separate the actual loss from the internal experience of malattachment and detachment.

Moreover, the point was made that we must distinguish, as with the concept of trauma, those conditions that precede the experience of loss, those that are part of the reaction to loss and those that prevail after the loss.

A significant finding reported in the paper, namely, that during the latency period changes seem to affect children's behavior most strikingly, was discussed. It was suggested that this was based on children's cognitive development, their capacity to see their roles more specifically, and thereby experience difficulties when confronted with a new social situation, specifically the entrance into a new school.

This led to the consideration of those findings that stress the child's capacity to find substitutes for the primary caretaker—the turning to the peer group and to other members of the extended family, particularly grandparents; the role of boarding schools for young children, and so forth. Some agreed that the heavier burden is carried by boys. Others felt that studies indicate that there is an increase of disorders in girls during the first six years and that later boys show a higher frequency. These findings rest on developmental processes and do not refer to those specific symptoms such as eneuresis, dyslexia, or speech disorders that have a decisive relationship to the gender of the child.

The discussion turned then to the characteristics of change; those that are looked for, and for which there is a preparation; and those that are positive rather than damaging. Thus the aim of the change gains significance in measuring the outcome. (This was seen in Israel and reviewed in relationship to migration to Australia.) The question had to do with the individual's family, group ideals, and aspirations, or those group experiences that victimize and render individuals and groups helpless.

The conditions of African family life and attachment and loss were considered specifically in reference to polygamy. Some offered the opinion that polygamy provides alternate caretakers and gives more than one person to be loved. Since often the first wife selects the other wife, there is no jealousy but mutual responsibility. Thus love has a different meaning in Nigeria. It is not exclusive and it encompasses more than a one-to-one relationship. Others disagreed with this notion of the abscence of rivalry and jealousy among members of a polygamous family. Various examples were given that indicate that women may leave their husbands.

As to other situations of loss and stress, reference was made to the increasing number of children in refugee camps. Much is done about food and preparation for new places, but no effort is addressed to the mental health of the children and their parents. One needs to be clear that social action, however useful, must be correlated to emotional repair and the often lasting effect of loss on development and adult adjustment. Later in life, under new stress, old hurts may become revitalized. Furthermore, it was suggested that the various degrees of loss will have to be related to separation and to individuation and to the various levels of conflicts dependent on stages of development. The impact of loss on cognition must include the emotional correlates.

This discussion stressed the usefulness of the paper and its clinical base. During the rest of the study group meetings, applications were made of the propositions of the paper and the extension and application of it to the Nigerian conditions.

Discussion of Dr. Sanda's Presentation

Chairman: Colette Chiland, M.D., Ph.D. (France)

Dr. Sanda confronted the I.S.G. with some of the specifics of Nigerian tradition and the results of Westernization in the sociocultural and socioeconomic spheres. According to him, the life of the individual was traditionally completely oriented toward the group. This viewpoint has been confirmed in studies of the extended family, of polygamous families, and of the lives of women who, in Nigeria, were mainly responsible for the education of the infants and toddlers, the socialization of the children, and for what has been called the famililization process. Even before the industrial and urban revolutions, changes had been brought about over the course of centuries by religious importations (both Christian and Islamic) and later by British colonization, which anglicized many aspects of daily life, as a result of which the traditional family inevitably found itself in some difficulty. All these influences had variable effects because of the multiplicity of ethnic and language groups.

Somewhat later, Dr. Binitie expressed some doubt about these ideas. In his opinion, the changes reported were often more apparent than real: traditional conceptions persisted more than was realized. For all Nigerians, death constituted a passage between life on earth and superterrestrial existence, so that families were in a stage of transition.

Our Nigerian colleagues did their best throughout the week to clarify the significance of various concerns that appeared in the group, for example, the continued prohibitions governing the sexual life of young people, the maintenance of status differences between male and female adolescents, the continuation of the practice of female circumcision (which, to some extent, has disappeared). The participants eventually were able to realize that violent changes were manifested above all in people of the middle classes, who subscribed to Western values and in the rural areas where, for various reasons, native traditions had been violently mobilized. From this point of view, it would not be unreasonable to speak of a psychosocial explosion (even if marriage continues to have greater influence than is believed), particularly among adolescent girls and young women. One of the members of the group referred to a truly double system of communication in which the most important parts of the message were based on traditions that were not often clearly expressed.

Discussion of Dr. Binitie's Presentation

Chairman: Lionel Hersov, M.D. (U.K.)

Professor Binitie's rich picture of the cultural factors, traditional patterns, and the impact of Western thinking as they influence adolescent development, adjustment, and clinical pictures was responded to in terms of their influence on adolescent psychopathology, personality evolution, comparisons with other changing cultures, and the impact of the sexual revolution.

Hersov opened the discussion by pointing out the relationship between Nigerian cosmology and the existential anxiety in the case reports. The conflict of cultures is responded to by individualistic patterns. These patterns were determined by identifications and modeling. One of the conflict areas stemmed from the motivation in schools and the resulting drive for self-improvement. It is in the professional families reported on by Dr. Binitie that the gaps between ethnic values and Western influences appears to be greatest, resulting in symptoms familiar in Western adolescent psychopathology.

Lebovici differentiated between school anxiety as a more surface manifestation and that which is better understood in terms of underlying psychopathology. It can also be understood as psychopathology in evolution. In the cases reported, it appears as marginal psychopathology arising from the individuals' not being in conformity with the major society.

Neubauer pointed out that the psychopathology reported here is similar to that throughout the world. It is colored by cultural conflicts reflecting external versus internal forces. The latter he related to developmental issues such as patterns of attachment and their relationship to loss of significant objects not uncommon in boarding schools. The psychopathology reported could be understood better by the interaction of the developmental processes with social and cultural forces. He also described individual adolescent differences in dealing with multiple values, some with elan, but some unable to adjust to double standards.

McCarthy felt that the pathology reported was similar to that found in Ireland. The approach to it was more like that of adult psychiatrists dealing with youth. The role and the fate of the sexual and aggressive drives must also be considered. He pointed out that one factor that should be considered in some African countries such as rural Zambia is the sexual freedom that results in missing many adolescent conflict areas.

Solnit also stressed that the psychopathology is best understood in developmental terms as the basis for treatment. He raised questions about the attitudes toward sexual drives and neurotic difficulties. At what level is the inner life of the individual patient dealt with by both the traditional healers and more modern therapies?

Lourie pointed out how cultural influences determine the type of psychopathology, using the Indo-Chinese as an example. Where Western culture has taken root and is in conflict with rural culture, the differences in adolescent and young adults in dating patterns, for example, can lead to depression when parents and grandparents are still insistent in selecting mates.

Jensen's question about what Nigerian colleagues saw as causation in Binitie's cases was answered by Sanda, who pointed out how in the third case, the sexual freedom reported was in conflict with Yoruba standards in which sex before marriage is not acceptable unless it leads to marriage. Also children are seen as children until their parents die, which leads to autonomy conflicts as well.

Mrs. Helen Nwagiou, a psychiatric social worker (University of Ibadan), pointed out that adolescent development was different in different areas of Nigeria and with different parental orientations. In the middle class, girls are confined to the house—for them virginity before marriage is required. There is less strictness imposed on boys, who are freer to experiment. Village children have much more freedom because parents are in the fields. However, there is more strictness for the girls, and "escorts" for them are not uncommon. The girls are circumcised (clitoridectomy) at two weeks of age, which is suspected as a basis for more frequent depressions in females. The girls are married any time from 12 to 19 years of age.

Homosexuality is not uncommon in boarding schools but is not carried on later.

Jegede pointed out that Nigerians are not a homogeneous society. The Yoruba tribes are not particularly permissive. Binitie's patients are from the Ado tribes, so generalizations are not possible. There are cultural differences not only within ethnic groups but also differences between religions, that is, Christian versus Muslim versus spirit gods. He also pointed out that adult psychiatrists in Africa in general are not oriented to internal thinking.

Jegede indicated that before Western influences were involved, there was no adolescent period as it is generally known. The early teenager became an apprentice to mother or father with no opportunity for experimentation as in the West. Traditional families do not discuss sexual matters, but the adolescents are now exposed to sexual information and stories in the media. Therefore, a form of hypocrisy is evolving in the young.

Graham traced the information on these themes to the studies of Boaz and Mead in the 1910s. Inner forces in the more primitive societies they reported on were not taught or communicated. This was apparently related to lack of privacy due to close living in such societies. A result is the somatization of anxiety and its sources.

General Comments

Colette Chiland, M.D., Ph.D.
Serge Lebovici (France)

It is difficult to convey an idea of the many themes evoked and developed and the richness of the material presented to the I.S.G. The fascination was in part due to the fact that we had, as it were, "dropped in" on a society in a state of transition and that this affected family and community life, continuity of contact, the clinical conditions of the children and some traditional approaches to them, and the development and delivery of mental health services.

The members of the I.S.G. had an opportunity to observe an amusing but highly meaningful theatrical performance that illuminated the transitional status of family structure and its impact on the people. The play *Our Husband Has Gone Crazy Again* dealt with the actualities and potentialities of the polygamous system and the complications involved in it. The wives abandon their husband for various reasons, but the situation is precipitated by the arrival of a liberated, American-born wife. The story ends happily but conventionally, although it is difficult to imagine that a young girl brought up in the United States would in any way submit to the traditional authority of a man dedicated to polygamy. The performance brought us, with heightened awareness, into contact with the average Nigerians and their outlook on life. The actors were remarkably effective in the vivid ways in which they expressed themselves in words, song, and body language. The audience was fully participant, agreeing or disagreeing with the action. The women present, mainly young students, were clearly in favor of the feminist position and utterly opposed to the practice of polygamy.

At the start of the week, much of the discussion addressed itself to the following question. Were there changes in the sociocultural traditions during this period of transition, and if there were, what effect was this having on personality development. The answers that we received were diverse and sometimes contradictory. This was to be expected, since observers are not only themselves part of the experimental field but located in different sections of it, and therefore with different perspectives.

One of the effects of transition was certainly present: the emergence of marginal types of individuals, with a psychosocial foot on both sides. For example, men who submit to a monogamous marriage may insist on the wife becoming pregnant before marriage. The average people, particularly those who have managerial roles, are heavily immersed in the present cultural context. Their family lives are often extremely troubled, and the fathers' disciplinary roles are in great jeopardy. More generally, family life is complicated by industrialization, and a tiny vignette illustrates this: for a child to get from home to school by bus takes about six hours in the morning!

Some of the participants insisted that the family group was largely responsible for the organization of the self, but, in spite of this, one remained unclear about the vicissitudes of the individuation–separation process. One would like to have known (but there seemed to be no answer to this) whether change induced an increase in subsequent separation anxiety. Our Nigerian colleagues felt that some of these questions were still speculative, and they had no verifiable answers as yet but it seemed to them that the transitional process brought about difficulties for every member of the family group at every level of development. There was some suggestion that the extended family had been idealized. One could perhaps evaluate this type of support system by examining its helpfulness in difficult clinical cases such as the ones presented by Dr. Binitie. It was difficult to reach agreements on many of these major issues, and even on the clinical plane it was hard to know if symptoms were expressive of internal conflict or external maladaptation to a changing culture. I would guess that the Nigerian people in general would tend to externalize their inner conflicts in the form of somatic or behavioral disorders. Other participants were inclined to think that the conflicts observed in this population are universal. One is reminded of the many discussions that have taken place on the role of the oedipal complex in primitive societies such as that of the Tobrianders questioned by Malinowski. In some African countries such as Senegal, the oedipal configuration has been described in the book *African Oedipus* by Ortigues [1] and the work by Parin and Morgenthaler [2] entitled *White People Talk Too Much*. In this same context (but on a psychotic level) the I.S.G. members were shown a case of schizophrenia—a type none of them had seen before. The patient manifested intense guilt regarding his father who had displaced God in his psyche and was punishing him mentally.

It seems to me that cultures and all socioeconomic classes make a contribution to clinical psychiatry and that there are some universal mechanisms at work. My personal experience of migrant adolescents belonging to disadvantaged families has convinced me that depression is central to the problem together with disillusionment with the father. These intrapsychic problems can be aggravated by the abuse of drugs. I have also seen young girls, belonging to the second generation of migrants from North Africa, attempting to emancipate themselves and their parents while their parents tried in return to maintain their influence and the illusion of the authoritarian father common to the country of origin (e.g. Algeria).

One would have expected that in a country undergoing so much shift, deprivation of all types would be rampant and would have dire consequences for the future. Among the malnourished children, a large number demonstrate emotional disturbances, and it is evident that there is a correlation between cognitive and affective difficulties.

The subject of trust and the rupturing of attachment bonds to the loved one drew an interesting research paper from the Mindes and Dr. Musisi. The discussion included an African sample as well as children who had survived concentration camp experiences and had been bottled up over a long period of time. In all such cases, the factor of vulnerability appeared to be linked to the sex of the child and, curiously enough, to the latency period when children are thought to be at their most stable. Our Nigerian colleagues furnished some of their impressions. They could cite cases in which the father had died and a number of father substitutes from the extended family began to fill the vacuum left by him. But even in the case of the extended family group, which seems especially constructed to deal with the problems of loss, institutional services are also required, since the group is not adequate by itself to deal with all the needs created by the situation. An interesting discussion arose around the question of whether loss constituted an example of stress and whether stress research, as undertaken by Lennart Levi in his special center in Stockholm, could be usefully applied to this predicament. Some of the participants felt that the term *stress* was too general and nebulous and that the questionnaire proposed by WHO was confusing. In any case, this type of concept and this type of approach does not take into account the subjective and intrapersonal life of the child.

All the participants were able to visit the clinical facilities in the area surrounding Ibadan. Some of us reacted to the plight of adolescent patients in chains but were not unfamiliar with it since we had seen the same thing in Senegal. Although not in any way defending such practices, Graham pointed to the fact that helpers of the mentally ill became familiar with it and worked for it. The patients were therefore not with strangers but with friends.

Under these conditions in Nigeria, one can certainly argue for an extension in the use of native healers, particularly in the more remote and inaccessible parts of the country. These "barefoot psychiatrists" do seem to have certain efficacy in some cases of neurosis. They make use of herbal medicines, the composition of which they keep strictly secret, but this is not unusual in the Western world where medicine guards its own turf and keeps its own secrets regarding diagnosis and treatment. One important element of traditional practice is that the whole family is seen in consultation, and this has always been done, so that what is now done frequently in the West is nothing new and may even be adopted from the "primitives!" The important part of traditional treatment is the participation of that family group. Such traditional techniques may be especially helpful in the treatment of certain adolescents who rebel against the notion of a clinician–patient dialogue in which they seem to feel at a great disadvantage.

At one point, the discussion turned around to the specific existence of intrapsychic problems. Some of the Nigerian participants thought that the rendered description of adolescence was an occidental invention. Do we create phases of the human life cycle in response to changing societal demands and needs? I was reminded here of Philippe Aries, whose work suggested that the child, as we know him, was born at some time in the eighteenth century! Stereotypes around the notion of adolescence grow up very rapidly, since the stage appeals to the theory makers.

The WHO National Care Study Exercise, in which Dr. Graham has been involved, has confirmed the absence of qualified personnel, the diversity of practice, and the absence of contact between the primary helpers and the people. How can one train them in six to ten weeks to understand the problems and deal with them? What else can one do? Teach medical students through their training to cope with their problems? Recruit, as in China, "barefoot doctors"? The goal would be to make effective contact with the community. Our Nigerian colleagues remarked that the WHO questionnaire had been helpful in some significant ways. For instance, they had learned that the extended family is not always as protective as it is made out to be; that education in itself is not preventive, since manifold difficulties have been found in educated families. They felt that what might be effective was a modified system that was not organized according to the English mode or the public health system. The educational system also required modification, such as the abolition of severe corporal punishment and the preparation of the academic examination as an end in itself. One also needed to extend education into the preschool years and educate the mother as part of the same process.

What was needed in Nigeria were certain imperatives that applied to all countries of the world: careful studies of the first year of life, the development of infant psychiatry, and cooperation between the different specialties that included pediatricians, social workers, and adults in the pursuit of better mental health for the children and their families. Toward the closing of the discussion, Serge Lebovici (France) made a few succinct comments. First of all, he took up the matter of social class, observing that the pieces dealt with by the psychiatrist all came from the middle class and it was therefore not surprising that the patients discussed at the conference had been middle-class patients. These are the ones that psychiatrists deal with for the most part. They are the ones who have energy and initiative to move up the social ladder, and once they get to the top, they are preoccupied with survival. However, from a comprehensive psychiatric point of view, the largest number of Nigerian patients would come from the lower classes. What they suffer from are the problems of impoverishment and deprivation which gain expression in delinquency, vandalism, and other antisocial forms of behavior. What they ask of us is not psychotherapy but a recognition of their psychosocial needs and hunger. (As Brecht might have said, you have to fill their stomachs before you treat their minds.) This group requires a large amount of the small resources available, mainly because of the intractability and widespread nature of their difficulties. As Lourie would put it, we need a social policy that aims at prevention, and the policymakers need to be reminded not only of the importance of the mother to the family but also the importance of the family to the mother. Lebovici felt very strongly that we should not attempt to present a Western model to an African country in view of the latter's very limited resources. Their major mental health task was to work with pediatricians, teachers, and others within a preventive framework. Change in itself, he reminds us, did not constitute a panacea. There could be great gains from change so that more people could be better fed, better educated, better housed, and have access to better recreation. But there is also a price to be paid for change: there is a danger in losing some of the inherent virtues of the people, some of the ennobling traditions of mutual help, and some of the faith that molds people together. In the past, we paid particular attention to the aspects of change that are linked with psychopathology. Our next task is to examine more positive aspects and work toward them.

References

1. Ortiegus, M.C. and Ortiegus, E.O. *Oedipe Africain.* Librairie Plon, Paris, 1966.
2. Parin, P. and Morgenthaler, F. Die Weiss Denken Zuviel. *Psychoanalyz.* Kindler, Muchen, 1972.

SITE VISITS

Aro: Village of the Past, Present, or Future?

Reimer Jensen (Denmark)

Aro Village is a psychiatric treatment center located near the town Abeokuta between Lagos, the capital of Nigeria, and Ibadan, a university town about 80 miles north of Lagos.

In 1954, Dr. Adeoye Lambo founded a day hospital in Aro offering mental health services to a widespread population. He had also built up a department of psychiatry at the University Hospital in Ibadan, but the services there could not be used by people living as far away as Aro.

In Aro, the mental health service developed into a psychiatric hospital with in-patient as well as out-patient clinics, together with a nursing school. Some of the patients were accommodated in nearby villages, and one of these is still functioning. This is Aro Village, considered to be an interesting and unusual experiment in meeting psychiatric needs. The idea involves the use of a social setting that is similar to the home community of the patient while providing at the same time a tolerant and stimulating environment. A modern hospital unit could seem very strange and frightening to people coming from villages in the bush.

Aro Village looks like a normal village in this part of the world, and it seems to function like an ordinary village, even though the inhabitants have certain special advantages, for instance with respect to the water supply and the possibility of finding work in the hospital nearby. However, on closer inspection, the settlement is very different from other villages in that almost every family has agreed to accommodate one, two, or three mentally ill patients. Each patient has a room where he or she can live with the relatives who accompany them to the treatment center. A fee of 50 naira must be paid when the patient is admitted to the village, and, in addition, each patient is charged 6 naira per month for room and board, and 1 naira is paid to the village administration. (One naira is the equivalent of U.S. $2 and roughly what a worker can earn in two weeks.)

Village life offers many possibilities for meaningful work. The patients are supposed to be engaged in daily activities, but during the visit of the international study group most of them were fairly inactive. They can also take part in more traditional occupational therapy and make products for personal use or for exhibition and sale. Their inactivity during our visit might have been a reaction to the intrusion of a strange group looking with curiosity into their daily lives, or it could be attributed to the mental illness itself.

All types of mentally disturbed patients can be admitted to the village. Probably psychoneurotic individuals could profit from the treatment in this social setting, but most of the patients appeared to be psychotic, with little ability to involve themselves in the realities of the moment. Attendants were on call day and night, and psychiatrists from the Ibadan University Hospital visited the village regularly. Facilities at the Aro hospital were also available.

The treatment in the village can be described as a wholehearted attempt to bridge the gap between modern psychiatry with its use of medication, individual and group psychotherapy, and so forth, and traditional modes based on divination, witchcraft, and magic potions that are indigenous in all parts of Africa.

The traditional healers were accepted in the village by the psychiatrists but any overlapping of treatments was not easily tolerated.

A number of psychiatrists, for instance, Lambo of WHO, who were trained in Europe or the United States, were open to the idea that the ancient therapies were not without significance in the total spectrum of treatment, buttressed as they were by deep-rooted religious beliefs and a profound understanding of supports to be derived from the family and the community. Traditional medicine was a comprehensive system that included interactions between the visible and invisible spirit worlds, with a hierarchy ranging from living beings to the gods above through the intermediaries of healers and ancestral ghosts, all working in the service of the patient.

Direct communication between the different levels in the hierarchy was not possible for ordinary men, but through Ifa, the god of divination, the healers could influence the bad spirits within the patient who caused the mental illness.

The traditional doctors made use of different diagnostic nosologies, but all their evaluations postulated the existence of curses and bad spirits acting together. The treatment was aimed at neutralizing these forces. The spirits were driven away by means of homemade drugs, sacrifices, special amulets, strong suggestions, and sometimes harsher and seemingly punitive interventions. Chains were occasionally employed to prevent patients from escaping, but shackles were not seen in the village.

Modern psychiatry as practiced in Africa is still interwoven with traditional approaches, so that even in the most advanced centers there is a detectable blending of the old and the new, although the modern doctors would be embarrassed to admit this. A host of quack practitioners operate profitably in the hiatus sometimes left between psychiatry and serious witchcraft, even when psychiatry or traditional resources are available to the patient.

Through the centuries, the traditional healer in Africa has attacked problems that could not be solved in any other way. In Nigeria, trained psychiatrists can today reach only a small portion of the mentally ill population. At present, there is one fully trained psychiatrist available for every half a million inhabitants. For this reason alone, the traditional healer meets a huge demand, and it is therefore understandable that he is accorded the status of a chief. He is an integral part of the community, in close touch with its everyday life, and he is sure that he approaches his therapeutic task *from the inside* with some confidence in what is wrong with his patients and what he can do for them.

We met a traditional healer in Ibadan who was chairman of an organization of healers in the city approved by the City Council, and had been in practice for more than 40 years. When we asked him whether he had ever referred a patient to a psychiatrist or psychiatric hospital, he answered without hesitation, "No. Why should I do that? I know exactly what to do to get my patients well!" His patients occupied the lower floor of his house, and many of them were in chains. Like all professional groups, even in the West, this one did not suffer unduly from modesty or self-criticism. And they are understood and accepted by a majority of the population, not only by the illiterate section but occasionally by the educated, who may turn to them regressively when they are under severe stress. Oddly enough, women do not ply this particular trade.

In spite of the fact that the two medical cultures have overlapping interests and activities, intrinsically the two approaches represent two very different worlds: one is based on superstitious beliefs and magical thinking, and the other tries to treat patients by way of careful observations and methodologies grounded in up-to-date scientific knowledge. Whereas the healer is convinced that he can cure all his patients and approaches them with an authority derived from a long line of predecessors in his business, the psychiatrist works tentatively and open-mindedly, ready to question and reexamine procedures. One can imagine illiterate peasants being more responsive to the voice of certainty than to the faltering tones of doubt.

The existence of Aro Village as a psychiatric treatment center indicates that a dual approach that seems unworkable in theory is not only feasible but successful in practice. However, the fact that it is the only village of its kind in operation also points to the difficulties of bridging the gap between the two cultures.

The psychiatric hospital is one mile away and there we were able to discuss psychiatric diagnoses with the staff. It has often been claimed that certain mental illnesses such as childhood psychosis, affective disorder, and psychoneurosis are not found in the undeveloped countries, but careful examinations of this issue have revealed an incidence of these conditions in the Third World (although not with the same frequency as in the developed areas, and sometimes with different symptomatic pictures). At the Aro mental hospital, depression was often seen hidden behind an agitated behavior or concealed by somatic complaints. Suicidal attempts were rarely reported. If patients were asked directly whether they had thoughts of committing suicide, they would rarely admit it, but if questioned less overtly, many would disclose wishes of giving up living but left it to the spirits or the gods to do something about it.

Aro Village is a fascinating experiment in the treatment of mental disorder. After all these years, it still remains an experiment, like Gheel, workable under certain conditions in certain countries. It also demonstrates the enormous problems that visit a developing country. Strong forces work to speed up progress and are counterbalanced by equally strong forces that slow down the process. The village probably represents a transitional phenomenon on the road to development, and with its going, some important assets may well be lost from the society.

On the way to Aro, the study group was received by King Lipede in his palace in Abeokuta, and this visit was a good illustration of a country in transition. As the bearer of tradition, the king is admired and respected by his people, especially because he has continued to foster old ways and values while at the same time opening up the society to the outside world. His palace displayed a large number of old masks and other African antiques symbolizing the everyday and religious lives of the people through the centuries. Juxtaposed with these were new acquisitions from Paris and other cities of the Western world that the king had picked up on his travels and which he looked upon with great ambivalence.

The psychiatric patients themselves are caught between the vanishing influence of old traditions and the emerging new perspectives and possibilities ensuing from contact and communication with the industrialized nations. Much work needs to be done to resolve the inevitable conflicts that are arising. Will child patients, when they are identified (as they are, in greater numbers) be subjected to the Aro dilemma, or will they be, from the beginning, the recipients of modern child psychiatric procedures? With the great scarcity of child psychiatrists in this area, this hardly seems possible at the present time.

Bibliography

Asuni, Tolani. The Dilemma of Traditional Healing with special Reference to Nigeria. *Soc. Sci. and Med.*, Vol 13B, Pergamon Press, 1979, pp. 33–39.

Avis, Dickinson. Psychiatrists and traditional doctors in Nigeria. *Bull. Brit. Psychol. Soc.* 33 (1980), 237–240.

Lancet. The Village of Aro. 5 September 1964, 513–514.

Laosebikan, Supo. Prospects and problems attendant on the use of modern psychotherapeutic techniques with Africans. Paper presented at the Nigerian Psychological Society Conference, University of Lagos, February 6–9, 1980.

Odejide, A.O. Cross-cultural psychiatry: A myth or reality. *Comp. Psychiatr.*, 20, 2 (1979).

Odejide, A.O. Traditional (native) psychiatric practice: Its role in modern psychiatry in a developing country. *Psychiat. J. Univ. Ottawa*, LV, 4 (1979).

Odejide, A.O. Olatawura, M.O., Sanda, A.O., and Oyeneye, A.O. Traditional healers and mental illness in the city of Ibadan. *J. Black Stud.*, 9, 2 (1978), 195–205.

Oyeneye, A.O. *Psychiatric Interview—An Experience with the Traditional Herbalists Treating Psychiatric Patients in Ibadan City.* Behavioral Sciences Research Unit, University of Ibadan, Nigeria,

A Home for Motherless Babies at Ibadan: A Site Visit by an International Study Group

Colette Chiland, M.D., Ph.D. (France)

It is hardly possible in a brief visit to appreciate what really takes place in an institution when the routine of its everyday life is disturbed by the arrival of 20 inquiring strangers.

We began by asking about the frequency of motherless babies in the city of Ibadan, since it seemed to us astonishing that, in a society in which polygamy and the extended family system have been preserved relatively unchanged, no maternal surrogates for such babies could be obtained. In addition to the public institution that could take up to 40 infants (there were 36 at the time of our visit), there were two private facilities that could each take about the same number. In view of the significant maternal mortality in Ibadan, the number of cots available might seem to be limited, but it is still surprising that any at all are needed in this country.

All the babies had identified fathers, and they were not accepted for admission unless the fathers contracted to visit the babies at least once a week if they lived in Ibadan or twice a month if they lived further away. In fact, the fathers came more often than required and were welcomed at all times. Custody is maintained by the father, who receives counseling when he takes over care of the child at any time between 18 months and two years.

The institute was staffed by twice as many personnel as basically necessary. Eight caretakers were on the morning shift, six were on the afternoon shift, and six came on duty at night.

We found the youngest infants in their cribs with a few toys that could be exchanged between them. When we were around, it seemed that the caretakers did not talk much to the babies but we wondered whether this was caused by the inhibiting effect of our presence. For the bigger and more mobile babies from six months onward, there did not seem to be enough space for social and group activities.

There were several twins in the home, pointing to the fact that multiple births are relatively frequent in Nigeria, especially among Yorubas. One of us was enchanted by the sight of apparently identical twins, only to be informed that they were of different sexes!

Very few of the infants are deserted. There were two such cases at the time of our visit. They would be kept for a time at the home and then sent to any family that would accept them. Legal adoption does not exist as such in Nigeria. The families are paid about U.S.$30 per month for each child.

The institution was founded in 1967 and appears to have no staffing problems. The director seemed very devoted. It was wonderful for us to see these Nigerian babies with their great black lustrous eyes fixed intently on the strangers in a very appealing way.

EPILOGUE

The Essential Human Child and His Cultural Counterparts: An Epilogue for an International Congress

E. James Anthony, M.D. (U.S.A.)

In this book, we have tried to represent the clinical ideas and skills of many different countries and cultures, ranging from the northernmost areas of the earth to the equatorial band. The different contributors have experienced different environments, different institutions for upbringing, and different languages in which to communicate their thoughts and feelings. As immigration continues, in spite of governmental attempts to restrict it, people are gradually becoming alike, if not physically, at least culturally, throughout the world. Nationalists in various places are struggling to preserve the "pure" cultures, but since cultural dissemination proceeds invisibly through space, it is hard to jam the transmitting waves on this shrinking planet. In many foreign and previously exotic countries, the same sounds of music are heard as in Liverpool and New York. One might even predict that in the not-too-distant future psychopathology itself will be universalized, and clinical anthropologists will find it more difficult to isolate mental disorders peculiar to a particular society.

In my own role of clinician in different parts of the world, I am becoming impressed by diminishing clinical differences. The developing countries are beginning to manifest the same nosographies as those used in the developed countries, and, in this stage of transition, developing psychopathologies are hard to distinguish from developed ones. For instance, it is interesting to encounter school phobias in primitive settings where formal education has been in existence for less than a decade. In fact, it is a sad commentary on our times that the developing countries are not only catching up industrially and technologically but also clinically. As their environments become more complicated and heterogeneous, their psychiatric illnesses take on a greater subtlety and sophistication.

The questions I pose in this final presentation have to do with three analytic tasks that may not be possible to accomplish at the present time with the crude psychological and clinical assessment tools we have in hand.

1. Is there an essential psychology and psychopathology that afflicts the human child irrespective of the shaping forces of the environment?
2. Is there a cultural coloration or discoloration that is added to the essential psychological and clinical picture?
3. Is there an accultural revision of the essential and cultural psychologies and psychopathologies that occurs when societies are in transition?

Since every child is born into a culture, lives in that culture, or shifts to a new culture, what is essential and universal may simply constitute a heuristic. One can, however, get down to the essentials of a culture where change is not a predominant factor and where two types of continuity are ensured: the continuity of traditional life and upbringing from the past into the present and future, and the continuity of development through the life cycle. If we are to explore the psychological and clinical essences, we should act quickly before a cultural equalization takes place on a worldwide scale. Some anthropologists have predicted a "coca-colonization" of the planet in the near future, but that was at a time when the United States appeared to be invading every corner of the globe economically, technologically, and culturally. This seemed a depressing prospect to those who relished the almost endless variety of humanity that stamped each child indelibly with its national characteristics, so that the child who was "made in Russia" presented distinct differences from children "made in Japan" or "made in France."

Is the essence of the child only apparent in the infant, and is every human infant a Renaissance character capable of accomplishments within every culture but who, by the time it reaches middle childhood, has already become culture-bound and limited? One possible thesis is that the essences persist beneath the cultural embellishments and that one has only to scratch a child from any particular culture to find the essential child. It could be the identity theme imprinted on it by parents and primary institutions, what Kardiner [7] termed the "basic personality," but this has already been culturally stereotyped even before exposure to secondary institutions and experiences. One of the tasks that I foresee for the future clinician dealing with emotional disturbances is an entrance into the child's life at a much earlier stage. In doing so, he or she not only will be able to disentangle uniquely human from uniquely cultural aspects, but perhaps also be able to help in the process of individuation when parents interfere with it. One should refrain particularly from clinical stereotyping that brings about further dedifferentiation. One's first clinical axiom should therefore be that childhood is not a static and passive state of being but a creative process of becoming. From this point of view, diagnosis is a cliché. One is dealing not with the essential child but with the way in which this particular child corresponds to a large number of children whose behavior falls under this special rubric. The clinician, therefore, should be alive to all these concurrent factors operating in the development of the child: its humanization, its culturation, and, under changing circumstances, its acculturation. The clinical factor becomes superimposed on these.

Let me try to illustrate the difference between the essentially human and the cultural. In the following example, provided by the anthropologist Ruth Benedict [1], the setting is an American Indian one, in which it is common for groups of elders to sit together as heads of households and discuss local affairs. Within this particular culture, the women are conspicuously absent from the realm of discourse, although they may be about, tending to the domestic aspects. This would also be true of the children, who would be quiet under such circumstances—seen but not heard. What happens next could happen in any culture. The head of the household turns to his little three-year-old granddaughter and asks her to close the door. It is a heavy one and hard to shut. The little girl tries but finds she cannot move it. On several occasions, the grandfather, gently and quietly, repeats his request to please close the door. The rest of the elders sit gravely until the child eventually succeeds and the grandfather courteously thanks her as if she had done something very special for him.

Let me try to convey the many different impressions that struck me when I first encountered this vignette.

First of all, I was impressed by the patience of the group of elders.

No one seemed to be in a hurry to help the little girl, and no one became restless, because they all seemed to understand that she was only a little girl. Clinicians can learn that the essential virtue in dealing with developing children, as well as children from developing countries, is to wait and give the child a chance to catch up with the situation. (I recall, when in Africa, finding a plant that was intriguingly called *wait-a-bit,* and I decided on the spot to make it my clinical symbol as a perpetual reminder not to be in a hurry when children were concerned. Like Freud, I learned to become therapeutically "interminable" and found it effective in many different cultures, even in those in which time was money.

The second aspect of the situation that impressed me was the intuitive understanding by the elders of the child's emerging capacities and competences. It seemed that everyone in the group knew that the girl was able to do what she was asked to do, if she was given the time to do it. In many parts of the world where I have traveled, I have encountered the same collective wisdom, derived not from experts or books but from shared experiences over generations. The wonder of folk psychology is that it has been edited and reedited over the centuries and built up on common sense, common lore, and the common touch that allows primitive peoples not only to get to know one another psychologically but also to deal with one another psychologically. This collective common sense unfortunately is fast becoming uncommon as societies develop and leave their ancient intuitions behind them.

The third feature that impressed me was the basic respect for the child as an individual in the course of finding a place for herself in the scheme of life. Erikson [2], has spoken of the inherent humiliation of being a child—of being small, relatively insignificant, less knowledgeable, and less efficient in carrying out ordinary tasks—and he reminds us to nurture the child's fragile self-esteem. Adults may often threaten this by wanting to do too much for the child, thus adding to feelings of powerlessness. The handicapped are often treated in the same way with equally detrimental effects on their feelings of competence. In the case of the little girl, the elders all recognize that it is her responsibility to do what has been asked of her, and none of them wish to take this away from her. Although she is not immediately successful, she is self-motivated to continue (apart from gentle appeals from her grandfather) without asking for help, breaking down in tears, or running away from the situation. For the child, it is a lesson in shouldering responsibility and persisting with duties until they have been accomplished.

My next impression related to what Winnicott [13] has described as the holding and facilitating environments. The group provided a good example of this. There can be no doubt that the little girl felt that she was among her own people, enfolded within their community, and supported in her autonomy. Her grandfather's quiet reiteration of his request informed her that she was not alone and that all of them could be counted upon had the task proved insuperable.

My fifth impression came at the point of the successful completion of the task. The outcome was treated without congratulations and without applause, but with special thanks. It was seen as a perfectly natural event in the life of a little girl, not as a developmental triumph that might easily imbue the child with a sense of false omnipotence. She also remained in the room with the elders as part of the community, already playing her part in its life.

My last impression was of the continuity in the progression from child to adult. In this setting, from infancy onward, the child was offered full participation in the everyday life of the household so that she would be able to grow into adulthood without the major discontinuities that beset the developmental pathways of children in highly developed societies. As the little girl closed the door, all the elders present were clearly cognizant of her continuing role within the span of a human life cycle. In a symbolic sense, she will one day close the door to the home that she establishes, and within which the village elders will sit with her and her children in council. The continuity is not perfect: At some time, a son becomes a father and a daughter a mother, but even the preparation for fatherhood and motherhood begins in childhood and is rehearsed right through to adult life.

The shift from play and fantasy to reality can also be encompassed in certain traditional cultures with a sense of the essential and with a minimum of discontinuity. Using again an Indian community as a paradigm [1], one can observe how play is used in the service of rehearsal. The culture may change, the implements may vary, but the developmental tasks remain the same. In this type of hunting economy, the newborn boy is presented with a toy bow, and as he grows and begins to run about, serviceable bows, suited to his size, are made for him by his father. As a growing child, he is gradually taught how to recognize and hunt for birds and animals, beginning with those that are most easily captured. As he brings in the first of each species, his family duly make a feast of it, accepting his contribution as seriously as the buffalo that his father brings in.

When he finally kills a buffalo, it represents only the final step of his childhood and not a new adult role with which his childhood experience has been at variance. Children from this type of culture are taught very early how to survive physically and to rely on their own resources, whereas in our overprotective societies, the young, except under ghetto conditions, languish in dependency and expect to have their every need catered to even into late adolescence. Even negativism and oppositional behavior are tolerated in primitive settings as positive reactions about which the father is able to boast. In such societies, docile children are expected to become weak and subservient adults and are regarded with some contempt.

Childhood Sexuality of the Essential Child

A great deal of hypocrisy is prevalent in advanced cultures where there is one standard of morality for the child and a very different one for the adult. Many technologically backward countries start with the basic assumption that sexual unions are sterile before puberty and fertile thereafter, and their attitudes and behavior regarding childhood sexuality are determined by this reality. "Sexual rehearsals" are regarded indulgently as experimental and innocuous. Once again, the collective wisdom of primitive peoples concludes that sexuality cannot be bad during childhood and then become good for the adult; it cannot be harmful and then become healthful; and it cannot be strictly forbidden until a certain age and then become licensed. If, as clinicians, we learned from them, we would postulate a second axiom: the child should be taught nothing that it must unlearn later in adult life.

This cardinal rule is flaunted in the Western world so that children learn that sexuality is dangerous and evil and continue to believe this as adults; as a result, they become prone to sexual maladjustment.

Let me illustrate the differences. According to Henry [6], Pilága children do not suffer from the psychiatric disorders seen in industrial societies. Thus they do not have night terrors, digestive disorders, or destructiveness. "They know naughty but not neurotic behavior. Most of the behavior traits which, in our society, lead a thoughtful parent to consider a child in need of psychiatric care, either do not occur or are ignored among the Pilága" (p. 70). The children pass each day in various sexual games in which they chase one another and attempt to touch each other's genitals. The play may go on for hours and is accompanied by the excited screams of the children. In much of the play, there is a blending of sexuality and violence. "Young children are permitted absolute sexual freedom. The adult sexual act is performed at night but without any attempt at concealment. Up to the age of five, boys masturbate and practice pederasty unashamedly in broad daylight. The girls masturbate against one another in public, and at five years they start taking little boys to bed with them and attempting coitus . . . [this may] continue until about the age of twelve. Children and adults joke constantly about sex" (p. 32). As far as the anthropologists could discern, sexual maladjustment is almost unknown.

Almost the reverse is true in highly civilized cultures that remain "repressed," according to Foucault [3], in spite of so-called sexual freedom. The subject is discussed very openly, but a great deal of this is talk, and the defense and denials are still prevalent. Foucault sees sexual education as an attempt to keep children talking rather than acting or experiencing.

Here are some comments from children living under such conditions. A teenage boy has this to say:

My parents thought it was wrong to show any affection in front of us children, and they would never allow us to watch any movies or television shows in which couples were making out. We could watch war pictures and fighting but no sex. Then one day, I walked into their bedroom when they were not expecting it and I saw something that frightened the pants off me. It was quite horrible, and it became worse because my father came roaring out to say that if I ever did that again, he would break my neck. It stuck in my mind so much that I could not sleep, and my dreams became quite frightening. I think it was almost a year before I could look them in the eyes again.

And a girl recalls once seeing her mother come out of the bedroom looking for the bathroom with the front of her nightgown soaked with blood.

It frightened me and puzzled me for a long time afterwards because I imagined her having cancer or a burst blood vessel. I felt too shy to speak about it to anyone else but it worried me for a very long time. It was not until I started my own periods that she explained it all to me.

Sexuality clearly can be a natural experience for a child and incorporated into play or a traumatic experience that reverberates within as a poorly understood threat.

The Malleability of the Essential Child

The essential infant emits a wide range of sounds during its babbling phase, and at this stage is capable of speaking in any language to which it is exposed (providing the brain areas related to speech are intact). Its mastery of its native language is so extraordinarily competent under ordinary circumstances that inherent linguistic structures have been postulated.

The mechanisms of imitation and identification are so subtle in their operation that the process of assimilating the behavioral patterns of a culture and accommodating to the rules and regulations governing them remains as psychobiologically improbable as the acquisition of speech, and yet they both happen within a relatively short period of time. The infant becomes, in a few years, a communicating and transacting member of the native environment. By the end of the first decade, the child's customary attitudes and behavior become relatively indistinguishable from those of others belonging to the same milieu.

Some anthropologists have come to believe that the child's masculinity and femininity, its temperamental introversion and extraversion, and its range of fantasy are also strongly determined by the society in which it lives. In fact, the entire life cycle is, to a great extent, a product of culturally determined child-rearing practices. For example, Manus [9] parents do not habitually play with their children or tell them stories, and as a consequence they are undeveloped imaginatively. Like many other developmental experiences, fantasy would seem to be a joint production of parent and child. As Mead [9] put it, "The majority of children will not imagine bears under the bed unless the parent provides the bear." The clinician is well aware of how often phobias and fears are shared between mother and child, so that the notion that the child's interior world is highly susceptible to what the parent feeds into it psychologically comes as no surprise. Haggard [5] provides supporting evidence in a study of children brought up in comparative isolation in the northern regions of Norway who provide very impoverished responses in Rorschach and TAT projective tests.

The well-known Whiting and Child study [12] carried out 30 years ago on 75 different societies also reached the conclusion that different cultures fixated the child's development at different psychosexual levels and consequently generated different psychopathologies. There were behaviors stemming from positive fixations as a result of gratifications and behaviors originating in negative fixations arising from prohibitions. In their initial approach to the problem, they hypothesized a relationship between the amount of anxiety involved in child rearing and the rate at which early indulgence gave place to later prohibitions. The subsequent findings showed a significant correlation between the degree of "socialization anxiety," the severity and frequency of punishment, and the seriousness of emotional disturbances in the child.

This shaping of the child's personality by child-rearing experiences peculiar to a particular culture has received some confirmation from the work of clinical researchers in the United States. For example, several decades ago, Frankel-Brunswik [4] found that children brought up under authoritarian regimes tended to develop authoritarian personalities that were rigid, prejudiced, affectionless, conforming, and controlled by strong taboos against sexual and aggressive drives. The children appeared to be seething internally with repressed hostility that was projected onto the outside environment, which they then saw as threatening and dangerous. In spite of their power orientation, their admiration for strong leaders, and their contempt for weakness, such children were inwardly insecure and weak. Whether extremist political settings, either right or left in orientation, contribute to the emergence of this type of personality still remains to be demonstrated. One would probably find a mixture of conformists and rebels, representing two sides of the same coin.

The Essential Child's Response to Cultural Change

The essential child is as attuned to its culture as it was to its mother as an infant, molding itself to its institutional contours, developing along with it, and changing when it undergoes change. A similar mirroring reaction occurs in the culture as in the family. Not only do these mirrors respond sensitively to the child but also enable it to monitor its beliefs and conduct in a close and comfortable correspondence with the total environment.

Fifty years ago, the Manus lived on pile dwellings on a lagoon, naked except for G-strings, and very much immersed in ancestor worship, magic, and divination. They were described as a submissive people with apathetic reactions and shallow affects, apparently incapable of intimate relationships. Today, they are a different people. They live in nice houses, wear ready-made clothes, and attend Christian churches. Even more striking, the children are different. They are now eager, competitive, exploratory, and quick to change their ways in response to innovations. Together with their parents, they have become part of an "achieving society" [9].

In sharp contrast, 50 years of technology have made little or no impact on social and personal structures in India. The Indian parents remain traditionally oriented and have been described as passive, conforming, indecisive, resigned, and unable to initiate changes or plans for the future. The family itself retains its solidarity, its dependence on the extended group, its respect for the elders, its religious orientation, its acceptance of fixed social stratification, and its mindless adherence to the disreputable caste system. We find predictably that Indian children closely reflect the culture and the family, being characteristically nonaggressive, nonassertive, inactive, and unquestioningly submissive to all authority. Psychoanalysts have pointed to the strong preoedipal attachment to the mother, the limited individuation, and the weak identity formations. Yet the psychosocial support systems are so good that the individual can remain confidently dependent on it for life.

When the culture in any area changes sharply as a result of modernization or when children are relocated within new cultures as a result of migration or war, the children generally adapt better to the new conditions than their parents or grandparents, who may attempt the difficult task of living psychologically in two cultural worlds that are geographically separated. When the families migrate together and remain together, the chances of adjustment are better, but if the children are isolated from their parents, or if the parents become ill as a result of the transition, syndromes of disorder appear typified by homesickness, insecurity, moodiness, bedwetting, psychosomatic gastrointestinal symptoms, delinquent behavior, a reduction in self-esteem, and hostility directed inward. With most children, these transitional disorders are temporary, and many of them are rapidly transformed from children of one culture to children of another, with the native culture soon becoming dimly remembered. The children are only too ready to forget their roots in their eagerness not to be considered "different," and this generally works to the advantage of the child unless the parents struggle to maintain the old ways against any encroachment from the new. When this happens, intergenerational conflicts and gaps make their appearance and break up families that were once well knit and cohesive. The psychopathology of immigration is one of the major psychiatric problems in the rapidly shifting world of today.

When the family moves from a simple rural setting to an urbanized one or upward from a lower social stratum to a higher and more demanding one, the children not only rapidly embrace the newer, more subtle and sophisticated ways of life but also newer, more subtle and sophisticated psychopathology. For example, in relatively simple societies where the group identity takes precedence to the ego identity, where loyalty is to the family and not to the individual, where the family structure is extended and not nuclear, where education is absent or minimally literate, where traditions are maintained from generation to generation so that development is consistent and continuous, adolescent turmoil is nonexistent. When families from such societies are exposed to a more complex and demanding type of environment, adolescent turmoil makes its appearance, creating much confusion and chaos on the domestic scene, since there is no precedent or preparation for it in the earlier history of the group.

Even such an essential phenomenon as bonding between the mother and her infant is highly susceptible to cultural influences. Under certain unpropitious circumstances, failures in attachment may occur, leading to avoidance behavior on the part of both mother and infant. The former may leave her baby for long periods of time, not responding to its crying signals and paying little attention to it beyond routine care; the latter may become highly aggressive or apathetically withdrawn and may soon begin to manifest such maladjusted behavior as rocking, self-injuring, uncontrolled tantrums, and sleep disturbances. Not only does the mother seem to reject the child, but the child rejects the mother. Under such conditions, it looks as if the essence of infancy and the essence of mothering are lost. This particular syndrome is prevalent in many different parts of the world, but more especially when cultural change impinges on traditional ways of life.

The Individual, the Group, and the Essential Child

What is striking about Western civilization over the past 600 years has been the increasingly intense cultivation of the individual, sometimes at the expense of the group. The focus today is on the processes of individuation, of identity formation, and on self-delineation. The setting for this "newer" psychology has been provided by the nuclear family that is generally regarded as short on psychosocial support but highly generative of neurotic conflict, particularly of the triadic variety.

In less developed societies, there would appear to be a relative weakness of the sense of self. Oriental traditions of thought, for example, have set much less store by the individual, and the belief in reincarnation has virtually excluded individuality as a desirable entity, since people are but a manifestation of the life within them, which will be reborn in another form after their apparent death. The self appears to be the special creation of modern, Western man.

During the child's development, in a nuclear family situation, the self is elaborated gradually in a dialectical process that first involves a grasp of consciousness, separating internal from external, and then a growing self-consciousness; that is, a self-regarding self encased within the body that reacts to others, interacts with others, grows to know right from wrong, feels sexual pleasures and experiences sexual fantasies, does things for itself, solves problems, takes responsibility, and works industriously. At the heart of this self is the self-image that involves all that one thinks of one's self and how one is perceived by others. The discovery of the self occurs late in childhood and is a grinding developmental task that is probably never completely accomplished. In certain children, under certain conditions, it becomes hypertrophied so that the child's sensitivity or self-consciousness becomes extreme and incapacitating. In the Western world, however, an individual is judged by the self that is presented to others.

How different all this is from the advice given to his son by a West African father: "Son, there is a certain form of behavior to observe, and certain ways of acting in order that the guiding spirit of our race may approach you also ... If you desire the guiding spirit of our race to visit you one day, if you desire to inherit it in your turn, you will have to conduct yourself in the self-same manner; from now on, it will be necessary for you to be more and more in my company" [8]. Clearly, this does not take into consideration the developing individuality of the son but only his relationship to the tribe and to the ancestral spirits. At times the group identity is fostered when the group is under threat, and this has been done systematically in the kibbutz where one can often listen to the collective mind in the making. For example, a little boy looks at the moon through the window and says (in typical Piaget style): "Look at the big moon in my sky," and the nurse at once corrects him, saying, "you mean, in *our* sky." In another group, the children asked the nurse to sing them a song before they went to bed, but one of them demanded something different. The nurse replied that she would do what the group asked her to do and not what *one* child wished [11]. In such ways is the group identity built up, providing the underpinning to interdependent living.

The Myth of the "National Character"

The essential child is hidden behind the culturated and the acculturated child; hidden behind the group identity; hidden behind the clinical label; and, finally, hidden behind the stereotype of the "national character." Every culture has a myth-making propensity and invents culture heroes and heroines who are used to provide the members of the culture with a sense of esteem, potency, and security. These sustaining culture heroes may degenerate in time into cult heroes who are often less than ideal representations. The essential child in a particular culture may try to live up to his or her heroic past and develop omnipotent illusions through identification or feelings of inferiority through comparison. Cult heroes with messianic purpose can be extremely dangerous to susceptible youth, especially when the cult hero is psychiatrically disordered.

Apart from creating its own stereotypes, the culture and its people may be stereotyped by other societies, and these can be disturbing to the individuals. As seen by others, Orientals are inscrutable, Americans are hearty and extroverted, Scandinavians are simple-minded sun lovers without a thought in their heads, and the British continue to act as if they still ruled a large part of the world. Such partisan characterizations frequently serve the purpose of propaganda and racism and can be used in subtle ways to deny basic human rights. The African mind is a case in point. A common white stereotype views blacks as immature, violent, undisciplined, and preoccupied with the thought of raping white women. The blacks have generated equally ugly images of the whites and may live in constant fear of their own self-creations. Children assimilate stereotypes very early on in life when their minds are suggestible and their critical powers limited. They grow into adults with the same stereotypes encapsulated almost unchanged within their minds, and may then behave as irrationally as if they had psychoanalytic transferences to these "bad objects."

Cultures, nevertheless, are different from one another both in form and content, and it is helpful to carry out transcultural research to define the similarities and differences more objectively. It is misleading to sum up an entire culture in a single word, but it is possible to study profiles of grapes that cluster together more frequently in one culture than in another. It is the presence of these clusters that gives the members of a particular society a family resemblance.

As an illustration of this kind of thinking, let me cite the well-known study comparing and contrasting American and Mexican children by a crosscultural team of investigators [6a]. It was found that the American children were more active, more ruggedly independent, more technologically minded, more aggressively assertive, and more complex in their thinking than Mexican children, who were, in contrast, more passive, more obedient, more family-centered, more cooperative rather than competitive, and more fatalistic in their outlook on life, which was often perceived as something to be endured rather than enjoyed.

It would seem from this summing up that American children had all the positives and the Mexican children all the negatives, but such a judgment would depend on the point of view of the judge. Furthermore, not all American children are "goal-getters" and certainly not all Mexican children are "pushovers." In some instances, class factors may have greater influence than national ones.

The Mexican poet Octavio Paz [10] did come to the conclusion that the North American system set a premium on the positive aspects of reality, and that from early childhood, the North American child is subjected to schemes of formulas that are endlessly repeated by the media. "A person," says Paz, "imprisoned by these schemes, it like a plant in a flower pot that is too small for it: He cannot grow or mature." This may result in violent individual rebelliousness. It would seem that the Mexican child is not channeled from the beginning but allowed to develop in a far more *laissez-faire* manner.

What is different from the overuse of destructive stereotypes are the tentative generalizations drawn by these researchers. They point out that anyone who meets Mexicans and North Americans in their homes and in their families, in various regions and at different levels of social class, will at once realize that such generalizations may be helpful in dealing educationally with children from different ethnic groups but that generalizations are also oversimplifications that ignore the variability open to the essential child exposed to a particular culture.

Some Final Thoughts Stimulated by the Ever-Stimulating International Scene

For some 50,000 years, it has been humankind's pride to find good answers to the difficulties of human living: good explanations of why the crops have failed; why the hurricanes came; why earthquakes took place; and why people died of plague and starvation. It is only more recently, within the scientific era, that we have stopped making up answers and have attempted instead to raise questions that could be answered through systematic investigation.

The transcultural clinician needs to learn from the anthropologist, from the ecologist, from the demographers and epidemiologists, from the historians, and from the geographers to understand why a terrain gives rise to certain kinds of people and certain family structures.

These other disciplines can teach us how to change our traditional techniques when approaching children from different cultures. In my own case, I have examined children with clinical disorders all over the world and have found that certain techniques are better able to cross borders. In my inquiries, I make use of what I have called my five D's:

1. Doll play with small, manipulable, acultural dolls can be used to learn about both the internal and external life of the child.

2. Dreams are of interest to all cultures, even when set in very different landscapes, because the essential conflicts underlying the manifest experiences are not dissimilar.

3. Drawings also seem to be acceptable to children of all cultures, who will do their best to represent the universe in which they live.

4. Dramatizations are the prevailing myths and legends of particular communities, and the children of these communities are only too eager to act out the dramas that often have so much meaning to their lives.

5. Dialogues need the help of a good interpreter, but once conversations are initiated, children from any culture can become funds of information not only about themselves and their families but also about the community. I carry these "little conversations" to areas of birth, life, sickness, poverty, marriage, death, and afterlife. It allows me to gauge the sense of continuity built up in the mind of the child I am interviewing.

A special crosscultural scientific tool is the myth, and we can learn about it from the play and dramatizations of the children, from the rituals in regular use, and from the folk stories that are passed from one generation to the next by word of mouth. I have learned that the myth is not merely a story told but a reality that is lived, and it fulfills in all cultures the indispensable function of relating human individuals in a meaningful way to their environment.

The essential child, girl or boy, can be seen *in statu nascendi* in all cultures throughout the centuries, although it is only in the last 300 years that we have become so aware of the child as being-in-itself. What is human seems to repeat itself throughout history, and the essential process of humanization has not changed in the different epochs.

Let me take you back to the early days of Mexico and describe the advice given by an Aztec mother to her young daughter [6]. It tells us that parenthood and the tenderness that motivates it has changed very little since those days and that through the mother's eyes we can reconstruct the essential girl as she once walked the streets of Mexico. By what the mother says to her daughter, it is clear that she is still very much in love with her husband: "My beloved, my very dear little dove, although you are a female, you are the very image of your father, and so what more can I say to you except a few words."

She then proceeds to share with her daughter a little of her personal and interpersonal wisdom, indicating that she would like the young girl to adopt a middle way in all her behavior. Her clothes should be becoming and neat, but she should not be underdressed or overdressed; her speech should be deliberate, calm, and gentle, and not mincing, forceful, or nasal; her gait should be neither hasty nor slow and not restless or draggy; her body should be poised with her head slightly inclined, and, if at any time she was obliged to jump over a pool of water (apparently a not unusual hazard on Aztec roads), she should do it lightly, adroitly, and decently, with a minimum of exposure; and she should wash herself and her clothes but with moderation and not too frequently since if she did it every day, others might accuse her of being "too delicate."

The mother ends her words of advice to this girl, who is on the verge of growing up, with a little allegory. "In this world," she says to her, "we travel by a very narrow, steep and dangerous road that passes over a lofty mountain ridge on whose top, it becomes a narrow path, on either side of which is a bottomless abyss. If you deviate from the path, you will fall disastrously and it is the better part of discretion to keep to the path."

Here we have an Aztec version of *The Pilgrim's Progress*. The mother is telling her child that adolescent development is not an easy time but that if one internalizes the precepts and practices of one's parents, one should be able to maneuver into adult life successfully.

She then adds something that immediately sets her in a class above the merely good-enough mother. She speaks directly from her heart to her child:

What I want to say to you is that I love you very much and that you are my dearest daughter. Remember the nine months that I bore you in my womb, and after you were born, the time you spent in my arms and then on my lap taking my milk into you. I am telling you this so that you will know that I and your father are the source of your very being and it is our words that are being received into you, and so I ask you to treasure them as you once treasured my breast and my milk.

When one speaks of the essential child and the quintessence of childhood, one should remember to include along with them, since they are inseparable, the essential parent and the quintessence of parenthood. If I were looking for a good example to convey to a class of expectant fathers and mothers in the United States of what having a child was all about, I could do no better than to select this Aztec illustration, not for what the mother says, which reflects that era, but for what she feels, and it is this that makes her an essential mother.

Let me summarize what I think underlies essential childhood. First, there are some universal propositions that relate to essential childhood, which include a universal symbolic language of dreams, myths, rituals, and dramatic play; second, basic conflicts involving nuclear family relationships that run a course during early childhood; third, common mental functions stemming from mental structures that involve conscious and unconscious fantasies, defenses, and coping devices, representations of the outer world, and modes of preoperational and operational thinking; fourth, fears, feelings, and fantasies about fundamental human experiences like eating, excreting, reproducing, sickening, and dying. Overlying these fundamental operations are the veneers of different cultures. This is in theory.

In practice, the essential human child in all cultures is one who feels well, plays well, works well, eats well, thinks well, copes well, enjoys well, and expects well. The essential human child is a hopeful child. He expects well not only of himself, but of his parents and of the world at large. He gives generously of himself and he takes uninhibitedly for himself. He is able to listen when others talk to him, and he is able to talk back. Most of all he knows where he came from and at each step of his development, he forms a better idea of where he is going. To all around, he radiates a sense of himself. All this essence is epitomized in the remark of an almost destitute boy from the Sioux tribe as it is quoted by Erikson [2, p. 129]: "The way you see me now is *the way I really am,* and it is the way of my forefathers" (italics added).

References

1. Benedict, Ruth F. Continuities and Discontinuities in cultural conditioning. *Psychiatry,* 1 (1938), 161–167.
2. Erikson, Erik H. *Childhood and Society,* 2nd Ed. Norton, New York 1963, 109–126.
3. Foucault, M. *The History of Sexuality, Vol. I, An Introduction* (translated by R. Hurley). Pantheon, New York, 1978.
4. Frankel-Brunswik, E. *Prejudice in children: An experimental approach.* Unpublished address, 1957.
5. Haggard, E.A., and Von der Lippa, A. Isolated families in the mountains of Norway. In Anthony, E.J., and Koupernik, C., *The Child and His Family* eds. John Wiley, New York, 1970, 465–488.
6. Henry, Jules and Zunia. Doll play of Pilaga Indian children. In *Research Monographs,* 4. American Orthopsychiatric Association, New York, 1944.
6a. Holtzman, W.H., Guerrero, R., and Swartz, Jon D. *Personality Development in Two Cultures.* University of Texas Press, Austin, 1975.
7. Kardiner. *The Individual and His Society..* Columbia University Press, New York, 1939.
8. Laye, Camara. *The Dark Child.* Farrar, Straus, & Giroux, New York, 1966.
9. Mead, Margaret. *New Lives for Old: Cultural Transformation—Manus, 1928–1953.* William Morrow, New York, 1956.
10. Paz, Octavio. *The Labyrinth of Solitude* (translated by L. Kemp). Grove Press, New York, 1961, 25.
11. Spiro, Melford. *Children of the Kibbutz.* Harvard University Press, Cambridge, Mass., 1958.
12. Whiting, J. W. M., and Child, I.L. *Child Training and Personality.* Yale University Press, New Haven, Conn., 1953.
13. Winnicott, Donald W. *The Maturational Processes and the Facilitating Environment.* Hogarth Press, London, 1965.

Index

Accidents:
    as masked suicidal attempts, 188
Adolescent problems in Nigeria, 261-275
    clinical problems, 266-269
Adoption and fostering as preventive
    measures, 171-179
    follow-up studies, 174-176
    negative outcome in foster children, 177
African theatre:
    "Our husband has gone crazy again," 291
Animal studies in stress, 44-47

Breast feeding and its significance, 50, 51

Cardiovascular studies in infancy, 57-62
Childhood hysteria, 186, 187
Children of alcoholic parents, 35-41
    differences between the sexes, 37
Children as patients, 3-23
    becoming patients, 9-13
    intermittent treatment with, 13-18
    as psychiatric patients, 5, 6
    as psychotherapeutic patients, 6-9
    as sufferers, 21

Day care for three-year-olds, 129-143
    effects of increased density of personnel, 133
    follow-up study, 138-139
    parental reports on current stresses, 129
    relation of density to conflict, adrenaline,
        and noradrenaline levels, 129
Diagnosis of hyperactivity in children, 190
Disruption of attachment systems in young
        children, 215-231
    Bowlby's attachment theory, 216-218
    family structure in relation to child rearing
        and "loss," 228-230
    levels of "loss," 218-219

transcultural studies, 220-231
uprooting of the family, 225-228
Drug abuse and alcoholism in children and
        adolescents, 153-160
    alcoholic children of alcoholics, difficulty
        in treating, 159
    alcoholic fathers "breed" alcoholic sons, 159
    child as father to narcoman, 160
    children of alcoholic fathers psychiatrically
        deficient, 158
    correlation with broken homes, 157
    decrease in users among students, 155
    early onset of drinking predisposing to
        alcoholism, 156
    noncooperation with families of drug
        users, 155
    ten-year follow-up, 153
    "treatment chain" with drug users, 155, 156

Effect of civil war on children, 69-79
    awareness of sectarian division, 70-74
    awareness of violence, 74-79
Essential human child in different cultures,
        309-326
    childhood sexuality, 314-315
    continuity and discontinuity, 311-313
    malleability, 315-317
    myth of the "national character," 321-325
    response to cultural change, 317-319

Family village in Stockholm, 181-183
    use for drug users, 182
Feeding disturbances in children, 191-193
Filicidal mothers, 27-33
    effect of incest on child, 32, 33
    guilt over childhood incest, 32
    relation to childhood incestuous
        experiences, 27, 28, 30

Gastric ulceration in the neonate, 48, 49

Infants under stress, 43-63
  experimental studies, 51-62
  role of cardiovascular systems, 46-48
  role of endocrine systems, 44-46
  stress syndromes in infancy, 48-51

Low birth weight, 49

Major stress factors and their assessment, 52, 53
Maternal blood pressure in pregnancy and its consequences. 51
Mental health of children in developing countries, 197-212
  emotional and behavioral disorder, 207-209
  lack of schooling, 209-210
  nutrition effects, 198-205
  patterns of professional services, 210-212
  sociocultural deprivation and retardation, 205, 206
Mental health in schools, 191

Nature of the African world, 261-266
Neonatal mother-infant contact, 105-125
  faulty anamnesis of mothers, 124
  relation of early interaction and subsequent development, 105
  techniques of observation, 112-115
Nigerian family in transition, 235-260
  change in family structure and function, 239-243
  effects of change for the Yoruba family, 243
  marital relationships, 255-256
  pre-colonial family, 236-239
  socioeconomic changes, 251-260
  status of women, 258
Nigerian home for motherless babies, 305-306

Psychosocial risk factors in children, 145-150
  advice to physicians, 150
  diagnostic profile of children at risk, 149-150
  relation to broken homes from divorce and death, 148
  social maladjustment an increasing problem, 145
  somatic symptoms without organic basis, 145-147

Social engineering and its problems, 189-190
Somatizing and "converting" psychological stress, 185
Suicidal behavior in children and adolescents, 163-169
  frequent cause of death in western countries, 164
  increasing rate of suicide in the young, 164
  motives for suicide, 163
  rate and social change, 165
  risk in young people, 166

Understanding children internally as well as externally, 85

Village of Aro, 299-303

Western society in turmoil, 93-103
  child rearing, 98-100
  family structure, 95-97
  increased stresses of welfare state, 93
  price paid for technological development, 93
  rise in psychosocial problems, 94, 95
  values and attitudes of young people, 101-103

WITHDRAWN
UST
Libraries